"SENSATIONS AS IF —"

A Repertory of Subjective Symptoms

By

HERBERT A. ROBERTS, *M.D.*

EX-CHAIRMAN, AMERICAN FOUNDATION FOR HOMOEOPATHY
HEAD OF DEPARTMENT OF HOMOEPATHIC PHILOSOPHY,
POSTGRADUATE SCHOOL OF THE AMERICAN FOUNDATION,
EX-PRESIDENT, INTERNATIONAL HAHNEMANNIAN ASSOCIATION

B. JAIN PUBLISHERS PVT. LTD.
NEW DELHI - 110 055

Price : Rs. 35.00

Reprint Edition : 1990
© Copyright with the Publisher
Published by :
B. Jain Publishers Pvt. Ltd.
1921, Street No. 10, Chuna Mandi
Paharganj, New Delhi - 110 055 (INDIA)
Printed at :
J. J. Offset Printers
Kishan Kunj, Delhi - 110 092

ISBN 81—7021—088—7

BOOK CODE B-2445

FOREWORD

THE possibilities of usefulness for any repertory are so varied, and the need for every form of index to our remedies for their use in individual cases is so imperative, that it has stimulated us to the task of enlarging that valuable little work on *Sensations As If* which was compiled some years ago by Dr. A. W. Holcomb and published under the auspices of *The Medical Advance* in 1894.

On the other hand, the possibilities of material in our materia medica for any repertorial index are so great that the margin of probable errors, and the certainty of omissions, are sufficiently appalling to daunt one's intention to offer such a work to a profession where careful comparison is so often necessary.

So it is with the greatest humility, and the complete consciousness of far too many errors, that these gleanings are offered to the homœopathic practitioner in the hope that this little work may serve a useful purpose in the healing of the sick.

Grateful acknowledgment is given to the late Dr. W. A. Yingling for the original impulse to compile such a work, and to the great help he proffered by sending the numerous symptoms he had collected for this purpose. His burden of years made the task impossible for him, but his interleaved copy of Holcomb's work, and his appreciation of and dependence upon the original work, nurtured the inspiration to develop it still further.

Besides these two sources, the basis of the material was secured from three major works: Hering's *Guiding Symptoms,* Clarke's *Dictionary* and Allen's *Handbook.* Frequent references have been made to Allen's *Encyclopædia.* Other volumes less well known, and including Anshutz's *New, Old and Forgotten Remedies,* have served in adding further symptoms.

In spite of scanning countless pages for over three years, many symptoms that properly belong here are missing. Errors must have crept into others, for careful checking of some obvious errors reveals mistakes in transcribing at some point in the assembling. For all these mistakes we must plead the frailty of human ability to turn out perfect work. Lack of time prevented checking back to its source every symptom after the transcript was completed, but wherever possible, outstanding inequalities have been carried back to the materia medica and proper corrections made. Some of the sources of information themselves have suffered from typographical errors, as comparisons have demonstrated; perhaps the most notable of these sources of error were the repertories already extant, and in particular Allen's *General Symptom Register*.

This must be our instruction to the one who uses this effort— the reassertion of an axiom in homœopathic teaching: *Let the single symptom be only a partial indication to the application of the materia medica. Beware the keynote that is not backed up by knowledge of, or reference to, the materia medica. No single symptom, no matter how "strange, rare and peculiar", can stand without the support of the well taken case, and the likeness of the whole patient to the remedy.*

It is true, however, that we may see cases where the regular course of repertorization fails to reveal the *simillimum*. It is in such a case as this that the special repertory may provide a clue to a remedy not included in the general repertory, or not so strikingly brought to our mind. This is the field of *Sensations As If*, as one possible indicator of the elusive *simillimum*.

Derby, Conn.
    January 10, 1937

H. A. ROBERTS.

CONTENTS

Sensations as if—

MIND AND SENSORIUM

Absent (forgetful)—*Bar. c.*
Accident would happen—*Mag. c., Mag. s.*
  —one were threatened with some fatal—*Alum.*
Accomplish her work, she cannot—*Bry.*
Accomplished, business never could be—*Med.*
Act, yet cannot (spellbound); all functions must—*Pop.*
Action and yet withheld from action, mind and body must be in—*Pop.*
Acts, mental, were performed in stomach—*Acon.*
  —there were one by his side duplicating his—*Ars.*
Afflicted, he had just been—*Cyc.*
Afraid of the first thing she sees—*Stram.*
Air itself were in tremulous motion (fever)—*Saba.*
  —he were in; on going to sleep quick drawing to feet wakens him—*Tell.*
  —he were entering cold—*Tarent.*
  —and busy himself, he must go into the—*Anac.*
  —she were so light she could float in—*Manc., Tep.*
  —she were floating in—*Cocaine, Nux m., Stict., Valer., Xanth.*
  —legs were floating in—*Stict.*
  —flying or swimming in—*Calc. ar., Manc., Valer.*
  —on going to sleep he were in—*Tell.*
  —when walking, he were gliding in—*Asar.*
  —when walking, he were walking on—*Asar., Chin., Coff., Lac c., Merc. i. f., Nat. m., Nux v., Op., Phos. ac., Phos., Rhus t., Spig., Stram., Stict., Thuj.*
  —hovering in, one were—*Manc., Nux m., Op., Stict., Valer.*
  —like a spirit (when walking in open air), he were hovering in —*Asar.*
  —and tormented by great anxiety lest slightest touch or motion make her fall from the height; she were being lifted high in—*Hyper.*
  —suspended in—*Sep.*
  —he were walking in—*Aur. m., Lact.*
Alarm, awakens in—*Agn.*

Alighted on floor, bed had gone out from under her and she had —*Ars.*

Alone and all about her were dead and still, she were—*Rhus t.*

Animal right through, she were—*Lach.*

Apoplexy, he would have—*Arg. m., Brom., Carb. v., Elaps, Ferr., Gas., Puls., Zinc.*

   –fear of having a stroke of—*Prim.*

   –struck with—*Kali cy., Tarent.*

   –were threatened—*Colch.*

Apparition, he would see an—*Brom.*

Approached and receded, everything—*Cic.*

Approaching catastrophe, someone were rapidly—*Tab.*

   –end were—*Zinc.*

Arms and legs, he had too many—*Pyrog.*

Around in a circle, head were going—*Tub.*

Arousing himself from a dream—*Carb. v.*

Arrest him (when door opens), someone were coming to—*Ruta, Tab.*

Arrested, ideas were—*Seneg.*

Asleep—*Rhus t., Ter.*

   –he were half—*Con., Rheum*

   –left half of head were—*Calad.*

   –when waking in morning, he had not been—*Trif.*

   –he were just falling—*Asar.*

Atmosphere in room were heavy and thick—*Agn.*

   –in a hot—*Puls.*

   –when eating, he were entering a warm—*Nux v.*

Attack him, severe disease were going to—*Arg. n.*

   –threatened with epileptic—*Alum.*

Attacked by paralytic stroke, he would be—*Carb. v.*

Attention must be centered on act of respiration, his whole—*Chlor.*

Awake all night, he had been—*Puls.*

   –she would never get—*Ang.*

Awakened, he had just been—*Cyc.*

Awakens in alarm—*Agn.*

   –in morning, she were friendless when she—*Lach.*

   –in fright—*Bell.*

Away from home—*Aster.*

Backward when in rocking chair, one were going over—*Tub.*

Bad, she had done something—*Alum.*

Balance his head (vertigo), he had to—*Æsc.*
Balancing himself to and fro—*Ferr.*
  –over water in crossing a bridge—*Ferr.*
  –to and fro when closing eyes, seat were—*Thuj.*
Balls of fire were rolling over bed-clothes—*Stram.*
Barrier between senses and external objects—*Æth.*
Beast under bed, some dreadful—*Cham.*
Bed were bouncing patient up and down—*Bell.*
  –something forces him out of—*Rhus t.*
  –by suction and unable to move, he were bound to—*Sars.*
  –she covered the whole—*Pyrog.*
  –head were falling out of—*Arg. m.*
  –one would fall out of—*Arg. n., Ars., Ars. s. f.*
  –were falling on her—*Stram.*
  –he were falling through—*Bell., Chin. s., Dulc., Lach., Rhus t., Sacc., Sec.*
  –were being drawn from under her—*Stram.*
  –had gone from under her and she had alighted on the floor— *Ars.*
  –were not large enough—*Sulph.*
  –were in motion, on awaking at night—*Lac c.*
  –were moving—*Clem.*
  –body were scattered about in—*Bapt.*
  –were sinking—*Lach.*
  –there were mice in—*Colch.*
  –she were sinking down deep in—*Bry.*
  –were sinking down on closing eyes—*Sec.*
  –were sinking from under her—*Kali c.*
  –everything were sinking down in—*Lyc.*
  –and of the person, sinking down of the—*Lach.*
  –sinking through—*Rhus t.*
  –he had sunken deep in—*Xanth.*
  –were swaying from side to side like a hammock—*Tub.*
  –when lying she did not touch—*Asar., Chin., Coff., Lac c., Nat. m., Nux v., Op., Phos. ac., Rhus t., Spig., Stict., Stram., Thuj.*
  –making a noise, something were under her—*Bell.*
  - turned about—*Nux v., Plb., Puls., Sin. n.*
  –were turning in a circle—*Con., Sol. n.*
Behind her, someone were—*Brom., Crot. h., Lach., Med., Sac. lac., Tub.*

Behind—*Continued*
  –him, someone were walking—*Calc. c.*
  –him when in bath tub, someone were—*Samars.*
Belong to her family, she did not—*Plat.*
  –to anyone, she did not—*Puls.*
Beside himself, he were—*Puls.*
  –himself with trifles—*Carl.*
  –him, someone were walking—*Calc. c.*
Bewildered—*Xanth.*
Black cloud settled over her—*Cimic.*
Blood ceased to flow (vertigo)—*Seneg.*
Boat, he were floating in a—*Bell.*
Body, he had no—*Psor.*
  –consciousness were outside of his—*Alum.*
  –in some way, she would become crazy if she could not get out
    of her—*Lac c.*
  –were greatly enlarged—*Bell.*
  –spirit had separated from—*Anac.*
  –mind were separated from—*Anac.*
  –were separated, soul and—*Thuj.*
  –were made of glass and easily broken—*Thuj.*
Bouncing patient up and down, bed were—*Bell.*
Bound to bed by suction and unable to move—*Sars.*
Boy, strange, were lying in bed with him—*Apis*
Brain were balanced on a slight point and likely at any moment
    to be turned over—*Camph.*
Brandy, he had taken—*Puls.*
Break if she lay too long in one position, she would—*Pyrog.*
  –the spell, she were charmed and could not—*Lach.*
  –in if alone, rowdies would—*Elaps*
  –down, she would—*Arg. m.*
Broken, whole body were made of glass and were easily—*Thuj.*
Buoyant—*Pip. m.*
Burning, he saw his neighbor's house—*Hep.*
Burst into tears, he would—*Cot.*
Business, he had much—*Phos.*
  –never could be accomplished—*Med.*
Busy himself, he must go into open air and—*Anac.*
Calamity were hanging over him, some overwhelming—*Calend.*
  –horrible, were impending—*Rhus t.*
Came toward her and frightened her, someone—*Sol*

Car, she were in a railroad—*Sang.*
Care what happened, he did not—*Sep.*
  –for her no one would—*Lil. t.*
Carousing, after—*Phys.*
Carried somewhere and conversed with another person, she were
    —*Raph.*
  –on wings when walking—*Thuj.*
Catastrophe, someone were rapidly approaching—*Tab.*
Chair were rising—*Phos.*
  –were standing in middle of bed, when half asleep—*Thuj.*
Changed, everything at home had—*Arg. n.*
Charmed and could not break the spell—*Lach.*
Child, she must have a—*Agar.*
  –he were a—*Cic.*
Circle, head were going around in a—*Tub.*
  –room were turning in a—*Nux v.*
Climbing a steep mountain, he were—*Prun.*
Clothes for a time, though near them could not get—*Caj.*
Cloud passed over him—*Samars.*
  –head were confused by a—*Crot. t.*
  –heavy, black, had settled over her—*Cimic.*
Clouds, ideas were floating in—*Datura a.*
Coal screen and whirled around, he had been placed in a—*Eup.
    per.*
Collect his sense, impossible to—*Hyos.*
Coming down on her, whole house seemed to be—*Saba.*
  –over her, overpowering giddiness were—*Con.*
  –up behind him, someone were—*Staph.*
  –up to meet him, stairs or ground were—*Pic. ac.*
Commingled, objects were—*Camph.*
Commit some horrible crime, one were impelled to—*Thea*
  –suicide, he were impelled to—*Thea*
  –suicide by drowning, he were impelled to—*Dros.*
  –suicide (on seeing knives) though she has a great aversion to
    it, she would—*Alum.*
Committed a crime, one had—*Alum., Am. c., Carb. v., Chel.,
    Cocc., Cyc., Dig., Ign., Merc., Nux v., Puls., Rheum, Rhus
    t., Verat. a., Zinc.*
  –a crime, conscious of having—*Zinc. ox.*
  –the unpardonable sin, she had—*Chel., Med.*
  –some evil, one had—*Cyc.*

Communing with self—*Op.*

Confined in too small a space—*Samars.*

Confused—*Samars., Tub., Verat. v.*

Confusion from insufficient sleep—*Sulph.*

　–smoke in head caused—*Sul. ac.*

Conscience, he had a bad—*Verat. a.*

Consciousness, he would lose—*Brom., Dig., Dios., Mag. m., Oxyt., Plat., Thea*

　–momentarily, he had lost—*Lyss.*

　–were outside of his body—*Alum.*

Conversed with another person, she were carried somewhere and —*Raph.*

Convulsion, going into a—*Pyrus*

　–she would have a—*Raph.*

Corner, something were creeping out of every—*Phos.*

　–of room, part of head fitted into each—*Cann. i.*

　–horrible faces were looking out of every—*Phos.*

Cotton, he were treading on—*Onos.*

Couch moved—*Plb.*

Covered the whole bed—*Pyrog.*

Country, and then in another, now in one—*Chlol.*

Crazy, she were—*Pall., Phys., Sulph.*

　–she were half—*Sanic.*

　–he were going—*Iod., Tarent.*

　–he would become—*Chlor., Cimic., Lac c., Lil. t., Manc., Med.*

　–if she did not hold herself, she would go—*Lil. t.*

　–snapping in head were nearly driving him—*Antip.*

　–she would go—*Ail.*

Creep into his own body, he would crouch together as much as he could and—*Cimx.*

Creeping out of every corner, something were—*Phos.*

Crime, he had committed a—*Carb. v., Chel., Chin. s., Cyc., Dig., Ign., Merc., Nux v., Puls., Rheum, Rhus t., Verat. a., Zinc.*

　–had been committed—*Am. c.*

　–one were impelled to commit some horrible—*Thea*

　–conscious of having committed—*Zinc. ox.*

Criminal, he were the greatest—*Saba.*

Crowded with arms and legs, he were—*Pyrog.*

Cruel, he would like to do something—*Abrot.*

Crush him, houses on both sides of street would approach and— *Arg. n.*

Crushed by bedclothes—*Pic. ac.*

  –by everybody's rushing—*Tub.*

Cry, he could—*Caj.*

  –he could do nothing but—*Apoc.*

Cured, he could not be—*Alum.*

Danced all night, he had—*Clem.*

  –several nights, he had—*Sabin.*

Dancing, he were—*Agar., Puls.*

  –up and down when walking—*Ars. s. f.*

Danger were impending—*Camph., Macrot.*

  –menaced him—*Fl. ac.*

Dazed, mind were—*Tub.*

Dead, one were—*Œna., Raph., Sil.*

  –and preparations were being made for her funeral—*Lach.*

  –and still, she were alone and all about her were—*Rhus t.*

  –and wishes someone would help her off, she were nearly—*Lach.*

Death were approaching—*Thea*

  –were close at hand—*Ant. t., Verat. a.*

  –were near—*Puls.*

  –must result (cardiac trouble)—*Pop.*

  –she dreaded—*Tab.*

Debauch, one had been up all night or after a—*Coniin., Nux v.*

  –after a—*Op.*

Deed, she had committed a wicked—*Cocc.*

  –which others knew; could not look anyone in the face, he were
     guilty of some—*Cob.*

Delicate and thin, whole body were—*Thuj.*

Delirious—*Nit. ac.*

  –she would become—*Gels.*

Demon sits on his neck prompting to offensive things—*Anac.*

Deprived of his senses, he would be—*Cyc.*

Deranged, she were going—*Lac c.*

Descending a mountain—*Cyc.*

Detached—*Samars.*

Devil on account of crimes he had never done, he were persecuted
    by men or the—*Zinc.*

  –she were a—*Kali br.*

Die, he would—*Am. c., Asaf., Asar., Gels., Glon., Lil. t., Med.,
    Mur. ac., Plat., Psor., Rhus t., Ruta, Sil., Sulph.*

  –she were going to—*Caps., Caust., Croc., Lyss., Magnol., Pyrus*

  –about to—*Glon., Lyc., Phos., Plat., Raph.*

Die—*Continued*

   —from exhaustion, she would—*Lach.*

   —from weakness, one would—*Asar., Lyc., Vinc.*

   —on going to sleep, she would—*Lach.*

   —before movement, about to—*Nat. h.*

   —a sudden death—*Thea*

   —she must—*Nux v.*

   —one would sink down and—*Asar.*

   —she must lie down and—*Kali c.*

   —than live, one would rather—*Xanth.*

Direction, vertigo moved now in one, now in another—*Coff. t.*

Disease, she were a loathsome, horrible mass of—*Lac c.*

Dissolved, body continuity would be—*Thuj.*

Dissolving and she were going crazy, brain were—*Calc. c.*

Distance, everything were at a great—*Magnol.*

Distant island, she were on a—*Phos.*

   —objects were too—*Anac.*

Disturb his sleep, someone would come and—*Agar.*

Divided into halves and left side did not belong to her, she were— *Sil.*

Dizzy—*Jug. r., Stram.*

   —he would become—*Malar.*

   —and lose consciousness, she would become—*Mag. m.*

Dizziness commenced in front of ears and pressed to vertex— *Salix p.*

Do anything yet something must be done, unable to—*Pop.*

   —nothing, he could—*Lyss.*

   —something dreadful while tremblings were on, he were going to—*Visc.*

Does everything that he does, someone by his side who—*Ars.*

Dogs surrounded him—*Bell.*

Done something bad she had—*Ferr.*

Double, one person were lying on the right side and another lying on the left, she were—*Pyrog.*

   —and fever would not run alike in both, she were—*Pyrog.*

   —the inner one a little smaller, the outside one loosely put on; when sitting or lying down the inner is all the time urging the outer to get up; she were—*Anac.*

   —existence, she had a—*Cann. i.*

   —one were—*Bapt.*

Drawing round in a circle and she could not hold head straight, something were—*Lyss.*

–her to the right in morning when walking, something were—*Sil.*

Drawn from under her, bed were—*Stram.*

–forth and wafted quickly in direction of legs—*Tell.*

–from floor, difficult to place foot to floor, one were—*Euon. atrop.*

Dreaded death—*Tab.*

–misfortune—*Rhus t.*

Dreadful while tremblings were on, she were going to do something—*Visc.*

–had happened, something—*Med.*

Dream, in a—*Ambr., Anac., Calc. c., Cann. i., Con., Med., Rheum, Sang., Sars., Stram., Valer., Verat. a., Ziz.*

–he were arousing himself from a—*Carb. v.*

Dreamed everything that happened during the day, one had—*Lach.*

Dreaming, he were—*Valer.*

Drinking, he had been—*Aran. s.*

Drop, she would—*Aran.*

–unconscious, he would—*Calc. c.*

Drugged—*Op.*

Drunk—see also INTOXICATED

Drunk—*Agar., Ant. cr., Arg. n., Asc. t., Aur., Bell., Bufo, Chlf., Cot., Croc., Kali br., Meph., Mez., Nux m., Œna., Op., Phys., Pip. m., Quer., Sil., Stram., Sulph., Suls. ac.*

–he had been—*Bapt.*

–all the time—*Arg. m.*

–for a week, he had been—*Onos.*

–the night before, he had been—*Bry.*

–partially—*Chlol.*

–affected side were—*Lat. k.*

–with cloudiness—*Alum.*

–giddy—*Ferr.*

–with nausea—*Acon.*

–with vertigo—*Ant. c.*

–with heavy head—*Acet. ac.*

–in head—*Calc. c.*

–on rising—*Graph.*

Drunken man were coming toward her and lying down beside her, a huge—*Cic.*

    –from smoke in brain—*Op.*

Dull from loss of sleep, head were—*Nicc.*

Dullness from taking liquor—*Saba.*

    –as after intoxication—*Squill.*

Duplicating his acts, there were one by his side—*Ars.*

Duty, he had not done his—*Cyc., Puls.*

Dying—*Acon., Apis, Cact., Chlf., Morph., Op., Podo., Ther., Thyroid., Vesp., Xanth.*

Earthquake, one were in an—*Fl. ac.*

Effort, she kept herself together only by a great—*Sac. lac.*

Elevated—*Phos., Rhus t., Sil.*

    –and would fall—*Mosch.*

    –and pressed forward—*Calc. c.*

Else and moves to edge of bed to make room, she were someone —*Valer.*

Emptiness around and under one on standing—*Kali br.*

    –behind one on turning around—*Kali c.*

Empty, head were—*Lact.*

End, gradually nearing his—*Verat. a.*

    –were near—*Graph.*

    –were approaching—*Zinc.*

Enemies allowed him no rest—*Dros.*

Engaged in a lawsuit, he were—*Nit. ac.*

Enjoyment, nothing could give her any—*Stram.*

Enormous size, one were of—*Cic.*

Enrage, with mirth, least provocation would—*Sumb.*

Estranged from him, objects about him were—*Valer.*

Epileptic spasm, she would have an—*Cina*

Ether in head, he had taken—*Cahin.*

Events that occurred in her dreams were not for hours, but for weeks' and months' duration—*Sang.*

Evil, he had done—*Zinc.*

    –power had control of the whole of him except will power— *Cann. s.*

    –were going to happen, some—*Alum., Meny.*

    –were impending—*Alum., Crot. h., Chin. s., Clem., Lach., Meny., Rumx.*

    –committed some—*Cyc., Zinc.*

Exalted—*Lac c., Plat.*

Excited after tea, brain were—*Hyper.*
    –and intoxicated—*Kali i.*
Exhausted—*Coca*
Exist any longer, she cannot—*Thuj.*
    –surroundings did not—*Puls.*
Existed around him, nothing—*Agn.*
Existence for her, outer world had no—*Nux m.*
    –he had only that moment begun his—*Camph.*
Expectant—*Coca*
Expecting unpleasant news—*Mez.*
Faces, horrible, were looking out of every corner—*Phos.*
Failed, memory—*Puls.*
Faint, he would—*Ang., Bry., Calc. c., Calend., Kali c., Lappa a.,*
        Med., Nat. m., Saba., Sep., Sil., Stann.
    –about to—*Cocc., Mag. c., Spong., Upas, Zing.*
    –about to (with qualmishness)—*Upas*
    –from emptiness of stomach, he would—*Bufo*
    –on lying down, he would—*Sulph.*
Fainted if he had any longer postponed waking, he would have—
        Carb. v.
Fainting, on the verge of—*Thea*
Faintness would occur—*Dig.*
Fall, one would—*Apis, Bell., Calc. c., Caust., Chen. a., Cup. m.,*
        Coloc., Equis., Lappa a., Lyss., Mag. m., Med., Puls.,
        Sabin., Sep., Spig., Stram., Visc., Wies., Zinc.
    –into a fire on walking past it, one would—*Onos.*
    –not unpleasantly, she would—*Lappa a.*
    –about to—*Mag. p. Ambo, Rhus t.*
    –out of bed, he would—*Arg. n., Ars., Ars. s. f.*
    –he were elevated and would—*Mosch.*
    –on dancing, he would—*Puls.*
    –headlong, he would—*Gels.*
    –if she did not hold onto something, she would—*Saba.*
    –if he looks down or on standing or walking, he would—*Spig.*
    –if he looks down on going downstairs, he would—*Onos.*
    –on looking up, he would—*Puls.*
    –from a seat, he would—*Alumn.*
    –from a height—*Calend.*
    –back on getting out of bed—*Rhus t.*
    –in open space, he would—*Ars.*
    –on standing, he would—*Oxyt., Samars.*

Fall—*Continued*
  –at every step, he would—*Dor.*
  –if he turns his head, he would—*Spig.*
  –if she walks—*Iod.*
  –when walking, he would—*Calc. c., Iod.*
  –backward, one would—*Chin., Dub., Spong., Staph.*
  –backward or to one side, he would—*Calc. c., Nux v.*
  –to left, she would—*Aur., Merl.*
  –to one side, he would—*Am. m., Calc. c., Rheum*
  –to one side, head would—*Spong.*
  –on one side on rising, he would—*Squill.*
  –from side to side, brain were loose and would—*Sul. ac.*
  –in all directions, head would—*Cann. s.*
  –to right, he would—*Itu, Sac. lac.*
  –to right side when at a height—*Zinc.*
  –to right when walking, he would—*Ruta*
  –to left, he would—*Calc. c., Dirc., Nat. m.*
  –forward, one would—*Chel., Chlf., Nat. m., Petr., Phos.*
      Ruta, Sil., Spig., Tarax.
  –forward, she must—*Nat. h.*
  –forward, head would—*Agn.*
  –forward and backward, she were going to—*Rhus t.*
  –forward on descending he would—*Samars.*
  –forward on rising from seat, he would—*Vib.*
  –forward when stooping, he would—*Berb., Puls.*
  –forward, turning around in head, head would—*Cupr.*
  –forward on walking, head would—*Calad., Hipp.*
  –over, he would—*Ars., Zinc.*
  –down on head, he would—*Chim. umb.*
  –on him, something would—*Tarent.*
Falling—*Bism., Med., Stram., Tub., Upas*
  –in children—*Gels.*
  –asleep, he were—*Asar., Mur. ac.*
  –when asleep—*Vib.*
  –when awakening—*Guaj., Sec.*
  –toward right side—*Camph.*
  –to left—*Eup. pur.*
  –if he turns to right or left—*Der.*
  –deep down—*Bell.*
  -forward—*Gels., Pic. ac., Xanth.*
  –backward—*Prim.*

Falling—*Continued*
 —off seat—*Stram.*
 —to pieces about her, room were—*Cann. i.*
 —backward through space—*Kali n.*
 —backward, head were—*Chin. s.*
 —from a height, she were—*Mosch.*
 —out of bed, head were—*Arg. m.*
 —through bed—*Bell., Dulc., Lach., Rhus t., Sacc.*
 —to pieces, whole body were—*Xanth.*
 —or sinking on closing eyes, bed were—*Sec.*
 —inward, walls of room were—*Arg. n., Carb. v.*
 —hole close by, into which he were in danger of—*Carb. s.*
 —on her, houses were—*Saba.*
Far off—*Med.*
 —in head—*Sec.*
Farewell to a near friend, she had bid—*Rhus t.*
Faster and faster, someone were reading after her so she must
  read—*Mag. m.*
Fatigue were forever banished—*Cann. s.*
Feeling for pins—*Sil.*
Feet would slip from under her—*Nicc.*
Fell, he suddenly—*Clem.*
Felt that things were near him even when not looking at them—
  Valer.
Fermenting, everything were—*Nux v.*
Fever, he had awakened from a—*Cic.*
 —were coming on—*Vichy*
Fit, she were going to have a—*Lyss.*
Fitted into each corner of room, part of head—*Cann. i.*
Float in air, she were so light she would—*Manc., Tep.*
 —to and fro on writing, things—*Anag.*
 —off, top of cranium were about to—*Nat. h.*
Floating—*Bell., Bry., Cocaine, Lach., Op., Pen., Xanth.*
 —in a boat—*Bell.*
 —over everything in the way—*Samars.*
 —body and limbs did not touch bed—*Stict.*
 —in air, she were—*Cocaine, Mosch., Nux m., Stict., Valer.*
 —off, head were—*Jug. r., Samars.*
 —in air, legs were—*Stict.*
 —in clouds, ideas were—*Datura a.*
 —outside his brain, ideas were—*Datura a.*

Floating—*Continued*
 –bed were—*Con.*
 –of images of fancy, head were moving up and down, with a
   similar—*Zinc.*
 –through air, when sitting—*Xanth.*
Floor were not there—*Samars.*
 –were sinking—*Lepi.*
 –were soft like wool, on walking—*Xanth.*
Fly, he were so light he could—*Camph.*
 –he were raised from ground and could—*Cann. i.*
 –he must—*Ars. s. f.*
 –away, she must—*Bell., Verat. a.*
 –she would—*Tub.*
 –(in female complaints) she would—*Lil. t.*
 –to pieces, he would—*Lact.*
Flying—*Jug. r., Op., Valer.*
 –round and round, head were—*Eup. pur.*
 –or swimming in air—*Calc. ar., Manc., Valer.*
Fog in brain—*Sulph.*
Forced him out of bed, something—*Rhus t.*
Forgetful, absent—*Bar. c.*
Forgotten something, he had—*Mill.*
 –something, he does not know what—*Iod.*
Forsaken by a near friend, she had been—*Rhus t.*
Frail and easily broken—*Thuj.*
Friendless and forsaken when awaking in morning—*Lach.*
Fright on waking, in a—*Bell.*
 –after sleep, in a—*Apis, Phys.*
Frightened—*Bor., Calc. p., Iber., Nat. a., Pæon., Psor., Sac. lac.,*
   Ter., Zinc.
 –he were terribly—*Stram.*
 –he had been—*Bapt., Calc. p., Merc.*
 –by a dream—*Bor.*
 –on waking—*Bell., Magnol., Mag. p. Aust., Samb., Sars.,*
   Zinc.
 –and indefinable dread with trembling—*Iber.*
 –by vision behind him—*Lach.*
Fumes of whiskey had gone to his head—*Ars. m.*
Functions must act, yet cannot (spell-bound)—*Pop.*
Gather ideas from afar, he had to—*Datura a.*

Gave way under him, everything—*Sanic.*
 —way under him, ground—*Kali br., Tep.*
Get out of her body in some way, she would become crazy if she could not—*Lac c.*
Giddiness, overpowering, were coming over her—*Con.*
Giddy—*Aml. n., Bell., Bufo, Gels., Sacc.*
 —(drunk)—*Ferr.*
Glass and easily broken, body were made of—*Thuj.*
Gliding along—*Bell.*
 —in air when walking—*Asar.*
Glittering, objects were too bright and—*Camph.*
Gnashing their teeth around his bed, he heard wild beasts—*Ars.*
Go round and round, brain seemed to—*Saba.*
 —from under him, legs would—*Staph.*
 —out of his mind, he would—*Kali br.*
Going up, feet were—*Phos. ac.*
 —out of mind—*Cot.*
Grasp any thought, he could not—*Phos.*
Grew larger and longer, one—*Plat.*
Grief, great, weighed upon him—*Con.*
 —or sorrow, laboring under some—*Am. m.*
Ground or stairs came up to meet him—*Pic. ac.*
 —gave way beneath his feet—*Dign., Kali br., Tep.*
 —were moving—*Clem.*
 —she would hardly touch—*Ars. m.*
 —were unsteady or sank—*Tep.*
 —on walking he did not touch—*Calc. ar., Camph., Peti., Tep., Thuj.*
 —he stood on wavering—*Sulph.*
 —were wavering on closing eyes—*Chlf.*
Guilt, great, weighed upon him—*Con.*
Guilty of some deed of which others knew; could not look one in the face—*Cob.*
Hammock, bed were swaying from side to side like a—*Tub.*
 —one were swinging above treetops in a—*Coff. t.*
Hand, delicate, were smoothing her—*Med.*
Hands of a stronger power, he were in—*Lach.*
Hanging over him, some overwhelming calamity were—*Calend.*
 —over a chair were a person, something—*Calc. c.*
 —with head downward, he were—*Glon.*

Happen, accident would—*Mag. c., Mag. s.*
  —something were going to—*Aml. n., Lappa a., Lyss., Mosch., Nat. a., Nat. m., Nicc., Pyrus, Xanth.*
  —something dreadful were going to—*Aml. n., Lappa a., Med., Thea*
  —some evil were going to—*Meny.*
  —something horrible were going to—*Elaps, Pall.*
  —some great misfortune were going to—*Calc. c., Ign., Rhus t., Vichy*
  —something unpleasant were going to—*Caust., Glon., Lyss., Mag. c., Mag. s.*
  —something were going to (with sense of horror)—*Tub.*
  —something terrible were going to—*Lyss., Onos., Pyrus*
Head were another strange head—*Ther.*
  —there were no—*Cocc.*
  —were on a pillow but did not know where rest of body was —*Pyrog.*
  —were falling out of bed—*Arg. m.*
Hears voices of people far away—*Anac.*
Heaven or hell, he did not care if he went to—*Med.*
  —with most wonderful visions, he were in—*Calc. ar.*
  —he were in—*Op.*
Heaviness of head—*Puls.*
Heavy and thick, atmosphere in room were—*Agn.*
  —for bed and it would break down unless supported, he were too—*Ovi g. p.*
Held up high when sitting, he were—*Rhus t.*
Hell or heaven, he did not care if he went to—*Med.*
Herself, she were not—*Puls.*
High building, stepped from a—*Dub.*
  —steps were too—*Tab.*
Higher than the houses, he were—*Camph.*
Hold her head straight, she could not—*Lyss.*
Hole close by into which he were in danger of falling—*Carb. s.*
Homesick, melancholy—*Sac. lac.*
House, he were not in his—*Op.*
  —burning, he saw his neighbor's—*Hep.*
  —were turned upside down (vertigo)—*Bufo*
Houses on both sides of street would approach and crush him—*Arg. n.*
  —were falling on her—*Saba.*

Houses—*Continued*
- −move as she walks—*Tep.*
- −at a distance turn bottom upward—*Eug.*

Hover in air, she would—*Manc.*

Hovering in air—*Manc., Nux m., Op., Stict., Valer.*
- −in air like a spirit (when walking in open air)—*Asar.*

Hurry, everything must be done in a—*Sul. ac.*

Ideas from afar, he had—*Datura a.*
- −were floating outside his brain—*Datura a.*
- −were floating in clouds—*Datura a.*
- −prevented him from completing work, a rush of—*Stann.*

Ill, he were going to be very—*Podo.*

Illness, severe, were impending—*Nicc.*

Ill-treated by everyone—*Sumb.*

Imminent, death were—*Puls.*

Impelled to commit some horrible crime—*Thea*
- −by an invisible agent, he slid along the ground—*Op.*
- −to commit suicide, he were—*Thea*
- −to commit suicide by drowning, he were—*Dros.*
- −to do reckless things—*Lyss.*

Impended, something unpleasant—*Agar., Caust.*

Impending, some horrible calamity were—*Rhus t.*
- −danger were—*Camph., Macrot.*
- −evil were—*Alum., Crot. h., Lach., Meny., Rumx.*
- −severe illness were—*Nicc.*
- −misfortune were—*Aster., Aur. m., Calc. c., Chin. s., Clem., Cyc., Graph., Kali p., Psor., Puls., Sanic., Sulph., Vichy*
- −some great misfortune were—*Sulph.*
- −trouble were—*Am. c.*
- −something were—*Nat. a.*

Imperative duties hurried her, with utter inability to perform them—*Lil. t.*

Impossible to think, it were—*Onos.*

Incline to right side, head would constantly—*Ferr.*

Inconsolable—*Stram.*

Individuals, she were two—*Lil. t.*

Inferior, persons about her were mentally and physically—*Plat.*

Inflated, head were (with confusion)—*Merl.*

Influenced him at the same time, two entirely different trains of thought—*Lyss.*

Insane, she were going—*Cann. i., Syph.*

Insensible in vertigo, he would become—*Nat. ntrs.*
Insulted, he had been—*Cham., Cocc., Sulph.*
Interest in anything, he felt no—*Nux v.*
Intelligence, he had received joyful—*Lyss.*
Intoxicated—see also Drunk.
Intoxicated—*Agar., Ang., Bufo, Carb. ac., Chin. s., Chlor., Cic., Cocc., Cor. r., Cot., Croc., Cur., Ferr., Gels., Glon., Hydr., Hyos., Jug. r., Kali br., Kali c., Lact., Lil. t., Lyc., Mag. p. Aust., Med., Merl., Mez., Mill., Nicc., Nux m., Nux v., Op., Petr., Phos. ac., Phos., Pip. m., Psor., Ptel., Puls., Ran. b., Raph., Rat., Rhod., Rhus t., Saba., Sec., Sep., Sol. n., Spig., Sulph., Suls. ac., Tab., Tarax., Thuj., Valer., Verat. a.*
  –when trying to move—*Gels.*
  –by degraded blood, brain were—*Crot. h.*
  –while undressing—*Sec.*
  –he had been—*Iodof., Kali c., Rheum*
  –he were pleasantly—*Oxyt.*
  –at 4 p.m. and in evening—*Cench.*
  –and excited—*Kali i.*
  –on seeing flowing water when walking—*Ferr.*
  –in room but not in open air—*Croc.*
Intoxication, dullness as after—*Squill.*
Island, she were on a distant—*Phos.*
Isolated from world—*Coca*
Jostling against everyone she meets—*Acon.*
Journey, after a long—*Chin. a.*
Jump out of window, one were impelled to—*Thea*
Kill people when in street, he ought to—*Camph.*
  –her, her mother wants to—*Sac. lac.*
Killed, she were being—*Sulph.*
Know where one were, one did not—*Cann. s., Glon., Merl.*
Laboring under grief or sorrow—*Am. m.*
Lady, she were a noble—*Phos.*
Large enough, bed were not—*Sulph.*
  –one were—*Arg. n., Caj., Par.*
  –sometimes very small and then very—*Sulph.*
  –room were too—*Tub.*
  –all things and persons were too small and too low, and he were too—*Plat.*
Larger and larger, one were growing—*Aur., Plat., Stram.*

Laughing at her whenever she goes into street, men were—*Bar. c.*

Lawsuit or dispute, causing uneasiness and anxiety, he were in a —*Nit. ac.*

Lazy to move, one were too—*Eucal.*

Learn anew everything she wished to do, she would have to—*Sep.* .

Legs and arms, he had too many—*Pyrog.*

  –he would stumble over his own—*Caj.*

  –were all over sidewalk—*Kali br.*

  –were going out from under him with slightest gust of wind—*Staph.*

Lie down, she must—*Nux m.*

  –down in street, she could—*Kali c.*

  –down all the time, she would like to—*Saba.*

Lies down beside him, another person—*Petr.*

Life in him, he had no (weakness)—*Dub.*

  –he wished to take his own—*Rhus t.*

  –were unreal—*Med.*

  –were in danger from assassination or poison—*Plb.*

Lifted from couch, she were being—*Stroph.*

  –high in air, she were being—*Hyper.*

Light—*Gels., Lach.*

  –head were—*Sarr.*

  –head were too—*Jab.*

  –body were very—*Mez.*

  –everything about body were too—*Dig.*

  –she could float in air, she were so—*Manc., Tep.*

  –and could fly, he were—*Camph.*

  –she did not touch ground when walking, she were so—*Tep.*

  –on walking, she were very—*Spig., Tep., Thuj.*

Lighter and could fly, not touching ground—*Camph.*

Limbs, she had no—*Stram.*

Liquor; dullness, he had taken—*Saba.*

  –he had taken—*Bapt.*

  –under the influence of—*Pip. m.*

Live, she could not—*Vib.*

Living, he could not make a—*Chlor.*

Locomotive, about to be run over by a—*Phos.*

Longer, time were—*Pall.*

  –and longer, he were growing—*Plat., Stram.*

Look one in face because of guilt (though not guilty), he could not—*Cob.*

Looking out of every corner, horrible faces were—*Phos.*
  –down, he were—*Phos.*
  –over her shoulder, strange persons were—*Brom.*
Loose, brain were—*Phos., Spig.*
Lose consciousness, he would—*Brom., Dig., Dios., Oxyt., Plat., Thea*
  –consciousness on lying down—*Agar.*
  –consciousness, she would become dizzy and—*Mag. m.*
  –all self-control, she would—*Gels., Samars.*
  –her reason, she would—*Acon., Cupr., Glon., Iris t., Lil. t., Phys.*
  –her senses, she would—*Calc. c., Cann. s., Gels., Nat. s., Psor., Sulph.*
Losing his reason, he were—*Kali bi., Merc.*
  –senses, she were gradually—*Sil.*
Lost (before headache)—*Cot.*
  –consciousness, he momentarily—*Lyss.*
  –her will power, she had partly—*Nit. ac.*
Lying, she did not touch bed when—*Asar., Chin., Coff., Lac c., Nat. m., Nux v., Op., Rhus t., Spig., Stram., Thuj.*
  –in bed, she were not—*Hyper.*
  –very heavy in bed—*Hyper.*
  –down, one would lose consciousness on—*Agar.*
  –on one side she were one person and when lying on other side another person—*Pyrog.*
  –on a large snake—*Lac c.*
  –in bed with him, a strange boy were—*Apis*
  –down beside her, a huge drunken man were coming toward her and—*Cic.*
Man were coming toward her and lying down beside her, a huge drunken—*Cic.*
  –were present who was not (delirium)—*Hyos.*
Marble statue, he were a—*Cann. i.*
Medicine or had been poisoned, he had taken—*Linar.*
Memory failed—*Puls.*
Men or devil on account of crimes he had never committed, he were persecuted by—*Zinc.*
  –were laughing at her on street—*Bar. c.*
Menaced him, danger—*Fl. ac.*
Mental acts were performed in stomach—*Acon.*
Mice in bed, there were—*Colch.*

Mind on anything, inability to fix—*Con.*

  –he would go out of his—*Kali br.*

  –he were going out of his—*Eup. per., Ham., Ol. j.*

  –on walking, he were going out of—*Cot.*

  –were separated from body—*Anac.*

Miscarries, everything—*Nux v.*

Misfortune, great, were going to happen—*Calc. c., Ign., Rhus t., Vichy*

  –were impending—*Aster., Aur. m., Calc. c., Clem., Cupr., Cyc., Kali p., Psor., Sanic., Sulph., Vichy*

  –he dreaded—*Rhus t.*

  –to himself, he foresaw a—*Spong.*

  –would overtake him, some—*Cupr.*

  –oppressed by some—*Hura*

  –would befall him, some personal—*Crot. t.*

Monster would come from under her chair, some horrid—*Lac c.*

Motion, air itself were in tremulous (fever)—*Saba.*

  –bed were in—*Lac c.*

  –all within head were in—*Verat. a.*

  –everything were in—*Saba.*

  –everything were making a see-saw—*Cyc.*

  –objects were in—*Kali cy., Mos., Sep., Thuj.*

Mountain, he were climbing a steep—*Prun.*

  –he were descending a—*Cyc.*

Mouse ran under her chair—*Cimic.*

Move, yet > by motion, she could not—*Homar.*

  –in all directions, everything about him began to—*Tab.*

Moved slowly, everything about him—*Hydr. ac.*

  –around him, objects—*Nux v., Sep.*

  –couch (vertigo)—*Plb.*

  –in a circle on stooping, everything—*Sol. n.*

  –rapidly and confusedly, all about her—*Sang.*

  –backward and forward, objects—*Carb. ac.*

  –to right, all objects—*Nat. sal.*

Moving in all directions, head were—*Eup. pur.*

  –around one, objects were—*Sep.*

  –to and fro when sitting and lying, he were—*Thuj.*

  –up and down with a similar floating of images of fancy, head were—*Zinc.*

  –brain were (vertigo)—*Cyc.*

  –around, everything were—*Anac.*

Moving—*Continued*
 –from side to side, everything were—*Cic.*
 –ground were—*Clem.*
 –when walking, all houses were—*Tep.*
 –to and fro, his seat were—*Thuj.*
 –in a circle when stooping, things were—*Sol. n.*
 –and jarring her, she were in railway car which was—*Sang.*
 –in a new world—*Camph.*
 –up and down, objects were—*Phos.*
Moves to and fro, everything—*Form.*
Muddled, brain were—*Coca*
Murder someone, he would—*Hep.*
 –him, someone were coming to—*Tab.*
Music, under influence of pleasant and quick—*Zinc. p.*
Net, in a—*Nat. m.*
New and he had never seen them, all things appear—*Stram.*
News, expecting joyful—*Lyss., Valer.*
 –bad, about to arrive—*Aster.*
 –unpleasant, he would hear—*Dros., Lyss.*
 –expecting unpleasant—*Lyss., Mez.*
 –agitated by unpleasant—*Alumn.*
Noble lady, she were a—*Phos.*
Nobody, he were a—*Agn.*
Nothing, he could do—*Lyss.*
 –existed around him—*Agn.*
 –could give her any enjoyment—*Stram.*
Objects about him were estranging him—*Valer.*
 –leave their place and follow her—*Coff. t.*
 –moved to right—*Nat. sal.*
 –reel—*Bell., Bry., Glon.*
 –run into each other—*Iris fœ.*
 –turned upside down—*Guan.*
 –waver—*Grat., Til.*
 –were in motion—*Kali cy., Mos., Sep., Thuj.*
 –were too far off (vertigo)—*Anac., Stann.*
Occurred a week ago, things done today—*Med.*
Opiate, he were under influence of an—*Cann. i.*
Oppressed—*Carb. v.*
 –by some misfortune—*Hura*
Outside patient, a second self—*Bapt.*
 –of herself and could see into herself—*Pyrus*

Paralyzed—*Agar., Cist., Cyc., Sacc., Sang.*
  –about to be—*Syph.*
  –will were—*Carb. v., Pop.*
  –after a short walk—*Con.*

Pass a certain point on walking without falling, he could not—*Arg. n.*

Passed over him, a cloud—*Samars.*

Pendulum, vertigo were like vibration of a—*Bell.*

Performed in stomach, mental acts were—*Acon.*

Persecuted by men or the devil on account of crimes he had never done—*Zinc.*
  –in visions—*Hyos.*

Person, she existed in another—*Pyrog.*
  –lies alongside him, another—*Petr.*
  –she were one person while lying on one side and some other person when lying on other side—*Pyrog.*
  –had seen what he saw and had said what he himself had said, another—*Alum.*
  –had touched him quietly on both sides—*Bapt.*

Persons were looking over her shoulder, strange—*Brom.*
  –about her were inferior—*Plat.*
  –two, lay in her bed and the body of the other overlapped hers by half—*Cyc.*
  –she were two—*Lil. t.*

Pieces and could not get them adjusted, he were in several—*Phos*
  –and it were only by a great effort she kept herself together; it would be a relief to fall to—*Sac. lac.*
  –whole body were falling to—*Xanth.*

Pillow, head were on a; but did not know where rest of his body was—*Pyrog.*

Pitch forward, he would—*Senec.*
  –forward on face when walking, he would—*Ter.*
  –every nerve were strung to highest—*Pip. m.*

Place, he were in a strange—*Cic., Tub.*

Poison, he had taken—*Caj., Euph.*

Poisoned, he had taken medicine or had been—*Linar.*

Power, she were in hands of a stronger—*Lach.*
  –of moving were lost—*Mag. p. Aust.*

Pregnant—*Verat. a.*

Pressed forward, he were elevated and—*Calc. c.*

Prevented him from completing work, a rush of ideas—*Stann.*

Projected from head that he could not see over, something—*Phel.*

Prompting to offensive things, a demon sits on neck—*Anac.*

Prostrated, extremely—*Eup. per.*

Provocation, least, would enrage (with mirth)—*Sumb.*

Pulled backward—*Samars.*

–backward, he were (with headache)—*Merc.*

Pulled and torn into threads—*Plat.*

Pursuing him, someone were—*Anac., Merc.*

Pushed forward, head were suddenly—*Ferr. p.*

Railroad car, she were in a—*Sang.*

Raised up, he were being—*Sil.*

–from ground and could fly—*Cann. i.*

Ran under her chair, a mouse—*Cimic.*

–against something—*Arg. m.*

Reach to clouds, arms, face, tongue, and forepart of brain seems to—*Pic. ac.*

Reading after her so that she must read faster and faster, someone were—*Mag. m.*

Real, things were not—*Cann. s.*

Reality, everything perceived had no—*Anac.*

Reason would leave him—*Tanac.*

–from pain, one were losing one's—*Kali bi.*

–were losing his—*Merc., Nat. m.*

–she would lose her—*Acon., Cupr., Glon., Iris t., Lil. t., Phys.*

Receded, everything approached and—*Cic.*

Reeled around her, things—*Merc. i. r.*

–to and fro, head—*Carb. v.*

Reeling—*Spig.*

–from side to side—*Gamb.*

–when at rest—*Tax.*

–all objects were—*Bell., Bry., Glon.*

Reproved, he expected to be—*Dig.*

Respiration, whole attention must be centered on act of—*Chlor.*

Rest, enemies allowed him no—*Dros.*

Reveling all night, he had been—*Rhod.*

Revolving on axis—*Nux v.*

Rid her mind of the torture, she must do something to—*Med.*

Riding when lying down, < closing eyes—*Ferr.*

–with closed eyes—*Cyc.*

Rise up again if one stooped, one could not—*Bry., Puls., Rhus t.*

Rising, chair on which he were sitting were—*Phos.*
   —before him, sidewalk were—*Spig.*
   —when walking, street were—*Sep.*
Rocked, one were being—*Bell., Calad., Nat. m.*
   —when lying down and closing eyes, he were—*Calad., Nat. m.*
Rolling about in head (vertigo), something were—*Sep.*
   —over like a ball—*Samars.*
   —over bed-clothes, balls of fire were—*Stram.*
Room were full of strange men, passing in and out, who wanted
     to take her away—*Bell.*
   —in it, someone would get into his bed and there would be no
     —*Nux v.*
   —were too large—*Tub.*
   —were too small—*Cyc.*
   —were falling to pieces about her—*Cann. i.*
   —went round—*Calc. caust., Cann. s., Cod., Dub., Grat., Kali bi.*
Round and round, brain whirled—*Saba.*
   —and round, objects were turning—*Laur.*
   —and round, head were flying—*Eup. pur.*
   —and round when looking at water, everything went—*Ferr.*
   —and round, objects go—*Psor.*
   —room went—*Calc. caust., Cann. s., Cod., Dub., Grat., Kali bi.*
Rouse him, someone were trying to—*Cur.*
Rousing him from a dream—*Carb. v.*
Rowdies would break in if alone—*Elaps*
Ruined, he will be—*Puls.*
Run as never before, he could—*Agar.*
   —a long way, he could—*Coca*
   —away, she had to—*Ars. m.*
   —backward, he were chased and had to—*Sep.*
   —up and down and scream, she would like to—*Calc. c.*
   —into each other, objects—*Iris fœ.*
Said it, another person had—*Alum.*
Scattered about—*Bapt.*
Scream, he must—*Lil. t.*
   —unless he held on to something, he would—*Sep.*
   —would like to run up and down and—*Calc. c.*
Sea, one were at—*Cocc.*
Seasick, one were—*Tab.*
   —after riding on horseback in dark—*Sanic.*
Seasickness (vertigo as from)—*Magnol.*

Seat were balancing to and fro when closing eyes—*Thuj.*
  –were tottering—*Chlf.*
  –were undulating when sitting up in bed in morning—*Zinc.*
Second self outside of patient, there were—*Tab.*
See something if he turned around, he would—*Brom.*
  –into herself, she were outside of herself and could—*Pyrus*
Seeking something, he were—*Stram.*
Seen what he had seen, and said what he himself had said, another person had—*Alum.*
Self-control, one would lose all—*Gels., Samars.*
  –consciousness were outside of body—*Alum.*
Self outside patient, a second—*Bapt.*
  –and is not sure which will conquer the other, there were another—*Op.*
Senses, impossible to collect his—*Cham., Hyos.*
  –she would lose her—*Agar., Calc. c., Cann. s., Sulph.*
  –when thinking long about anything, she would lose her—*Ars.*
  –one would lose one's—*Brom., Cupr., Gels., Nat. s., Psor.*
  –she were gradually losing her—*Sil.*
  –would vanish—*Plat., Ran. b.*
  –deprived of his—*Cyc.*
Separate from him, strange thoughts were—*Saba.*
Separated from body, spirit were—*Anac.*
  –from body, mind were—*Anac.*
  –soul and body were—*Cann. i., Thuj.*
  –from himself in evening—*Saba.*
  –from whole world, he were—*Anac.*
Settled over her, heavy black cloud had—*Cimic.*
Shocks, he fell suddenly from electric—*Clem.*
Shoved forward when driving—*Ferr.*
  –forward when lying down—*Ferr.*
Shut in a dark cellar (anxiety)—*Nat. p.*
Sick—*Tarax.*
  –persons, two, in bed, one of whom recovered and the other did not—*Sec.*
Sidewalk were rising before him—*Spig.*
Side who does everything he does, someone by his—*Ars.*
Sin, she had committed the unpardonable—*Chel., Med.*
Sink away, she were going to—*Lyss.*
  –down and die, he would—*Asar.*
  –through bed, she would—*Chin. s.*

Sinking down in bed, everything were—*Lyc.*

–deep down in bed, she were—*Bry.*

–through bed—*Bell., Dulc., Lach., Rhus t.*

–from under her, bed were—*Kali c.*

–or falling on closing eyes; bed and all were going down—*Sec.*

–down, bed and patient were—*Lach.*

–when working in a hot room—*Glon.*

–and would die—*Asar.*

–through floor, he were—*Phos.*

Sitting too high—*Aloe*

–in wet—*Morph.*

Sits on his neck prompting to offensive things, a demon—*Anac.*

Sleep, deprived of—*Rhus t.*

–he would die on going to—*Lach.*

–loss of—*Merl., Zinc.*

–he had too little—*Rheum*

–just awakened from—*Mang.*

–going to—*Lappa a., Plat.*

–were in air, on going to—*Tell.*

–going into a state of deep—*Camph.*

–in a stupid—*Ant. t.*

–(confusion) he ought to—*Ant. t.*

–in a sound—*Visc.*

–someone would disturb his—*Agar.*

Sleepy—*Merl., Nat. m., Nux m.*

Slept enough, he had not—*Ars., Bapt., Bell., Calc. c., Colch.,
Coniin., Dig., Eucal., Luna, Magnol., Nicc., Nux v., Phos.,
Ran. b., Ruta, Sulph., Thuj.*

–he had not—*Lac. ac., Rhus t.*

–in morning, he had not—*Bell., Ham.*

–all night, he had—*Euph., Linar.*

Slid along ground impelled by an invisible agent—*Op.*

Slip from under her, feet would—*Nicc.*

Slipped back and forth beneath her, ground—*Tep.*

Small, everything around her were very—*Plat.*

–and sometimes very large, sometimes very—*Sulph.*

–room were too—*Cyc.*

Smaller than they really were, objects were—*Stram.*

–one were—*Carb. v.*

–everything were—*Plat.*

Smoke on brain—*Op.*

Smoothing her, a delicate hand were—*Med.*
Smother on falling asleep, she would—*Arum t.*
Snake, she were lying on a—*Lac c.*
Snakes, he were surrounded by myriads of—*Lac c.*
Sneaking up behind her, someone were—*Sanic.*
Soft like wool on walking, floor were—*Xanth.*
Someone else, she were—*Cann. s., Lach.*
  —else and in hands of a stronger power—*Lach.*
  —would get into his bed and there would be no room in it—
    Nux v.
  —were behind one—*Brom., Crot. h., Lach., Med., Sac. lac.,*
    Tub.
  —were behind him when in bathtub—*Samars.*
  —were coming up behind him—*Staph.*
  —would come and disturb his sleep—*Agar.*
  —by his side who does everything he does—*Ars.*
  —had sold his bed—*Nux v.*
  —were pursuing him—*Anac.*
  —were reading after her so that she must read faster and faster
    —*Mag. m.*
  —were sneaking up behind him—*Sanic.*
  —else were speaking—*Cann. s.*
  —were walking beside her—*Calc. c.*
Something were under bed making a noise—*Bell.*
  —forced him out of bed nights—*Rhus t.*
  —hanging over a chair were a person—*Calc. c.*
Sorrow or grief, laboring under some—*Am. m.*
Soul and body were separated—*Cann. i., Thuj.*
Speaking, someone else were—*Cann. s.*
Spell, she were charmed and could not break the—*Lach.*
  —bound; all functions must act yet cannot—*Pop.*
Spirit had separated from body—*Anac.*
Staggering—*Carb. ac.*
  —(too weak)—*Olnd.*
Stairs or ground were coming up to meet him—*Pic. ac.*
Stand up, when sitting she must—*Sep.*
Standing, faintness would occur while—*Dig.*
  —on head—*Phos. ac.*
  —on wavering ground—*Sulph.*
  —securely, he were not—*Asar., Calc. ac.*

Stepped from a high building—*Dub.*
    –on empty space—*Dub.*
Stepping on air—*Nat. m.*
    –on down when walking—*Der.*
Steps as easy as one, she could take ten—*Pulx.*
Stimulant had been taken—*Nux v., Saba.*
Stones were sinking under his feet when crossing a stone bridge
    —*Nat. m.*
Stood alone in world, she were left entirely to herself and—*Plat.*
    –on wavering ground—*Sulph.*
Stool, he would be obliged to go to (vertigo)—*Spig.*
Strain herself, she could easily—*Sep.*
Strange boy lying in bed with him—*Apis*
    –head, head were another—*Ther.*
    –person were at his side—*Thuj.*
    –place, he were in a—*Cic., Tub.*
    –everything in room were strange—*Tub.*
    –and horrible, everything were—*Plat.*
    –thoughts were separate from him—*Saba.*
    –objects were—*Cann. s.*
    –well-known street were—*Glon.*
Stranger were beside him—*Anac.*
Strangers, he were in midst of—*Aster.*
Street were strange, a well-known—*Glon.*
    –were rising when walking—*Sep.*
Strength were failing, all his—*Coloc.*
Strike anyone in face who spoke to him, he would like to—*Nux v.*
Struck with apoplexy—*Kali cy., Tarent.*
Strung to highest pitch, nerves were—*Pip. m.*
Study, head were dull from too much—*Nat. n.*
Stumble over his own legs, he would—*Caj.*
Stunned—*Laur.*
Stupefied—*Nux v., Olnd., Rhus t., Staph.*
    –head were—*Rheum*
    –in morning—*Thuj.*
    –from coal gas—*Zinc.*
    –from night reveling—*Nux v.*
    –as after tobacco smoking—*Spig.*
Stupid if head were held erect—*Nux v.*
    –in left half of head—*Psor.*
    –after a debauch—*Psor.*

Suction, bound to bed by—*Sars.*
Suicide, impelled to commit—*Thea*
   —by drowning, impelled to commit—*Dros.*
   —though she has a great aversion to it, she would commit (on seeing knives)—*Alum.*
Sun pushed her down and she had to rest in shade in order to walk on—*Psor.*
Sunk deep in bed, he had—*Xanth.*
Superior power, under influence of a—*Thuj.*
Support himself, he could not—*Tab.*
Surrounded by dogs, he were—*Bell.*
   —by myriads of snakes, he were—*Lac c.*
Surrounding objects were very small and he were very large—*Stram.*
Surroundings did not exist—*Puls.*
   —whirled with her—*Aloe*
   —or self tottered—*Anac.*
Suspended in air—*Sep.*
   —and not lying in bed—*Hyper.*
Suspicious of those about him—*Hyos.*
Swashing in brain when walking—*Spig.*
Swayed to and fro, objects around him—*Bell., Form.*
Swaying in head when walking—*Daph.*
   —to and fro when sitting, whole body were—*Paraf.*
   —back and forth, head were constantly—*Zinc.*
   —back and forth, bed were—*Zinc.*
   —from side to side like a hammock, bed were—*Tub.*
   —about on chair—*Spong.*
Swimming in head—*Ars. h.*
   —brain were—*Sol. n.*
   —when lying down—*Ox. ac.*
   —or flying in air—*Calc. ar., Lact., Manc., Valer.*
Swing, one were in a—*Merc.*
   —one were swung to and fro in a—*Ign.*
Swinging—*Sulph.*
   —in bed—*Camph., Lact.*
   —from behind forward, head were—*Pall.*
   —above tree tops into clouds (in hammock)—*Coff. t.*
Swung to and fro in a swing or cradle—*Ign.*
   —from behind forward, head were—*Pall.*
Take his own life, he wished to—*Rhus t.*

Taken medicine, he had—*Linar.*
 –poison, he had—*Linar.*
 –from him, objects around him had been—*Valer.*
 –stimulant, he had—*Nux v., Saba.*
Talked very rapidly, all around her—*Sang.*
Tall, very—*Neosin, Stram.*
Taller, he had grown—*Pall.*
Tea, brain were excited after—*Hyper.*
Tears, he would burst into—*Aster., Cot.*
Teeming with live things whirling around it, head were—*Sil.*
Telling truth, she were not—*Macrot.*
Temper, he were in a bad—*Zinc.*
Terrified on waking—*Lyc.*
Thicker than natural, everything he touched were—*Coc. c.*
Thin and delicate, whole body were—*Thuj.*
Think outside of himself, he cannot—*Crot. t.*
Threads, torn and pulled into—*Plat.*
Things done today occurred a week ago—*Med.*
 –were not real—*Cann. s.*
 –wrong with him, he had a million—*Samars.*
Think of words, he could not—*Verat. a.*
 –outside of himself, he cannot—*Crot. t.*
 –it were impossible to—*Onos.*
 –about something, he knows not what; he ought to—*Iod.*
Thought influenced him at same time, two entirely different trains
 of—*Lyss.*
Thoughts, strange, were separate from him—*Saba.*
 –would suddenly vanish—*Croc., Kali c.*
Threatened with epileptic attack—*Alum.*
 –with fatal accident—*Alum.*
Time to arise, it were—*Dig.*
Tipping over when sitting or walking—*Euon. atrop.*
Tipsy—*Spong.*
Tired, spoke as if—*Cann. i.*
Tobacco, vertigo were from—*Rhod.*
Together, could not get himself—*Caj.*
 –and it would be a relief to fall to pieces; only by a great
 effort she kept herself—*Sac. lac.*
Top-heavy, head were—*Cham.*
Topsy-turvy on walking, head were—*Cham.*
Torture, she must do something to rid herself of the—*Med.*

Tossed up from below in every direction, objects were—*Lac d.*

Tossing on a rough sea—*Lac. ac., Sac. lac.*

Tottering, surroundings were—*Anac.*

　　–seat were—*Chlf.*

Touch anything, she could not—*Pall.*

　　–bed when lying down, he did not—*Asar., Chin., Coff., Lac c., Nat. m., Nux v., Op., Phos. ac., Rhus t., Spig., Stram., Stict., Thuj.*

　　–bed, body and limbs were floating and did not—*Stict.*

　　–ground, feet did not—*Calc. ar.*

　　–ground, he were lighter and did not—*Camph.*

　　–ground when walking, he does not—*Peti.*

　　–ground on walking, she were so light she could not—*Tep.*

　　–ground, she would hardly—*Ars. m.*

Touched earth with his feet, he scarcely—*Datura a.*

　　–him quietly on both sides, some person had—*Bapt.*

Transfer himself into another and only then could see, he could—*Alum.*

Tread lightly to avoid injuring or disturbing his companions, he must—*Cupr.*

Treading on cotton—*Onos.*

Trembled and turned in a circle, everything—*Plb.*

　　–and wavered, everything—*Aml. n.*

　　–but without trembling—*Carb. s., Med., Sul. ac., Zinc.*

Trifles, beside himself with—*Carl.*

Trouble were impending—*Am. c.*

　　–every trifle would lead into great—*Anac.*

Truth, she were not telling—*Macrot.*

Tumble, he would—*Calc. c.*

Turn in a circle, head would—*Bry.*

　　–in a circle about her, objects—*Coff. t.*

　　–bottom upward, houses at a distance—*Eug.*

　　–around, she would (fainting, nausea)—*Alum.*

　　–around with him on closing eyes, objects—*Cod.*

Turned around, one were being—*Bry.*

　　–backward and around—*Ang.*

　　–around with her, everything—*Phos.*

　　–about, bed—*Nux v., Plb., Puls., Sin. n.*

　　–in a circle, everything—*Agn., Bell., Cyc., Laur., Nat. m.*

　　–in a circle, everything in front of her (when walking)—*Nat. m.*

Turned—*Continued*

–in a half-circle, everything—*Staph.*

–in a circle for a long time, he had—*Puls.*

–round and round, everything—*Laur.*

–in a circle, bed—*Con.*

–so rapidly that he perceived a current of air produced by the motion, he were—*Mosch.*

–upside down, house were—*Bufo*

–upside down, objects—*Guan.*

–in a circle, everything trembled and—*Plb.*

–around, he would see something if he—*Brom.*

Turning around, body or objects were—*Cyc., Saba.*

–around, everything were—*Alum., Lyc., Mag. c., Valer.*

–around, brain were—*Bry.*

–around, occiput were—*Iber.*

–around each other, things were—*Saba.*

–around in head and would fall forward—*Cupr.*

–in a circle—*Alum., Anac., Arg. n., Aur., Carl., Chel., Merc., Ruta, Tub.*

–in a circle, head were—*Bry.*

–around, he were—*Agar.*

–in a circle, he were—*Con.*

–in a circle, he had been—*Thuj.*

–in a circle, everything were—*Bell., Chel., Cyc., Verat. a., Zinc.*

–in a circle during rest—*Juncus*

–in a circle when stooping—*Aur. m.*

–rapidly in a circle, bed were—*Sol. n.*

–in a circle, room were—*Nux v.*

–with him in a circle, surroundings were—*Am. c.*

–on sitting up, everything were—*Chel.*

–with her, things were—*Aloe, Anac., Arn., Calc. c., Ferr.*

–round and round, objects were—*Laur.*

–to left, he were—*Anac.*

–into urine, she were—*Lac. ac.*

Two persons, she were—*Lil. t.*

Unable to collect his senses—*Cham.*

Unconscious, he would drop—*Calc. c.*

Unconsciousness might follow confusion—*Syph.*

–going into a state of—*Camph.*

Understand anything, she could not—*Sep.*

Undulating in whole head—*Indg.*
   —when sitting up in bed in morning, seat were—*Zinc.*
   —in head and whole body—*Stroph.*
Unhampered by a material body—*Cinch. b.*
Unpardonable sin, she had committed the—*Chel., Med.*
Unpleasant news, he had heard—*Lyss.*
   —news, he would soon hear—*Mez., Lyss.*
   —were going to happen, something—*Agar., Glon.*
Unreal, life were—*Med.*
   —everything were—*Aml. n.*
Urine, she were turning into—*Lac. ac.*
Vanish, senses would—*Plat., Ran. b.*
   —thoughts had—*Kali c.*
   —thought would—*Croc.*
   —from her, everything would—*Lyc.*
Vanished, all senses had—*Spira.*
   —thoughts had—*Kali c.*
Vehicle which was moving and jarring her, she were in some—*Sang.*
Vertigo would come on—*Brom.*
   —proceeded from stomach—*Kali c.*
   —started from left eye—*Lob.*
   —were from seasickness—*Magnol.*
Visions of delight filled his brain all night—*Op.*
   —are real—*Lach.*
Voices of absent persons, he heard—*Cham.*
   —of persons far off or dead, he hears—*Anac.*
Wafted and drawn forth quickly in direction of legs, always waking him—*Tell.*
Waking from a heavy sleep—*Rheum*
Walk forever, she could—*Fl. ac.*
Walked a long journey, she had—*Eup. pur.*
   —a great distance and were tired, one had—*Lac. ac.*
   —too far—*Verat. a.*
Walking on air—*Asar., Chin., Lac c., Nat. m., Nux v., Op., Phos., Rhus t., Thuj.*
   —backward when walking forward, he were—*Sil.*
   —beside him, someone were—*Calc. c.*
   —up and down rooms in his dreams—*Agar.*
Walls of room were falling inward—*Arg. n., Carb. v.*
Watching, after long night—*Op., Vib.*

Waver, objects—*Grat., Til.*
Wavered, everything trembled and—*Aml. n.*
Wavering, brain were—*Phos., Sul. ac.*
  –in brain when walking—*Phys.*
  –on closing eyes, ground were—*Chlf.*
  –ground, he stood on—*Sulph.*
  –objects were—*Cyc.*
  –and revolving, brain were—*Nux v.*
Waving lengthwise while lying—*Merc.*
Way home were too long—*Glon.*
Weighed upon him, a great grief—*Con.*
Weight, without—*Hyos.*
Went round and round on looking at water, everything—*Ferr.*
  –around with her, everything—*Ferr.*
  –round, room—*Calc. caust., Cann. s., Cod., Dub., Grat., Kali bi.*
Where he was, he did not know—*Cann. s., Glon., Merl.*
  –she was or what to do on waking, she could not tell—*Vib.*
Whirled around, he had been placed in a coal screen and—*Eup. per.*
  –round and round, brain—*Saba.*
  –about him when standing, everything—*Bry.*
  –around, everything in head—*Viol. o.*
  –around, everything—*Alum.*
  –with her, everything—*Aloe, Rhus t.*
  –around in head, something—*Sec.*
  –with her, surroundings—*Aloe*
  –in a circle, things—*Verat. a.*
Whirling in head—*Chel., Chlf., Ovi g. p.*
  –in head like a millwheel—*Chin. s.*
  –in head when thinking—*Coff.*
  –around it, head were teeming with live things—*Sil.*
  –around, everything were—*Zinc.*
  –in opposite direction if he shuts eyes—*Saba.*
  –around with her, bed were—*Nux v.*
  –room were—*Nux v.*
  –with everything round him—*Op.*
Wicked deed, she had committed a—*Cocc.*
Wild, he would go—*Lob.*
Will power, she had partly lost her—*Nit. ac.*
  –were paralyzed—*Pop.*

Wills, one commanding what other forbids, he had two—*Anac.*
Wings, when walking she were carried on—*Thuj.*
Wine, he had taken—*Saba.*
Wished to take his own life, he—*Rhus t.*
Withheld from action, mind and body must be in action, and yet
    —*Pop.*
Wobble to and fro, brain seems to—*Cyc., Spira.*
Wobbling in brain—*Ars.*
Wood and couldn't think, back of brain were made of—*Staph.*
Wool, on walking floor were soft like—*Xanth.*
Work without fatigue, he could—*Pip. m.*
  –she could not accomplish her—*Bry.*
World, outer, had no existence for her—*Nux m.*
  –rested upon him (weakness)—*Tab.*
Wrong, something were—*Kali br., Samars.*
  –one had done something—*Ign., Nux m., Ruta*
  –with him, he had a million things—*Samars.*

HEAD

Abscess in head—*Acon., Ars., Bor., Bov., Bufo, Carb. v., Nux v., Petr., Rhod., Sep.*

    –were forming in head—*Hep.*

    –were forming in brain—*Cupr.*

    –would form on left forehead—*Colch.*

Accumulating at top of head when stooping, blood were—*Am. c.*

Ache, head would—*Cimx.*

    –on waking, head were about to—*Cur.*

Aching were in periosteum of right brow—*Ol. j.*

Adhered too closely to cranium, scalp—*Mag. p. Arct.*

Adherent to bone and almost immovable, scalp of forehead and occiput were—*Par.*

    –to bones of skull, scalp were—*Sin.*

Agitated with boiling water, brain were—*Acon.*

Air were in head—*Aur., Benz. ac.*

    –head were filled to bursting with—*Lyss.*

    –head were floating in—*Jug. r.*

    –head were full of compressed—*Aur.*

    –rushed through head, current of—*Aur.*

    –head were surrounded by hot—*Aster.*

    –headache were from cold—*Coloc., Tarent.*

    –cold, passed over brain—*Anan.*

    –forced itself into frontal sinuses—*Zinc.*

    –in contact with brain, every inhalation seems to bring cold—*Cimic.*

    –across forehead, draft of—*Laur.*

    –on forehead as from going from cold to warm room—*Carb. an.*

    –blowing on forehead, < night—*Sil.*

    –on left forehead, current of—*Bor.*

    –ascended from occiput, current of—*Thuj.*

    –in occiput, draft of cold—*Coc. c.*

    –vertex opened and let in cold—*Cimic.*

    –cold, blowing on left side of scalp—*Yuc.*

Alive, everything in head were—*Petr., Sil.*

    –were in head, something—*Crot. t., Sil.*

    –were walking inside of head in a circle, something—*Crot. c.*

37

Alive—*Continued*

 —in brain, something were—*Hyper.*

 —in forehead, something were—*Tarax.*

 —with pulsation of arteries, temples and scalp were—*Sang.*

Ant-hill and they were burrowing, brain were an—*Agar.*

Ants were crawling over scalp in spots—*Bar. c.*

Ants' nest, head were in an—*Mez.*

Apoplectic stroke, he might have—*Arg. m.*

Apoplexy, he were attacked by—*Elaps*

 —he were seized with incipient—*Ran. gl.*

 —he would have—*Ferr., Puls., Zinc.*

 —struck by—*Kali cy.*

 —he would be struck by—*Fl. ac., Tarent.*

Arrows of steel pierced from forehead to occiput—*Anan.*

Ascended from occiput, current of air—*Thuj.*

Asleep—see MIND AND SENSORIUM

Asleep, brain were—*Con.*

 —head were—*Nit. ac., Nitro. o., Sep.*

 —when lying down, head were—*Merc.*

 —left half of head were—*Calad.*

 —after debauch, head were—*Op.*

 —forehead were—*Mur. ac.*

 —in vertex—*Cupr. s.*

 —occiput were—*Cast. eq.*

 —in bones of skull—*All. c.*

Atmosphere, one were staying in a room with thick, heavy—*Agn.*

Awl had been forced through temple—*Thuj.*

Balancing to and fro, brain were—*Aphis, Chin.*

 —head were—*Æsc., Bell., Glon., Lyc.*

Ball in head, inflated like a—*Carb. ac.*

 —of lead which would not loosen in spot behind middle of head —*Staph.*

 —elastic, in head and spine, pressed like—*Benz. ac.*

 —were mounting in head—*Acon.*

 —moved about in head—*Anan.*

 —brain were compressed into a—*Cocc., Chin.*

 —were rolling in brain, a small leaden—*Lyss.*

 —were rising from throat to brain—*Plb.*

 —in forehead—*Lach., Staph., Verat. a.*

 —of fire in forehead—*Caust.*

 —of pain were in forehead—*Lac d.*

Ball—*Continued*

–in center of forehead, a round—*Lac d.*

–or wedge of wood in forehead—*Staph.*

–of fire were in each temple—*Lac v.*

–were driven from neck to vertex—*Cimic.*

–were beating against skull, with shattering in brain—*Plat.*

Band around head above ears—*Osm.*

–around head with fullness in skull, a cold—*Helod.*

–head were constricted by a—*Merc., Stann.*

–tightly encircled head—*Vacc., Vario.*

–enclosed head and at times crushed it—*Carb. ac.*

–head were enclosed in an iron—*Juni., Tab.*

–of hat were too tight around head and forehead—*Sars.*

–about head—*Acon., Am. br., Aml. n., Brom., Carb. ac., Carb. v., Chel., Cinnb., Clem., Cupr. s., Cyc., Dios., Franc., Gels., Helod., Hyos., Iod., Iris, Juni., Merc., Nit. ac., Osm., Phys., Raph., Rhus v., Sars., Spig., Spira., Spire., Tab., Ter., Tub., Vario., Xanth.*

–around head, an iron—*Tab.*

–around head, a hot iron—*Acon.*

–of iron, two inches wide, around head just above ears, growing tighter and tighter—*Berb. a.*

–narrow, all around head—*Cupr. s.*

–head were pressed with a—*Clem., Glon.*

–head were tied with a—*Dios., Merc.*

–tied around head above ears, pressing—*Am. br., Gels.*

–surrounded head, a tight—*Xanth.*

–were squeezed in an iron—*Tub.*

–around brain—*Sulph.*

–at base of brain—*Sulph.*

–across forehead—*Carb. ac., Chel., Indg., Iod., Mill., Phos., Tarent.*

–around forehead—*Bapt., Con., Helon., Indg., Sang., Sulph., Sul. i.*

–of India rubber around forehead—*Carb. ac., Plat., Sulph.*

–around forehead above eyes—*Carb. o., Chel., Merc.*

–around forehead and occiput—*Con.*

–above eyes—*Chel., Kali p., Thuj.*

–cold, around forehead—*Carb. s.*

–compressing forehead—*Ant. t., Gels., Nit. ac., Merc., Sulph.*

–crossed forehead and occiput—*Prim.*

Band—*Continued*

—hot, were drawn across forehead from temple to temple over eyes, and burning ring around each eye—*Chlol.*

—stretched over forehead, a rubber—*Carb. ac., Coca, Lil. t.*

—of ribbon stretched over forehead—*Lil. t.*

—tight across forehead—*Ant. t., Bapt., Chel., Indg., Med., Merc. i. r., Sang., Sulph.*

—tied tightly about forehead—*Sulph.*

—tightened around forehead, a rubber—*Samars.*

—pressing in root of nose and over and around ears—*Ther.*

—an inch wide, drawn from temple to temple—*Helon.*

—along right parietal eminence—*Pic. ac.*

—from nape of neck to ear, a tense—*Anac.*

—from ear to ear through occiput, weight of an iron—*Ferr.*

Bandage, head were compressed by—*Cocc.*

—constricted head—*Phys.*

Bandaged, head were—*Mag. s., Merc., Raph.*

—in forehead—*Merc.*

Bands were holding temples, two iron—*Bufo*

Bar in head—*Bell., Paull.*

Bare, brain were laid—*Anan.*

Barrel, whizzing in head and sounds as in empty—*Pimp.*

Bashed in, head had been—*Sulph.*

Beat head to pieces because of throbbing, she could—*Nit. ac.*

—of heart were felt all over head—*Parth.*

—against skull, brain—*Sulph.*

Beaten, head were—*Coff., Con., Euph., Rat., Ruta, Sil., Thuj.*

—to pieces, head were—*Con.*

—or bruised, head were—*Ruta*

—or torn on coughing, head were—*Sulph.*

—in right half of head—*Syph.*

—forehead were—*Ang.*

—brain were—*Ign., Nux v., Tell.*

—in, upper part of skull were—*Thuj.*

—scalp had been—*Sulph.*

Beating against obstacles, arteries of head were—*Spig.*

—against skull with shattering in brain, ball were—*Plat.*

—painfully against skull, external portion of brain were inflamed and—*Daph. o.*

—against skull, brain were—*Ars., Chin., Sulph.*

—in waves against skull, brain were—*Chin., Glon.*

Beating—*Continued*

   –on spot on right side of head, wave were—*Zinc.*

   –against skull, brain were loose and—*Stann.*

   –right side of forehead, hailstones were—*Amph.*

   –from within out, a hammer were—*Vinc.*

   –in head, little hammers were—*Nat. m., Psor.*

   –on skull, waves of water were—*Dig.*

Bed were too hard for head—*Sulph.*

   –were too hard for occiput—*Laur.*

Bee were humming in head—*Carb. v.*

   –had stung her on left temple—*Apis*

Bees in a great hollow in his head, he had—*Op.*

   –in head, sounds of a swarm of—*Sal. ac.*

Bell had been struck in head, causing a buzzing—*Sars.*

Belonged to someone else, head—*Ther.*

Bewildered with pain in back of head—*Xanth.*

Big as a bushel, head were—*Gels., Par.*

   –front of head were—*Parth.*

Bigger, head were—*Cund.*

Biting in occiput, leeches were—*Coc. c.*

Blanket, head were enveloped in a—*Sang.*

Blister had been applied to frontal region—*Sulph.*

Blood were accumulating at top of head when stooping—*Am. c.*

   –would burst out of forehead or eyes—*Lac. ac.*

   –ceased to flow to head—*Seneg.*

   –could not circulate in head—*Bar. c.*

   –collected in head and stood still—*Elaps*

   –in head were coursing upward and outward—*Ox. ac.*

   –head were filled with—*Ign., Lil. t., Nit. ac., Pic. ac., Sulph.*

   –sinciput were filled with—*Ran. b.*

   –were flowing to head—*Uran.*

   –were forced through a contracted vessel in head with buzzing
     —*Sal. ac.*

   –in head, there were too much—*Phos., Sulph.*

   –in head on ascending steps, there were too much—*Sulph.*

   –had left head, all—*Spire.*

   –mounted to head—*Glon., Mill., Puls., Spong.*

   –were pressing down in head—*Con.*

   –pressure in head from too much—*Merl., Nux m., Rhus v.*

   –rushed to head—*Calc. c., Cinch., Ferr., Glon., Meli., Phos.,
     Sac. lac., Sulph., Valer., Verat. a., Upas*

Blood—*Continued*

–rushed to head, vanishing thought—*Ran. b.*

–rushed to heart, then head—*Nux m.*

–into head and face, rushing of all the—*Cur., Ferr. s.*

–rushing into head and ears, all—*Aml. n., Mill.*

–all streamed from head into body—*Elaps*

–suddenly whole head were crowded with—*Glon.*

–were rushing through brain—*Con.*

–in brain there were too much—*Staph.*

–had left brain, all—*Ox. ac.*

–vessels in brain would give way—*Meli.*

–rushed to forehead and temples—*Phys.*

–trickling from forehead down to back of head—*Lac. ac.*

–rushed to occiput, all—*Ol. an.*

Blow on head—*Dol., Guare., Sul. ac.*

–in head, sudden—*Pyrog.*

–headache came from—*Nat. m.*

–on forehead—*Sol. n.*

–on forehead, heavy, waking from sleep—*Psor.*

–on vertex, a violent—*Valer.*

–in occiput—*Arg. m., Crot. h.*

–on occiput—*Hell.*

–on back of head, heavy—*Cann. i.*

–with hand upon left parietal portion of head, which then grasped hair and pulled it out by the roots—*Sep.*

Blowing on head, cold wind were—*Laur., Meny., Petr.*

–through head, cold wind were—*Nat. m., Verat. a.*

–through head on shaking head, wind were—*Cor. r.*

–on forehead, < night, cold air were—*Sil.*

–on left side of scalp, cold air were—*Yuc.*

Blown off, top of head were—*Cham., Anth.*

–up, head were—*Spong.*

Blows in right side of head, severe—*Acon.*

Board across head—*Cocc.*

–in front of head—*Calc. c., Sulph., Zinc.*

–before head—*Æsc., Dulc., Lyc.*

–lay upon head—*Calc. c.*

–lying on right side of head, heavy—*Eug.*

–pressing through head—*Zing.*

–across forehead—*Cocc., Kreos.*

–were before forehead—*Acon., Bell., Sel.*

Board—*Continued*
  –were screwed together and over forehead—*Sulph.*
  –were pressing against forehead—*Dulc., Plat.*
  –strapped or pressed to forehead—*Dulc., Plat., Rhus t.*
  –were on head—*Æsc.*
  –on vertex—*Tab.*
  –were bound to occiput—*Cere. b.*
Body in right half of brain, a foreign—*Con.*
  –under skull, a foreign—*Con.*
  –wobbling, were pressing head—*Asar.*
  –hot, descended into forehead when stooping—*Kali c.*
  –blunt, forced slowly into right temple—*Cocc.*
  –foreign, had been forced into occiput—*Rhod.*
  –hard, as large as an egg behind each ear—*Graph.*
Boil on parietal bone—*Ruta*
Boiling over and lifting cranial arch, brain were—*Cann. i.*
  –water, brain were moved by—*Acon.*
  –water in head, humming from—*Bar. c.*
Bolt were driven from neck to vertex—*Cimic.*
  –were pressing from temple to temple and tightly screwed—*Ham.*
  –or iron rod through from temple to temple were screwed tighter and tighter—*Phos.*
  –were run through head above tip of ears—*Dulc.*
  –or iron rod were thrust from right eyebrow to lower part of occiput—*Syph.*
Bored out, brain were being—*Tab.*
Boring in left temple, a gimlet were—*Culx.*
Bothered in occiput—*Hyper.*
Bound up, head were—*All. c., Cocc., Cyc., Gymn., Nit. ac., Spig.*
  –up with a cloth, head were—*Carb. v.*
  –up with a warm cloth, head were—*Peti.*
  –tight by a cord, head were—*Cocc., Merc. i. r.*
  –with a hot iron ring, head were—*Acon.*
  –head were tightly—*Colch., Nit. ac., Spig., Verat. v.*
  –up, brain were—*Æth.*
  –together, brains were—*Camph.*
  –by a tight cord in frontal region—*Merc. i. f., Tub.*
  –temples were—*Lith.*
  –temples were too tightly—*Plat.*
  –with a cord, vertex were—*Kalm.*

Bound—*Continued*

 –to occiput, board were—*Cere. b.*

 –with a cord, occiput were—*Chin.*

 –to occiput, something hard were tightly—*Phys.*

Bounding, brain were—*Lepi.*

Break during chill, head would—*Puls.*

 –skull would—*Aster.*

Breaking in head, something were—*Carl.*

 –forehead were—*Nat. s.*

Breeze, cold, were blowing on head—*Petr.*

Bristled, hair on head—*Sil., Zinc.*

Broad and high, forehead were very—*Cund.*

Broke in head on turning it, something—*Sep.*

Broken, brains were—*Verat. a.*

 –in sides of head—*Tab.*

 –in two, vertex were—*Am. m.*

 –bones of skull were—*Aur.*

 –off from rest of skull, occiput were fastened to pillow and —*Chel.*

Bruise on back part of head—*Nux v.*

Bruised, head were—*Acon., Alumn., Aur., Bell., Bon., Bov., Cham., Chin., Con., Cupr. ar., Euphr., Gins., Glon., Graph., Gymn., Hell., Kali n., Led., Mag. p. Ambo, Manc., Nat. c., Nux v., Petr., Plan., Rat., Ruta, Sil., Sulph., Tarent.*

 –and torn on coughing, head were—*Sulph.*

 –in bones of head—*Ip.*

 –in periosteum—*Ruta*

 –outer head were—*Hell.*

 –skin of head were—*Nux v.*

 –cerebellum were—*Rhus t.*

 –brain were—*Camph., Coff., Gels., Ign., Ip., Lepi., Mur. ac., Phos., Phys., Phyt., Rumx.*

 –in forehead—*Ant. t., Ars., Bapt., Cob., Glon., Hep., Hipp., Indg., Lil. t., Mag. s., Merc. i. f., Na. m., Plan., Puls., Ran. b., Rumx., Sol. n., Thuj.*

 –in left frontal eminence—*Arn., Lach., Plan.*

 –above eyes—*Cann. i., Gels., Plat.*

 –in temple—*Raph.*

 –sides of head were—*Ars., Benz. ac., Bov., Chin., Con., Crot. h., Grat., Kali i., Laur., Mag. c., Merc. i. f., Nit. ac., Plan., Plat., Sulph.*

Bruised—*Continued*

    –vertex were—*Chel., Gamb.*

    –occiput were—*Æsc., Agar., Alum., Cann. i., Chel., Crot. c., Crot. h., Gins., Hell., Ind., Merc. i. f., Nicc., Nit. ac., Phyt., Plan., Spig., Tarent., Valer., Zinc.*

    –left side of occiput—*Euph., Grat.*

    –right side of occiput were—*Caust.*

    –skull were—*Caps.*

    –hair were wounded or—*Sulph.*

Brush something off from head, trying to—*Nux v.*

Bubble burst in forehead and ran around to left side—*Form.*

Bubbles burst in forehead—*Stry.*

Bubbling in brain, something were—*Berb.*

    –in center of brain—*Med.*

    –in head at night—*Par., Puls.*

    –passed from center to circumference of head—*Med.*

    –in vertex—*Kreos.*

    –in right occiput—*Juncus*

Bulging at forehead and eyes, contents of head were—*Hell.*

Burning in brain—*Verat. a.*

    –like fire, thick feeling in lengthwise strip extending from frontal eminence to right side of vertex—*Sac. lac.*

    –like cayenne pepper, scalp were—*Iris t.*

Burrowing as if brain were an ant-hill—*Agar.*

    –above eyes—*Plat.*

Burst, head would—*Æsc., Ant. c., Ars., Ars. m., Bell., Bry., Calc. c., Cedr., Cham., Chin., Chin. a., Clem., Cob., Daph., Dios., Euphr., Ferr., Glon., Ham., Ip., Kali bi., Lac. ac., Lac d., Lyc., Lyss., Mag. m., Merc., Morph., Nat. m., Nux m., Petr., Phos., Phos. ac., Pic. ac., Ptel., Puls., Pyrus, Rat., Sal. ac., Samars., Sang., Sep., Sil., Sol. n., Sol. t. æ., Spig., Stann., Staph., Stram., Sulph., Sul. ac., Tab., Verat. a., Verat. v., Zinc.*

    –head must—*Sang.*

    –head and chest would—*Bry.*

    –from inward blows, head would—*Stann.*

    –during cough, head would—*Calc. c.*

    –from fullness and heaviness, head would—*Sul. ac.*

    –head, headache would—*Æsc.*

    –with suppression of menses, head would—*Bry.*

    –at stool, head would—*Sanic.*

Burst—*Continued*

   —when talking, head would—*Ign.*
   —with throbbing internally and externally at the same time, head would—*Sil.*
   —on waking, head would—*Cham.*
   —brain would—*Alumn., Ars. m., Con., Nux v., Puls., Sol. t. æ., Verat. a.*
   —brain were about to—*Mag. p. Arct.*
   —and fall out, brain would—*Puls.*
   —from forehead, brain would—*Sol. n.*
   —skull, brain would—*Glon., Lach., Zinc. s.*
   —forehead would—*Am. c., Bry., Calc. c., Cann. i., Ferr., Lac c., Nat. c., Nat. s., Sang.*
   —while coughing, forehead would—*Nat. m.*
   —above ear when vomiting, head would—*Asar.*
   —out forehead or eyes, blood would—*Lac. ac.*
   —in forehead, a bubble—*Stry.*
   —in forehead and ran around to left side, a bubble—*Form.*
   —temples—*Usn. bar.*
   —in right temple when coughing, head would—*Chin., Cina*
   —skull would—*Berb., Chin., Hep., Lach., Nux v., Phos. ac., Puls., Spig., Spong.*
   —skull, everything would press out and—*Sil.*
   —on coughing, skull would—*Caps., Nux v.*
   —from pain, skull would—*Cact., Hep.*
   —at vertex, head would—*Lac. ac., Pip. n.*
   —if she did not scream, top of head would—*Tub.*

Bursting, head were—*Æsc., Aml. n., Anil., Apis, Arg. n., Aster., Bell., Berb., Brom., Calad., Caps., Cham., Clem., Cinch., Cob., Coch., Dios., Fago., Glon., Gymn., Ham., Hep., Hydrs., Kali n., Kalm., Lac. ac., Lyss., Meni., Merc., Morph., Naj., Nat. m., Phos., Pic. ac., Pyrus, Rat., Rhus t., Sang., Sep., Sil., Spig., Stry.*

   —with air, head were filled to—*Lyss.*
   —right side of head were—*Zinc.*
   —when straining at stool, head were—*Sanic.*
   —head were enlarged to—*Pip. m.*
   —right parietal bone were—*Zinc.*
   —in head, something were—*Aml. n.*
   —in brain, water-pipes were—*Sil.*
   —vertex were—*Am. m., Lac. ac., Stront.*

Bursting—*Continued*

    –in forehead and ran to left side, bubble were—*Form.*

    –forehead were—*Am. c., Aml. n., Calad., Caps., Chin. s., Dulc., Ferr., Graph., Hell., Hydrs., Indg., Kali c., Merc., Olnd., Rat.*

Bushel, head were as big as a—*Gels., Par.*

    –and walls were too thin, head were a—*Par.*

Button, convex, pressing on left side of head—*Thuj.*

Buzzing in interior of brain, from forcing blood through a contracted vessel—*Sal. ac.*

    –from striking of a large bell in head—*Sars.*

    –in forehead—*Nux v., Verat. a.*

    –and humming from hornets' nest in occiput—*Carb. v.*

Cap were on head—*Merc., Pyrog., Stel.*

    –skin of head and face were covered with a—*Berb.*

    –and then struck, head were covered with a leaden—*Paull.*

    –on head, iron—*Stry.*

    –iron, were screwed on head—*Clem.*

    –were compressing vertex—*Acon.*

    –or iron helmet pressed down on head—*Crot. c.*

    –tight, were pressed down as far as temples—*Phys.*

    –tight, compressed head—*Carb. s.*

    –on head, a tight rubber—*Stel.*

    –filled with water drawn tightly over head—*Phys.*

Cast were fitted over vertex and pressed down—*Lyss.*

Catarrh would set in—*Rhod.*

Cats were tearing brain to pieces—*Ars.*

Cavity in head were closing up—*Gels.*

Ceased to flow to head, blood—*Seneg.*

Ceiling, head from eyes up were on—*Cocaine*

Charred after sensation of red hot iron passing up spine to atlas, around occiput and head—*Cann. i.*

Chills were creeping along convolutions of brain—*Abrot.*

Chilly in occiput—*Nux v.*

Chirping of locusts in head—*Bry.*

Choked up, head were—*Cub.*

Circle, head were going around in a—*Tub.*

    –something alive were walking inside of head in a—*Crot. c.*

Circled through head and around crown, pain—*Med.*

Circles, everything in head were going in slow—*Coff. t.*

Circulate in head, blood could not—*Bar. c.*

Clasped by a hand and were being twisted, brain were—*Mur. ac.*
Clear, head were—*Alco., Chlor., Coca*
Cleft with an axe, brain were—*Nux v.*
Clock were ticking in forehead—*Mag. s.*
Clogged, head were—*Sumb.*
Closed eyes with headache, something—*Cocc., Sulph.*
Closing up, cavity in head were—*Gels.*
Cloth, brain were enveloped in—*Cyc.*
Cloud settled down on head—*Samars.*
Clutched and drawn to one point of a circle, scalp were—*Chin.*
Cobweb over face, temples and scalp—*Bar. c.*
Cold in head, she had a bad—*Æsc., Eup. pur.*
  –would come on—*Ambr.*
  –ran over whole head, something—*Carl.*
  –air, headache were from—*Coloc., Tarent.*
  –air in contact with brain, every inhalation seems to bring—*Cimic.*
  –air passed over brain—*Anan.*
  –cloth around brain—*Sanic.*
  –inside of forehead—*Cist.*
  –forehead were icy—*Lachn.*
  –wind in forehead, from—*Phos. ac.*
  –spot in head opposite center of forehead—*Bell.*
  –water were poured over forehead—*Tarent.*
  –thumb in small spot on forehead, someone touched him with—*Arn.*
  –from wind in right frontal eminence—*Arg. n.*
  –in right side of frontal bone although warm to touch—*Agar.*
  –in right temple—*Berb.*
  –wet cloth in left temple—*Gamb.*
  –whole side of head were—*Mez.*
  –in vertex from pressure of hand or hat, icy—*Valer.*
  –air in occiput, draft of—*Coc. c.*
  –and hot at same time, scalp were—*Verat. a.*
Collected in head, all blood were—*Elaps*
Collided with skull, brain—*Sil.*
Come out, everything in head would—*Plat., Rhod.*
  –out of head on stooping, everything would—*Corn. a.*
  –out at forehead, everything would—*Olnd., Staph.*
  –out of forehead, everything would—*Hep.*
  –out of right side of forehead, everything would—*Am. c.*

Come—*Continued*

   —out of forehead, something would—*Paraf.*

   —out through forehead, front half of brain would—*Med.*

   —off, top of head would—*Cob., Cupr. s., Passi., Sang., Syph.*

   —off when laughing, stooping or rising from bed, top of head would—*Cupr. s.*

   —off at every jar, top of head would—*Cob.*

Compressed, head were—*Bry., Camph., Cocc., Coloc., Daph., Fl. ac.*

   —by a bandage, head were—*Cocc.*

   —from both sides, head were—*Lycpr.*

   —head were tightly—*Cocc.*

   —strongly above and behind—*Æth.*

   —in a vise, head were—*Bar. c., Cact., Rat., Zinc. s.*

   —brain were—*Asaf., Bell., Camph., Cham., Hyper., Staph.*

   —by a cloth in occiput, brain were—*Asaf.*

   —into a small ball, brain were—*Cocc.*

   —from both sides, brain were—*Kali i., Staph.*

   —brain, an iron helmet—*Crot. c.*

   —in anterior part of head—*Thuj.*

   —forehead were—*Acon.*

   —from margin of orbit to temple, forehead were—*Cann. s.*

   —by an iron ring, forehead were—*Fuc. ves.*

   —temples were—*Con.*

   —together, temples would be—*Sars.*

   —sides of head were—*Kali i.*

   —internally and externally, occiput were—*Staph.*

   —air, head were full of—*Aur.*

Compressing head, screw behind each ear were—*Ox. ac.*

   —forehead, a band were—*Ant. t., Gels., Merc., Nit. ac., Sulph.*

   —vertex, a cap were—*Acon.*

Confined in too small a space, cranial contents were—*Scut.*

Congested in front part of brain—*Crot. h.*

   —in forehead—*Cinnb.*

   —in top of head—*Abies c.*

Congesting head, cold were—*Merc. i. r.*

   —congestion, pressure in head were caused by—*Dig.*

Constricted, head were—*Cham., Crot. h.*

   —about head—*Merc., Phys., Stann.*

   —by a band, head were—*Merc., Stann.*

   —by a bandage, head were—*Phys.*

Constricted—*Continued*
    –by a tape, head were—*Gels., Nit. ac., Sulph.*
    –brain were—*Camph., Cocc., Merc.*
    –by a cord, brain were—*Cocc., Tub.*
    –by a ligature, brain were—*Cocc.*
    –on all sides by pressure, brain were—*Tarax.*
    –in forehead—*Plat.*
    –temples were—*Puls.*
    –in occiput—*Graph.*
    –scalp were—*Arg. n., Card. m., Sanic.*
    –scalp would be—*Plat.*
Constricting head, iron skull-cap were—*Cann. i.*
Constriction were slowly increasing and decreasing in vertex—
    Stann.
Contracted and relaxed, alternately, inner head were—*Calc. c.,*
    Lac c., Med.
    –brain were—*Crot. h., Grat., Plat., Sumb.*
    –and grew smaller, brain—*Grat.*
    –muscles of forehead and eyes were—*Bell.*
    –on forehead, skin—*Caul.*
    –skin of forehead were spasmodically—*Arn.*
    –on middle of forehead, skin—*Gels.*
    –whole side of head were—*Caust.*
    –skull at vertex became—*Kali bi.*
    –and bones scraped, scalp were—*Par.*
    –scalp would be—*Arg. n., Carb. v., Coc. c., Plat.*
    –and caused headaches, scalp—*Carb. v.*
    –to vertex, scalp from back and forepart of head were—*Sanic.*
Contracting, small spot in forehead were—*Arg. n.*
    –across back of head, scalp were—*Alet.*
    –scalp were—*Sanic.*
Contraction and expansion of inner head, there were alternate—
    Exal.
Cord around head—*Sulph.*
    –were frequently drawn and tightened to cut head in two—
    Mosch.
    –brain were constricted by—*Cocc., Tub.*
    –in frontal region, bound by a tight—*Merc. i. f., Tub.*
    –in forehead—*Merc. i. r., Nat. c.*
    –vertex were bound by—*Kalm.*

Cord—*Continued*

   –around skin of occiput—*Psor.*

   –especially at occiput, head were bound with—*Chin.*

Cords were drawn to each other, there were three points of tension in head and large—*Med.*

Cork and elongated upward, head were pithy like—*Graph.*

Corner, brain were pressed against a sharp—*Saba.*

   –sharp, were pressed against top of head—*Prun.*

Coryza in head—*Carb. v.*

   –would come on (in head)—*Dign., Ign., Jug. c., Nit. ac., Ox. ac., Sang.*

Coursing upward and outward, blood in head were—*Ox. ac.*

Cover, large, were drawn very tight over head—*Helod.*

Covered with a leaden cap, head were—*Paull.*

   –with a cap, skin of head and face were—*Berb.*

   –with parchment, head were—*Bar. ac.*

Crack on coughing, head would—*Puls.*

Cracking in head, metal plates were—*Merc., Phel.*

   –skull were—*Merc. i. f.*

Crackling, temples, forehead and nose were—*Acon.*

   –in vertex—*Coff.*

Crashing in forehead—*Stann.*

Crawl out at forehead, everything would—*Glon.*

Crawling on top of head, something were—*Arg. n., Cupr.*

   –on top of brain, something were—*Lac f.*

   –through forehead, worm were—*Sulph.*

   –from occiput to forehead, insects were—*Zinc.*

   –in vertex—*Cupr.*

   –on occiput, something were—*Crot. t.*

   –beneath skin of occiput—*Brom.*

   –over scalp in spots, ants were—*Bar. c.*

   –in scalp—*Coc. c.*

   –in hair, something were—*Thuj.*

   –in hair, something were running and—*Cast. eq.*

Crazy feeling in brain—*Vacc., Vario.*

Creeping along convolutions of brain, chills were—*Abrot.*

   –in scalp of vertex, something were—*Nat. s.*

Crepitation in forehead—*Acon.*

Crossed forehead and occiput, a band—*Prim.*

   –over each other, cranial bones were being—*Nat. h.*

Crowded with blood, whole head were suddenly—*Glon.*

Crush itself down over eyes, forehead would—*Sol*

Crushed, head were—*Anan.*

  –head were (felt even at root of tongue)—*Ip.*

  –head were being—*Aml. n.*

  –it, head were enclosed in a band which at times—*Carb. ac.*

  –when resting hand on it, head were—*Dios.*

  –head would be—*Dios.*

  –inward, head would be—*Syph.*

  –brain were torn or—*Coff., Phos. ac., Sep.*

  –on shaking head, brain were—*Squill.*

  –in a vise, base of brain were—*Nat. s.*

  –and pinched together with pincers, articulate eminences of frontal bone were violently—*Verb.*

  –forehead were—*Glon.*

  –forehead were being—*Ip.*

  –by violent concussions, forehead were—*Arn.*

  –together, temples would be—*Caul.*

  –left side of head were—*Paraf.*

  –in vertex—*Phel.*

Current of air rushed through head—*Aur.*

  –of air on left forehead—*Bor.*

  –galvanic, through head—*Nux m.*

  –electric, passing through head—*Sang.*

  –galvanic, extended from head into fingers and feet—*Glon.*

  –passed through left side of head into limbs, electric—*Ail.*

Cushion and someone were pressing two fingers into it at occiput, head were in—*Sil.*

Cut off at septum and middle of forehead, head were—*Chel.*

  –head in two, a cord were frequently drawn and tightened to —*Mosch.*

  –out of head, eyes would be—*Samb.*

  –to pieces on stooping, brain were—*Nicc.*

  –by a fine instrument, nerves in temples and forehead were being—*Spig.*

  –in left temporal ridge—*Hedo.*

  –off, part of right side of head were—*Lach.*

  –through, skull were—*Mosch.*

  –and reunited, skin of scalp were—*Ol. an.*

  –off near roots, hair were—*Sep.*

Cutting head off, pain were—*Phys.*

   –the body off from head at base of brain and he would fall forward—*Phys.*

Cyst would form on forehead—*Eupi.*

Dashed to pieces, brain were—*Æth., Coff., Nux v.*

Dead, occipital bone were—*Caust.*

Deep in head, eyes were—*Elect., Zinc.*

Descended into forehead when stooping, a hot body—*Kali c.*

Detached in head, something had become—*Con.*

   –and loose, brain were—*Guaj.*

   –from head, skin were (extending to neck)—*Calc. c.*

Digging into left side of brain, something were—*Kali i.*

Dilating, head were—*Cann. i., Carb. ac.*

Diminished in weight, whole contents of head had greatly—*Momor.*

Dislocated, head were—*Plb.*

Displacement had taken place in head—*Nat. m.*

Dissolving, brain were—*Calc. c.*

Distend or enlarge at temples and occiput, brain would—*Cocc. s.*

Distended, head were—*Arn., Bar. c., Cedr., Indg., Lact., Meph., Merl., Par., Ran. b., Ran. s., Sulph.*

   –from within out, head were being—*Arn., Stront.*

   –brain were—*Tarax., Thuj.*

   –vertex were—*Dign.*

Distending in center, brain were—*Indg.*

Distorted on motion, head were—*Phel.*

Down, brain went up and—*Cob.*

Draft of air across forehead—*Laur.*

Dragged by hair in vertex—*Acon.*

Dragging head down, weight fell forward into forehead (on stooping)—*Rhus t.*

   –in occiput—*Ery. a., Gels.*

Draw head backward, weight in occiput would; and neck had not enough strength to prevent it—*Alet.*

Drawing head toward shoulders, something were—*Lyss.*

   –from magnet in forehead—*Ictod.*

   –in middle of forehead—*Agar., Croc., Laur., Rat., Thuj.*

   –were in brain—*Arg. m.*

Drawn asunder in head—*Caust.*

   –backward, head were—*Cast., Stram.*

   –backward, head would be—*Nat. c., Spig., Zinc.*

Drawn—*Continued*

-forcibly backward, head were—*Chel.*

-backward by weight on nape of neck, head would be—*Phel.*

-backward, tendons were too short and head would be—*Laur.*

-backward and downward, head were—*Sulph.*

-forward, head would be—*Sang.*

-together, everything in head were—*Eug.*

-up in left side of head, all—*Sac. lac.*

-upward, head were—*Camph.*

-and tightened to cut head in two, cord were frequently—
   Mosch.

-tight on head, skin were—*Med.*

-very tight, large cover over head were—*Helod.*

-tightly from ear to ear, tape were—*Anac.*

-through head transversely from left side, knife were—*Arn.*

-from middle of forehead to occiput, thread had been—*Saba.*

-tightly through eyes to middle of head, a thread were—*Par.*

-through head, threads had been—*Meph.*

-up, all nerves of head were—*Camph.*

-up tightly, nerves of head were—*Cocc.*

-to each other, there were three points of tension in head and
   large cords were—*Med.*

-down, brain were—*Dirc.*

-down to root of tongue, brain were—*Ip.*

-over brain, skin were—*Ang.*

-through whole substance of brain, net were—*Cinch. s.*

-tight over brain, < occiput, dura mater were—*Par.*

-forward toward frontal sinuses, lobes of cerebrum were—
   Dirc.

-tightly about forehead, strap were—*Carb. v.*

-into folds, skin of forehead were—*Graph.*

-up, forehead were—*Colch.*

-across forehead from temple to temple over eyes, a hot band
   were—*Chlol.*

-over temples and forehead, something were very lightly—
   Bar. c.

-from temple to temple, an inch wide band were—*Helon.*

-around head tighter and tighter, rope were—*Nat. m.*

-in, temple would be—*Asar.*

-so tight it would snap, right temple were—*Am. c.*

-upward, skin on temples were—*Sep.*

Drawn—*Continued*
    –close together, bones of occiput were—*Coc. c.*
    –tightly over skull, something were—*Arg. n.*
    –toward vertex, all skin were—*Stront.*
    –up to vertex, scalp were all—*Sanic.*
    –to one point of a circle, scalp were clutched and—*Chin.*
    –forward on top of head, scalp were—*Colch.*
    –tight, scalp were—*Arg. n.*
    –tight over skull, scalp were—*Cocc., Helod.*
    –together in one spot, scalp were—*Zinc.*
    –upward, hair were—*Mur. ac.*
Dried on forehead, glue—*Alum.*
Driven into head, nails or needles were being—*Der.*
    –into head over nose, nail were—*Ign.*
    –asunder, head were—*Caust., Ran. b.*
    –into head, nail were—*Coff., Mag. p. Ambo, Ptel., Ruta*
    –into brain, nail were—*Asaf., Ptel.*
    –from left forehead into brain, nail were—*Sang.*
    –into forehead, nail were—*Ign.*
    –into frontal eminence, nail were—*Thuj.*
    –into right temple, screw were being—*Nat. s.*
    –into side of head near left eye, nail were—*Am. br.*
    –into right side of head, plug were—*Mez.*
    –into left side of head, nail were—*Nat. m.*
    –out through side of head, nail were—*Ign.*
    –into right parietal bone, nail were—*Lycpr., Thuj.*
    –into temple, wedge were—*Thuj.*
    –into parietal bone, nail were—*Coff., Thuj.*
    –into middle of head, nail were—*Paull.*
    –in vertex, nail were—*Hell., Hura, Manc., Nicc., Nux v.*
    –into vertex with a jerk, nail were—*Thuj.*
    –from within out in vertex, nail were—*Thuj.*
    –into left vertex, nail were being—*Paraf.*
    –from neck to vertex, bolt were—*Cimic.*
    –in on one side of occiput, nail were—*Puls.*
    –into occiput, nail were—*Tarent.*
    –into occiput and temples, plug were being—*Hep.*
    –asunder, bones of skull were being—*Lyc.*
Driving him crazy, snapping in head were nearly—*Antip.*
Drop to pieces if shaken, head would—*Glon.*
    –of cold water had fallen on left parietal bone—*Croc.*

Drop—*Continued*

　–from one side to the other, head were too heavy and would—*Fl. ac.*

　–of water (not cool) running down temple—*Verat. a.*

Drops of water were falling on brain—*Cann. s.*

Dull plug on left side of vertex—*Anac.*

　–stick in temple—*Asaf.*

Eaten too much and caused headache, he had—*Puls.*

Eating too much, he had been (felt in head)—*Glon.*

Electric current passed from head into limbs—*Ail.*

　–current passing through head—*Sang.*

　–spark in forehead—*Ol. an.*

　–machine were snapping in occiput—*Calc. c.*

Electrified, bunch of hair were—*Verat. a.*

Elevated after unconsciousness, head must be—*Glon.*

Elongated upward like a conical hat, head had suddenly—*Hyper.*

　–upward, head were pithy like cork and—*Graph.*

Else were upon head, something—*Thea*

Empty, head were—*Aster., Carb. v., Cor. r., Merl., Ment. pu, Nux m., Phos. ac., Sin., Thuj., Zing.*

　–space between brain and forehead—*Caust.*

　–forehead were—*Cedr., Clem., Croc., Hell.*

　–vertex were—*Sin.*

　–occiput were—*Hell., Mang., Nat. c., Sep., Sulph.*

　–while brain in front were too large, occiput were—*Hell.*

Emptiness in base of brain—*Staph.*

　–caused headache—*Nux v.*

Encircled head, a band tightly—*Vacc., Vario.*

　–by a hoop, forehead were—*Thuj.*

Enclosed in a band which at times crushed it, head were—*Carb. ac.*

　–in an iron band, head were—*Juni.*

Enlarge or distend at temples and occiput, brain would—*Cocc. s.*

Enlarged, head were—*Agar., Ant. t., Aran., Arg. n., Ars. i., Berb., Bov., Carb. ac., Chin. s., Coll., Com., Cor. r., Dulc., Gels., Gent. l., Gins., Glon., Lachn., Laur., Manc., Mang., Meph., Merc., Mimos., Nat. c., Nux m., Nux v., Pip. m., Plat., Ran. b., Sulph., Syph.*

　–head and face were—*Stry.*

　–to bursting, head were—*Pip. m.*

　–head would be—*Meph., Ran. b.*

Enlarged—*Continued*
--head were enormously—*Ars. i.*
--head were much—*Arg. n.*
--three times its size, head were—*Kali i.*
--brain would become—*Cocc. s.*
--cerebellum were—*Dulc.*
--forehead were—*Agar., Merc., Pip. m.*
--upper part of forehead were—*Cund.*
--vertex were—*Lachn., Phys.*
--occipital protuberance were—*Med.*

Enlargement of head—*Pip. m.*

Enlarging, head were—*Bov.*

Enveloped in a blanket, head were—*Sang.*
--in ice, head were—*Passi.*

Epileptic fit would approach—*Arg. n.*

Erect, hair were—*Sulph. i.*

Excited after tea, brain were—*Hyper.*

Expand if it were not for cranial bones, brain would—*Kali p.*

Expanded, head were—*Lact., Nux m.*
--from within, head were—*Stront.*
--in head, blood vessels were—*Ferr.*
--brain were—*Cupr. ar., Glon.*
--and pressed against skull, brain were—*Cupr. ar.*
--forehead were—*Datura a.*

Expanding in frontal region, head were—*Ery. a.*
--brain were—*Glon.*

Expansion and contraction of inner head, there were alternate—*Exal.*

Exploded in brain, something had really—*Phos.*

Exposed to sun, head had been—*Manc.*

Extended upward, vertex—*Lachn.*

Extravasated into scalp, blood were—*Ferr.*

Fall backward, head would—*Æth., Agar., Chin., Colch., Dios., Glon., Led., Œna., Op., Rhod., Spig., Tarent.*
--backward while walking, head would—*Chin., Phel.*
--in all directions, head would—*Cann. s., Con.*
--to one side, head would—*Ang., Aml. n., Arn., Ars., Cann. s., Cina, Dios., Ether., Ferr., Fl. ac., Kali i., Nux m., Op., Prun., Sulph.*
--to left during breakfast, head would—*Sil.*
--to left, head would—*Eup. per.*

Fall—*Continued*

  –forward, head would—*Agn., Bar. c., Calc. c., Clem., Cupr., Equis., Eth. n., Gels., Hipp., Hydr. ac., Ign., Itu, Lepi., Lyc., Nat. m., Nux m., Œna., Op., Par., Paull., Pic. ac., Phos. ac., Phos., Plb., Puls., Sars., Staph., Sulph., Tab., Thuj., Viol. t.*

  –forward because of pressure, head would—*Agn.*

  –forward on walking, head would—*Hipp.*

  –forward in head, something would—*Mag. s.*

  –forward, something were cutting head off from body and he would—*Phys.*

  –to pieces, head would—*Glon., Sil.*

  –apart, brain would—*Saba.*

  –out, brain would—*Rat.*

  –out of forehead, brain would—*Chel.*

  –out, brain would burst and—*Puls.*

  –out of right side of head when stooping, brain would—*Chel.*

  –out on motion, brain would—*Staph.*

  –forward, brain would—*Berb., Carb. ac., Carb. an., Grat., Guare.*

  –toward left temple, brain would—*Nat. s.*

  –out, forehead would—*Puls., Thuj.*

  –out of forehead, everything would—*Acon., Bar. c., Hep., Mag. s., Sep., Thuj.*

  –out, piece of forehead would—*Nux v.*

  –out, frontal bone would—*Coch.*

  –in periosteum of temporal bones, pain from a—*Ruta*

  –with pain in vertex, one would—*Con.*

  –forward, occiput would—*Hell.*

  –out of skull on stooping, everything would—*Bry.*

  –out, hair would—*Sil.*

Fallen on left parietal bone, drop of cold water had—*Croc.*

  –on right frontal bone, drop of cold water had—*Croc.*

Falling off, head were—*Sil.*

  –to left, head were—*Eup. pur.*

  –on brain, drops of water were—*Cann. s.*

  –forward, brain were—*Guare.*

  –from side to side, brain were loose and—*Sul. ac.*

  –from left side of head to forehead, something were—*Laur.*

  –from one side of head to other, when moving it, something were—*Tep.*

Falling—*Continued*

    –outward, forehead were—*Chel., Thuj.*

    –forward in forehead on motion, lump were—*Cham.*

    –out, weight in forehead were—*Chel.*

    –on vertex, tremendous weight were—*Bry., Sil.*

    –forward, occiput were—*Ant. t., Phys.*

    –forward during emptiness of forehead, occiput were—*Hell.*

Fast, skin on forehead had grown—*Sabi.*

Fastened to shoulder by long peg, head were—*Cupr.*

    –to pillow and broken off from rest of skull, occiput were—*Chel.*

Feeling, habitual, had disappeared from a place in vertex—*Lyss.*

Feet were in brain—*Amph.*

Fell forward, head—*Phys.*

    –from one side to other when moving head, something—*Tep.*

    –forward, brain—*Sul. ac.*

    –into forehead, brain—*Laur.*

    –forward and came through brain—*Sul. ac.*

    –forward and pressed against forehead, brain—*Coff.*

    –forward in brain, something—*Dig., Mag. s.*

    –forward in brain on stooping, something—*Ant. t.*

    –forward and came up again, brain—*Sul. ac.*

    –toward side he stoops, brain—*Am. c., Sul. ac.*

    –in forehead at every step, brain rose and—*Bell.*

    –toward left temple, brain—*Nat. s.*

    –into forehead, something heavy—*Nux v.*

    –forward into forehead, dragging head down on stooping, weight—*Rhus t.*

    –toward forehead when leaning forward, weight—*Paraf.*

    –from left side into forehead, something—*Laur.*

    –forward in occiput when stooping, something—*Ant. t.*

Filled to bursting with air, head were—*Lyss.*

    –with blood, head were—*Ign., Lil. t., Nit. ac., Pic. ac., Sulph.*

    –with fluid, head were—*Coff.*

    –with a heavy lump, head were—*Urea*

    –with blood, sinciput were—*Ran. b.*

    –with smoke, one side of head were—*Sul. ac.*

    –with lead, occiput were—*Lach., Mur. ac., Petr.*

Finger pressed at point where head and neck unite—*Rheum*

    –tips on head, pressure from—*Pall.*

Fingers in left temple, pressure of—*Staph.*

   –pressing on back of head—*Meph.*

   –on forehead, pressure of—*Cham.*

   –were pressing into occiput as into a cushion—*Sil.*

Fire in forehead, a ball of—*Caust.*

   –a thick feeling extending in strip from frontal eminence to right side of vertex, burning like—*Sac. lac.*

Fired in head, pistol were—*Dig.*

Firm in head, nothing were—*Verat. a.*

Fitted over vertex and pressed down, cast were—*Lyss.*

Flap when moving head, brain seems to—*Ars., Rhus t.*

Flashes of throb-like pain, top of head would be taken off by—*Xanth.*

Flattened by pressure, forehead were—*Cor. r.*

Float off, top of head would—*Nat. h.*

Floating in air, head were—*Jug. r.*

   –in brain, liquid were—*Arn.*

Flow to head, blood ceased to—*Seneg.*

Flowing into head, blood were—*Rhus t.*

   –to head, blood were—*Uran.*

   –through head too rapidly, blood were—*Spire.*

Fluctuating in brain on exertion, liquid were—*Arn., Cur.*

Fluid, head were filled with—*Coff.*

   –filled brain—*Cur.*

   –were injected paroxysmally into a small blood vessel—*Coc. c.*

   –were rushing through head from right to left—*Lil. t.*

Fluttering in brain that disappears when touched—*Pall.*

   –in sacrum rising gradually to occiput—*Ol. j.*

Fly apart, head would—*Pic. ac.*

   –to pieces if she moved, head would—*Coff.*

   –to pieces with cough, head would—*Bry., Caps., Rumx.*

   –off, top of head would—*Alum., Bapt., Cact., Cann. s., Carb. an., Cimic., Cob., Cupr., Ferr., Iris, Kali bi., Lach., Lith., Sanic., Syph.*

   –off from downward motion, top of head would—*Sanic.*

Foam were rising in head—*Myric.*

Fog, brain were wrapped in—*Petr.*

Folded on itself in occipital bone, something were—*Kiss.*

Folds, skin of forehead were drawn into—*Graph.*

Force head asunder, lever were applied to—*Bell.*

Force—*Continued*
 –brain out at forehead, pressure in occiput would—*Caps.*
 –out of forehead, everything would—*Rhod.*
Forced apart in pieces, head were separated or—*Arg. n., Bufo, Glon., Kali bi., Lyc., Mez.*
 –asunder, head would be—*Kali i., Sil.*
 –forward, head were—*Nit. ac.*
 –through every opening, contents of head would be—*Lil. t.*
 –asunder, brain were—*Stann.*
 –forward, brain would be—*Sil.*
 –out beneath frontal bones, brain would be—*Lycpr.*
 –out when at stool, whole brain would be—*Rat.*
 –through forehead, brain would be—*Kreos.*
 –out through right nostril, brain would be—*Bor.*
 –through longitudinal sinus, liquids were being—*Glon.*
 –through a contracted vessel in brain with buzzing, blood were —*Sal. ac.*
 –asunder, parietal bones were—*Cor. r.*
 –downward deeper and deeper into parietal bone, nail were— *Ign., Nux v.*
 –asunder on both sides from without, skull would be—*Nux v.*
 –itself into frontal sinuses, air—*Zinc.*
 –through temple, awl had been—*Thuj.*
 –slowly into right temple, a blunt body were—*Cocc.*
 –into occiput, a foreign body had been—*Rhod.*
Forcing itself out just above nose, brain were—*Am. c.*
Form on left forehead, an abscess would—*Colch.*
Formication in head—*Psor.*
Forming in head, abscess were—*Hep.*
 –in brain, abscess were—*Cupr.*
Freer in air, head were—*Phos.*
 –after sneezing, head were—*Tab.*
Frozen, head were—*Indg.*
Full, head were—*Dig., Sul. ac.*
 –head were too—*Æsc. g., Æsc., Apis, Calc. c., Con., Daph., Eupi., Gent. c., Nat. p., Ran. s, Sul. ac.*
 –of compressed air, head were—*Aur.*
 –of water, head were—*Bell.*
 –brain were too—*Caps., Coff., Con.*
 –for head, brain were too—*Bry.*

Full—*Continued*
    –and pressed outward, brain were too—*Bry.*
    –and throbbing, a vein in head were too—*Ferr.*
    –skull were too—*Helod., Nat. p.*
    –on vertex, skull were too—*Helon.*
Fullness and heaviness would burst head—*Sul. ac.*
    –in skull, a cold band around head with—*Helod.*
    –were pressing upward in forehead—*Meph.*
Furnace, head were in a—*Kali br.*
Furry, occiput were—*Ammc.*
Furuncles, small, would form—*Eupi.*
Galvanic current in head—*Nux m.*
    –current extending from head to fingers and feet—*Glon.*
Gathered into a ball, brain were—*Chin.*
Gathering in temple—*Nit. ac.*
Gimlet boring in left temple—*Culx.*
    –were piercing skull—*Puls.*
    –thrust into right temple—*Puls.*
Give way, blood vessels in brain would—*Meli.*
Glass and shattered at a blow, brain were made of—*Dig.*
Gloomy in forehead—*Agn., Plect.*
Glue had dried on forehead—*Alum.*
Gnawing in periosteum of outer head—*Ant. c.*
    –at base of brain, something were—*Nat. s.*
    –in forehead—*Merc. i. r., Sulph., Zinc.*
    –at small spot on vertex—*Ran. s.*
    –in occiput, temples and ears, something were—*Led.*
    –in occipital protuberance, a mouse were—*Zinc.*
Gone, top of head were—*Mez.*
Grabbing head during confusion, something were—*Hell.*
Grasped, hair were roughly—*Chin.*
    –by a hand and twisted, brain were—*Mur. ac.*
    –hair and pulled it out by roots, hand struck left parietal region
        and—*Sep.*
Grasping in head—*Ars.*
    –in vertex and occiput—*Verat. v.*
Grinding in vertex—*Myric.*
Griping in forehead came from stomach—*Con.*
Growing externally, head were—*Lac d.*
Grown fast, skin on forehead had—*Sabi.*

Gurgling behind upper portion of frontal bones, water were—
    Asaf.
Hacked with hatchet, head were—*Ammc., Phos. ac.*
    –to pieces, bone on left side of head were—*Calc. c.*
Hacking in head—*Kali n.*
Hailstones were beating right side of forehead—*Amph.*
Hair, he were pulled by—*Rhus t.*
    –hanging in middle of forehead which he wished to brush
        away—*Grat.*
    –were pulled out of occiput—*Arn.*
    –were too tight on occiput—*Lach.*
    –pins were sticking into her head—*Kali p.*
Hammer, palpitations in head were like a—*Glon.*
    –were beating in vertex from within out—*Vinc.*
    –on top of head, struck with—*Sal. ac., Sars.*
    –throbbing in cerebellum from—*Camph.*
    –on right side of head when walking, struck with a—*Tab.*
    –struck on occiput with a—*Tarent.*
Hammers, little, beating in head—*Nat. m., Psor.*
    –striking head from within outward—*Psor.*
    –striking on back of head, invisible—*Lyss.*
Hammering with flat instrument on head—*Am. c.*
Hand, touched on forehead by an icy cold—*Hyper.*
    –pressed on left parietal bone—*Kali ar.*
    –grasped hair and pulled it out by roots—*Sep.*
Handkerchief were tied around head—*Carb. v.*
Hanging down for a long time, head had been—*Op.*
    –head downward, he were—*Glon.*
    –by piece of skin at nape, head were—*Sil.*
    –in middle of forehead which he wished to brush away, hair
        were—*Grat.*
Hard in head, bed were too—*Sulph.*
    –head were lying on something—*Manc.*
    –behind right brow, something—*Staph.*
    –body as large as an egg behind each ear—*Graph.*
    –in occiput, bed were too—*Laur.*
    –were tightly bound to occiput, something—*Phys.*
    –substance pressing on skull—*Staph.*
Hat on, he had his—*Calc. c., Crat. ox.*
    –on his head, he could not get his—*Ars. m.*
    –head were suddenly elongated upward like a conical—*Hyper.*

Hatchet, head were being hacked with a—*Ammc., Phos. ac.*
Headache were approaching, sick—*Chr. ac., Phyt.*
  —might return—*Ign.*
  —were under dura mater—*Tus. p.*
Heat on vertex when hand were applied—*Lac v.*
  —and cold in scalp at same time—*Verat. a.*
Heaviness and fullness in brain, head would burst from—*Sul. ac.*
Heavier and heavier, head became—*Calc. ar.*
Heavy, head were too—*Am. m., Nat. m., Puls.*
  —from weight of blood, head were—*Ign., Lil. t.*
  —as from passage of storm cloud, head were—*Hyper.*
  —and would drop from one side to other, head were too—*Fl. ac.*
  —sinking down in head, something—*Nux v.*
  —brain were too—*Glon.*
  —and too large, brain were too—*Form., Glon., Hell., Mag. p.*
  —were pressing out of brain, something—*Phys.*
  —and tight in brain, it were too—*Merc.*
  —pressing on temples, something—*Iodof., Phaseo.*
  —on top of head, something were—*Lac v.*
  —and swollen on crown of head—*All. c.*
Held tight in left occiput (in confusion)—*Crot. t.*
  —in a vise, occiput were—*Coca*
Helmet or cap of iron pressed down on head—*Crot. c.*
High in forehead, very broad and—*Cund.*
Higher than the right, left side of forehead were—*Cund.*
Hit with a hammer on top of head—*Sars.*
  —against skull, brain were loose and—*Rhus t.*
Hold head up, she could not—*Sil., Stann.*
  —head still when sitting, she could not—*Squill.*
  —his head all the time, he must—*Saba.*
  —it together, head were pressed asunder in vertex and she must
    —*Carb. an.*
Hole were there and brain were touched—*Stram.*
Hollow, head were—*Acon. c., Ammc., Anac., Ant. c., Arg. m.,
  Arn., Berb., Bov., Cact., Calc. c., Caps., Chin. s., Chlor.,
  Cina, Cocc., Cor. r., Cyc., Euphr., Ferr., Gent. l., Glon.,
  Graph., Hell., Hipp., Ign., Jab., Kiss., Lyc., Manc., Meny.,
  Myric., Naj., Nat. m., Nat. p., Nux m., Ox. ac., Pic. ac.,
  Polyg., Polyp. o., Puls., Seneg., Sec., Sin. a., Spig., Stram.,
  Sulph., Tarent., Verat. a., Zing.*
  —in head, bees were humming in a great—*Op.*

Hollow—*Continued*
 –head were; brain were not enough for space—*Staph.*
 –forehead were—*Puls.*
 –occiput were—*Staph., Sulph.*
 –and ulcerated, occiput were—*Sep.*
Hoop around head—*Merc., Stann., Sulph., Ther.*
 –around head, a tight iron—*Tub.*
 –encircled forehead, a tight—*Thuj.*
Hornets' nest in occiput, buzzing and humming from—*Carb. v.*
Hot and cold at same time, scalp were—*Verat. a.*
 –iron were around head—*Acon.*
Humming of bees in head—*Carb. v., Op.*
 –of boiling water in head—*Bar. c.*
Hungry, head felt as if he were—*Glon.*
Ice on head—*Verat. a.*
 –head were enveloped in—*Passi.*
 –touched head, sharp points of—*Agar.*
 –lying against various parts of head especially on right side,
   pieces of—*Calc. c.*
 –on top of head—*Arn., Sep.*
 –on vertex, a lump of—*Verat. a.*
 –lay on vertex, then on forehead, nape of neck to small of
   back—*Laur.*
 –posterior half of head lay on—*Cast. eq.*
 –were lying in upper occiput—*Calc. p.*
 –had lain on occipital protuberance—*Podo.*
 –about four inches square in back of head—*Gels.*
Icy cold in vertex from pressure of hat—*Valer.*
Immovable, scalp of forehead and occiput were adherent to bone
   and almost—*Par.*
Increasing and decreasing in vertex, constriction were—*Stann.*
Inflamed and beating painfully against skull, external portion of
   brain were—*Daph. o.*
Inflated like a ball in head—*Carb. ac.*
Inhalation seems to bring cold air in contact with brain, every—
   Cimic.
Injected paroxysmally into a small blood vessel, fluid were—
   Coc. c.
 –into sinuses, water had been—*Lach.*
Insects crawling from occiput to forehead—*Zinc.*
 –on temples and occiput—*Thuj.*

Insects—*Continued*
 —caused itching on occiput or behind ears—*Sep.*
Insensible, parts of head would become—*Lyss.*
Instrument, dull, pressed on vertex—*Ran. s.*
 —dull, were pressing inward—*Asaf., Olnd.*
Iron band around head—*Tab.*
 —cap on head—*Stry.*
 —helmet or cap pressed down on head—*Crot. c.*
 —ring, hot, binding head—*Acon.*
 —band from ear to ear through occiput, weight of—*Ferr.*
 —skull cap constricting head—*Cann. i.*
 —band, brain were squeezed in—*Tub.*
 —band around head just above ears, and growing tighter and
     tighter—*Berb. a.*
 —ring, forehead were compressed by an—*Fuc. ves.*
 —bands were holding temples—*Bufo*
 —rod or bolt through from temple to temple and screwed tighter
     and tighter—*Phos.*
 —were stuck into vertex, a red-hot—*Crot. c.*
 —rod passing up spine to atlas, around occiput and head; head
     were charred after sensation of red-hot—*Cann. i.*
 —rod or bolt were thrust from right eyebrow to lower part of
     occiput—*Syph.*
Irons, pointed, were thrust in temples—*Anan.*
Issue from forehead and eyes, everything would—*Sep.*
 —though forehead, everything would—*Bell., Bry., Glon., Verb.*
Itching from lice on scalp—*Olnd.*
 —from insects on occiput and behind ears—*Scp.*
Jagging in head, sword were—*Carb. ac.*
Jerk in head from before backward when talking—*Cic.*
Jerked forward, scalp were—*Aml. n.*
Jerking down from head to jaw—*Calc. ar.*
Jolting in occiput at every step, weight were—*Bell.*
 —had caused headache—*Sep.*
Knife plunged into head—*Nux m.*
 —were drawn transversely through head from left side—*Arn.*
 —sharp, thrust from side to side in head—*Arg. m.*
 —sticking in temples, a pen—*Ferr.*
 —just above right temple, stitches of—*Verb.*
 —stabs under right temporal bone—*Paraf.*
 —stabbing from temple to temple—*Bell.*

Knife—*Continued*

  –sticking in forehead—*Ter.*

  –were stitching in forehead—*Ferr., Lact.*

  –thrust from occiput to forehead—*Gels.*

  –stitching in occiput—*Nat. m.*

  –at every pulsation, occiput were pierced with—*Con.*

Knives were tearing around in brain—*Thuj.*

  –were being thrust into brow—*Lach.*

  –forehead, eyes and ears were stabbed with—*Thuj.*

  –stitching in occiput—*Nat. m.*

Knock on head, he received a—*Sarr.*

Knocked in morning, head were—*Tarent.*

  –to pieces, bones of head were being—*Thuj.*

Laced, head had been—*Mosch.*

  –head and neck had been—*Glon.*

  –together in cerebellum and glabella—*Camph.*

  –skull were tightly—*Acon.*

Lacerated, brain were—*Puls., Sul. ac.*

Lain on occipital protuberances, ice had—*Podo.*

Lance, head were transfixed with a—*Opun.*

Lantern, head were a—*Ars., Puls.*

Large, head were too—*Apis, Arg. n., Arn., Ars., Bapt., Bell., Berb., Caj., Caps., Cimic., Cob., Coll., Cor. r., Glon., Hyper., Jug. c., Kali i., Lach., Lact., Lac v., Lith., Mang., Mim., Nat. c., Nux m., Phel., Ptel., Ran. b., Ran. s., Rhus t., Sac. lac., Sil., Spig., Spire., Til., Tong., Trif. p., Zing.*

  –she could not get her hat on, head were so—*Ars. m.*

  –head were immensely—*Par.*

  –head were suddenly too—*Ars. m.*

  –as a half bushel, head were—*Caj.*

  –as a church, head were—*Nux v.*

  –when toothache stops, head were—*Com.*

  –that it occupied whole room, head were so—*Antif.*

  –during stool, head grew—*Cob.*

  –internally, head were growing—*Lac d.*

  –brain were too—*Arg. n., Ars. m., Berb., Cean., Cimic., Hell., Lac. ac.*

  –for skull, brain were too—*Arg. n., Berb., Cimic., Glon., Still.*

  –occiput were empty but brain in forehead were too—*Hell.*

  –brain were too heavy and too—*Form., Glon., Hell., Mag. p.*

  –with every beat of heart, brain were too—*Echin.*

Large—*Continued*
 —enough for space, brain were not—*Staph.*
 —again and pressed out, forehead were as—*Nux v.*
Larger, head were—*Kali ar., Mang.*
 —head were growing—*Berb., Merc.*
 —head were slowly growing—*Bapt.*
 —than body ; head were large as a church—*Nux v.*
Lay upon vertex, something else—*Ther.*
 —on vertex, forehead, nape of neck to small of back, ice—
     Laur.
 —on ice, posterior part of head—*Cast. eq.*
Lead, oppression in head were—*Rhod.*
 —ball, small, rolling about in brain—*Lyss.*
 —in brain on turning head, there were—*Thuj.*
 —which would not loosen in spot behind middle of head, a ball
     of—*Staph.*
 —on top of head, there were a lump of—*Phel.*
 —in occiput—*Lach., Mur. ac., Petr.*
 —in occiput, causing head to fall backward—*Op.*
Leaden ball, small, were rolling in brain—*Lyss.*
 —cap and then struck, head were covered with—*Paull.*
Leaping in skull on motion, brain were—*Sol. t. æ.*
Leeches were biting in occiput—*Coc. c.*
Lever applied to force head asunder—*Bell.*
Lice on scalp, itching from—*Olnd.*
 —were running over scalp—*Caps., Pedi.*
Lift head from pillow, he could not—*Iodof.*
 —it off, vertex were separated from rest of head or she could
     —*Ther.*
 —off, top of head seemed to—*Passi.*
Lifted off in two pieces, crown of head were—*Gels.*
 —off, top of head were—*Dios., Lac d.*
 —off, top of head could be—*Ther.*
 —and raised about five inches and brains were coming out, top
     of head were—*Lac d.*
 —brain boiled over and calvarium were—*Cann. i.*
 —up by blood vessels, bones of forehead were—*Bell.*
 —up, bones of head were—*Bell.*
 —up, skull were—*Puls.*
 —off, scalp would be (with giddiness)—*Hydr.*
 —by hair, she had been—*Pedi., Sep., Sil.*

Lifting off, head were—*Ust.*
   –cranial arch, brain were boiling over and—*Cann. i.*
   –off, top of head were—*Lac. ac.*
   –up from adjoining parts, vertex were—*Eup. pur.*
Ligated, vessels of brain (especially base of brain) were full from being—*Pip. m.*
Ligature, brain were constricted by a—*Cocc.*
Light, occiput were—*Sec.*
Lightning in head—*Thuj.*
   –something shot through head like—*Morph.*
   –ran from body up into head—*Form.*
   –through brain down neck, something rushed like—*Chin. a.*
Liquid moving in head, by jerks—*Coc. c.*
   –were floating in brain—*Arn.*
   –fluctuating in brain on exertion—*Arn., Cur.*
Liquids were being forced through longitudinal sinus—*Glon.*
   –moving in head—*Glon.*
Live things whirling around it, head were teeming with—*Sil.*
Living were in brain, something—*Hyper.*
Load in head—*Ars. h.*
   –were pressing down in head—*Con.*
   –in brain were pushed from occiput to forehead with each expiration—*Pall.*
   –in morning, brain were oppressed by—*Ars., Ip.*
   –were lying on forehead, a heavy—*Eug.*
   –on vertex, a heavy—*Indg., Plat., Sulph., Zinc.*
   –were on upper part of head, an immense—*Ferr. t.*
Loaded, brain were—*Rhus t.*
Locust were chirping in head—*Bry.*
Loose in head when turning it, something were—*Kali c., Kalm.*
   –in head diagonally across top, something were—*Kalm.*
   –in head, turning and twisting toward forehead, something were—*Kali c.*
   –brain were—*Am. c., Bar. c., Bell., Bry., Carb. ac., Carb. an., Caust., Chin., Cic., Croc., Cyc., Dig., Elaps, Genist., Guaj., Hyos., Lact., Laur., Mur. ac., Nat. s., Nux m., Parth., Rhus t., Rumx., Spig., Sulph., Sul. ac., Thlaspi, Xanth.*
   –and beating against skull, brain were—*Stann.*
   –brain were detached and—*Guaj.*
   –and would fall from side to side, brain were—*Sul. ac.*
   –and would fall out, brain were—*Mez., Mosch.*

Loose—*Continued*

—and fell to side toward which he leaned, brain were—*Am. c., Sul. ac.*

—and hit against skull, brain were—*Rhus t.*

—and moved to and fro, brain were—*Bar. c.*

—in skull, brain were pressed together and lying—*Staph.*

—and rolling from side to side, brain were—*Tub.*

—on stepping, brain were—*Rhus t.*

—in brain when coughing, something tore—*Sep.*

—in forehead on shaking head—*Con.*

—in left side of forehead—*Nat. m.*

—in occiput, everything were—*Con.*

—from rest of skull, occiput were broken—*Chel.*

—on cranium, flesh were—*Sulph.*

—scalp were—*Sang.*

Loosen, ball of lead in middle of head which would not—*Staph.*

Loosened from back of head, scalp were—*Calc. c.*

Low a position no matter how high it were placed, head were placed in too—*Lach.*

Lower than body, head were—*Bry., Glon., Phos. ac.*

Lump, head were filled with a heavy—*Urea*

—brain were in one—*Ant. t.*

—in brain, large heavy—*Con.*

—brain were rolled up in a—*Ant. t., Arn., Cocc.*

—were falling forward in forehead on motion—*Cham.*

—in forehead that cannot be shaken loose—*Staph.*

—in forehead—*Cham., Pip. m.*

—or stone on top of head—*Ang., Phel., Nux v.*

Luxated, right side of occiput were—*Psor.*

Lying on something hard, head were—*Manc.*

—with head too low, he had been—*Phos.*

—in an unnatural position at night, head were—*Lyc.*

—with head in an uncomfortable position, he had been—*Cimx., Clem.*

—against various parts of head, pieces of ice were—*Calc. c.*

—loose within skull, brain were pressed together and—*Staph.*

—on brain, something were—*Grat.*

—on brain, weight were—*Pall., Sulph.*

—on forehead, heavy load were—*Eug.*

—on parietal bone, something were—*Fl. ac.*

Lying—*Continued*

   —on head about ear, something were—*Plan.*

   —upon a stone, in parietes—*Plat.*

   —on right side of head, heavy board were—*Eug.*

   —on vertex, heavy weight were—*Plat.*

   —in upper occiput, ice were—*Calc. p.*

   —across back of head, piece of wood were—*Psor.*

   —held firmly by neck, head moved forward while occiput remained—*Chel.*

Machine snapping in occiput, electric—*Calc. c.*

Magnet in forehead, drawing from—*Ictod.*

Marbles, two, striking each other over ear when walking—*Ars.*

Mashed, brain were—*Ip., Phos. ac., Sep.*

Measles, forehead were pressed as in—*Nat. m.*

Melody were ground on an organ in head and after a few turns it snapped off—*Merc.*

Metal plates were cracking in head—*Merc., Phel.*

Mill wheel whirling in head—*Chin. s.*

Motion, head were in—*Sep.*

   —all within head were in—*Verat. a.*

   —when leaning against something, brain were in—*Cyc.*

   —hairs of head were in—*Carb. v.*

Mounted to head, blood—*Glon., Mill., Puls., Spong.*

Mounting in head, a ball were—*Acon.*

Mouse were gnawing in occipital protuberance—*Zinc.*

Moved forward while occiput remained lying held firmly by neck, head (when raising it at night)—*Chel.*

   —about in head, a ball—*Anan.*

   —to and fro in head, something—*Sil.*

   —to and fro in head on raising it, a weight—*Op.*

   —in waves to head, something—*Glon.*

   —and beat upon skull, brain—*Ars.*

   —by boiling water, brain were—*Acon.*

   —to and fro, brain were loose and—*Bar. c.*

   —about vertex loosely, brain—*Thuj.*

   —when moving, brain—*Acon.*

   —on moving head, brain—*Sep.*

   —or raised, brain were—*Acon., Agar., Rheum*

   —when standing, brain—*Rheum*

   —and wanted to get out of skull, brain—*Prim.*

Moved—*Continued*

   –in waves of hunger, brain—*Sep.*

   –on vertex, a hair—*Stann.*

   –hair on vertex, someone—*Spong.*

Moving to and fro, head were—*Azad., Phel.*

   –in head by jerks, liquid were—*Coc. c.*

   –in head, liquids were—*Glon.*

   –in waves in head, something were—*Glon.*

   –in head, brain were—*Glon.*

   –about, brain were—*Ang., Lyc.*

   –in cranium, brain were—*Cyc.*

   –in forehead, something were—*Lyss.*

   –on top of head, something were—*Cupr.*

Nail were driven into head—*Acon., Coff., Der., Mag. p. Ambo, Ptel., Ruta*

   –were driven into middle of head—*Paull.*

   –were pricking in head and other parts—*Asc. t.*

   –were driven into brain—*Asaf., Ptel.*

   –pressed into brain—*Nux v.*

   –or plug pressing in one-half of brain—*Hep.*

   –were driven into head over nose—*Ign.*

   –were driven from left forehead into brain—*Sang.*

   –were driven into left frontal eminence—*Thuj.*

   –were pressed into forehead—*Puls. n.*

   –were thrust into temple—*Arn.*

   –were driven into side of head near left eye—*Am. br.*

   –were driven out through side of head—*Ign.*

   –were driven into left side of head—*Nat. m.*

   –were driven into parietal bone—*Coff., Thuj.*

   –were driven into right parietal bone—*Lycpr., Thuj.*

   –were forced downward deeper and deeper into parietal bone —*Ign., Nux v.*

   –were thrust into right side of head—*Agar., Lycpr.*

   –were driven into vertex—*Hell., Hura, Manc., Nicc., Nux v., Paraf., Thuj.*

   –were driven into vertex with a jerk—*Thuj.*

   –were driven from within out in vertex—*Thuj.*

   –were being driven into left vertex—*Paraf.*

   –were pressed into right side of head near vertex—*Euon.*

   –were pressing in vertex—*Form., Hell., Thuj.*

   –were sticking in vertex—*Nicc.*

Nail—*Continued*

  —or plug were driven in occiput—*Hep.*

  —were driven into occiput—*Tarent.*

  —driven in on one side of occiput—*Puls.*

  —pressed in occiput and point pierced brain—*Mosch.*

  —in bones of right side of head—*Kiss.*

Nailed to parietal bones, a piece of head were—*Coff. t.*

  —up, <in warm room, brain were—*Acon.*

Nails in head—*Asc. t.*

  —were being driven into head—*Der.*

  —in temples and root of nose, meeting at edge of hair at top of forehead—*Gymn.*

Narrow, forehead were too—*Gels.*

Needle pierced through brain over right eye—*Ign.*

  —were sticking in left side of forehead—*Verb.*

  —stitch in left temple—*Tarax.*

  —bones in vertex repeatedly pierced with—*Thuj.*

Needles in head—*Sep.*

  —or nails were being driven into head—*Der.*

  —sticking into head until head was turned toward side, a number of (associated with chest symptoms)—*Pip. n.*

  —ice cold, touched head or pierced it—*Agar.*

  —were pricking into brain, a thousand—*Tarent.*

  —were pushed through orbit into brain—*Ign.*

  —were running into brain—*Lyss.*

  —and pins in forehead—*Stram.*

  —were stuck into forehead—*All. c., Caul.*

  —were sticking in left temple—*Staph.*

  —fine, were stitching in vertex—*Staph.*

  —were sticking in middle of vertex—*Cic.*

Net were drawn through whole substance of brain—*Cinch. s.*

  —head were encompassed by—*Nat. m.*

No head, he had—*Asar., Calc. i., Cocc., Nit. ac.*

Nodes under scalp, there were painful—*Phos.*

Noise inside of head, there were—*Tarent.*

Numb, head were—*Graph., Nit. ac., Sarr.*

  —head would become—*Lyss.*

  —in left side of head—*Ol. an.*

  —brain were—*Bell.*

  —in bones of left side of head—*Daph. o.*

Numb—*Continued*
  –forehead were—*Bapt., Brom., Coll., Itu, Mag. m., Merc., Nat. a., Plat., Sil.*
  –top of head were—*Phys.*
Numbed in occiput—*Caust.*
Off shoulders, head were—*Puls.*
Ooze out through forehead, brain would—*Am. c.*
Open, head were—*Chin., Guare., Sil.*
  –and wind went through, head were—*Sanic.*
  –brain were—*Carb. an.*
  –and uncovered, upper part of head were—*Arum t.*
  –top of head would—*Nat. p.*
  –along vertex—*Spig.*
  –membranes were tense and pushing skull—*Meny.*
Opened and pain shot into abdomen on swallowing, head—*Lyc.*
  –and let in cold air, vertex—*Cimic.*
  –and shut, top of head—*Cann. i., Cimic., Cocc.*
  –and shut and calvarium were lifted, top of head—*Cann. i.*
  –and shut like a door, occiput—*Bell., Cann. i., Cimic., Cocc., Sep.*
Opening and shutting in right temple and vertex—*Cann. s.*
  –and shutting in vertex—*Cann. i.*
  –and shutting in left parietal region—*Vib.*
  –and shutting in occiput—*Cocc.*
Oscillating to and fro, brain were—*Lyc.*
Outward, blood in head were coursing upward and—*Ox. ac.*
Overfilled, brain were—*Wild.*
Packed in front of head, brain were—*Equis.*
Pain were caused by wrong position—*Lyc.*
  –circled through head and around crown—*Med.*
  –every step or sudden movement of head would cause pain (but it did not)—*Gels.*
  –were cutting head off—*Phys.*
  –were over surface of brain—*Nux v.*
  –in brain were pressing head forward—*Olnd.*
  –in right side of head, there would be a violent—*Crot. h.*
  –in back of head, bewildered with—*Xanth.*
Painful on touch, hair were—*Par.*
Paper, skull were as thin as—*Bell., Par.*
Paralyzed, brain were—*Chim. umb.*
  –when talking, brain would be—*Calc. c.*

Paralyzed—*Continued*
  –forehead were—*Sep.*
  –in occiput—*Phys.*
  –at occiput—*Atham.*
  –right side of head were—*Sil.*
  –left half of face and head were—*Stry.*
Parchment, head were covered with—*Bar. ac.*
Passage of storm cloud, head were heavy as from—*Hyper.*
Passed over brain, cold air—*Anan.*
  –through left side of head into limbs, electric current—*Ail.*
Peg, head were fastened to shoulder by a long—*Cupr.*
Penetrate skull to brain, cold air seems to—*Cimic.*
Penetrated by sharp wind, left occiput were—*Sabi.*
Penetrating brain, hot water on scalp were—*Peti.*
Pepper, scalp were burning like cayenne—*Iris t.*
Photographer's head-rest, head rested in—*Nat. a.*
Pieces, head were separated or forced apart in—*Arg. n., Bufo, Glon., Kali bi., Lyc., Mez.*
  –bones on left side of head were hacked to—*Calc. c.*
  –if shaken, head would drop in—*Glon.*
  –with cough, head would fly to—*Bry., Caps., Rumx.*
  –if she moved, head would fly to—*Coff.*
  –cats were tearing brain to—*Ars.*
  –brain were dashed to—*Æth., Coff., Nux v.*
Pierced it, ice-cold needles touched head or—*Agar.*
  –through into brain over right eye, needle—*Ign.*
  –brain, nail pressed into occiput and point—*Mosch.*
  –from forehead to occiput, steel arrows—*Anan.*
  –by a needle, bones in vertex were repeatedly—*Thuj.*
  –with a knife in occiput at every heart beat—*Con.*
Piercing skull, gimlet were—*Puls.*
Pinched together with pincers, forehead and temples were violently crushed and—*Verb.*
  –forehead were being—*Acon., Anac., Calc. c., Eug., Mez., Nit. ac., Nux m., Op., Psor., Til., Verat. a.*
Pincers, parts over zygomatic arch were seized with—*Puls.*
Pin sticking in brain—*Nux v.*
Pinned to head, ears were—*Vib.*
Pins and needles in forehead—*Stram.*
  –pricking in forehead—*Aur m., Calad.*
  –in vertex, number of—*Æsc.*

Pistol were fired in head—*Dig.*

Pithy like cork and elongated upward, head were—*Graph.*
 –upper part of head were—*Mez.*

Plug, skull would be pressed outward by sharp—*Prun.*
 –were thrust quickly by increasingly severe blows into head—*Sul. ac.*
 –were driven into right side of head—*Mez.*
 –were driven into brain—*Asaf.*
 –or nail pressing in one-half of brain or in occiput—*Hep.*
 –were pressing on right side of forehead—*Jac.*
 –pointed, were pressing inward in left temple—*Asaf.*
 –were sticking in right temple—*Plat.*
 –in right parietal bone—*Asaf.*
 –dull, on left side of vertex—*Anac.*
 –in right side of occiput—*Con.*
 –were being driven into occiput and temples—*Hep.*

Plunged into head, knife were—*Nux m.*

Point, dull, were pressing in forehead—*Rhus t.*
 –sharp, pressed against right frontal eminence—*Par.*

Points of ice touched head, sharp—*Agar.*

Position, head had been held in an uncomfortable—*Zinc.*

Poultices on head, cold—*Mosch.*

Pounded, head had been—*Cimic.*

Poured over forehead, cold water were—*Tarent.*

Pouring down inside of forehead, warm water were—*Glon.*

Press out of forehead, everything would—*Spong., Verb.*
 –forward, brain would—*Ip., Kali c.*
 –out and burst skull, everything would—*Sil.*

Pressed against pillow by a warm hand, head were—*Sel.*
 –asunder, head were—*Con., Euph., Fago., Juncus, Hyper., Lyc., Phyt., Prun., Saba., Sil.*
 –asunder, everything in head would be—*Mez.*
 –by a band, head were—*Clem., Glon.*
 –by too much blood, head were—*Con., Merl., Nux m., Rhus v.*
 –down, head were—*Senn., Zing.*
 –down on head, cap or iron helmet were—*Crot. c.*
 –head, a tight cap—*Carb. s.*
 –down, a cast were fitted over vertex and—*Lyss.*
 –down with a weight, head were—*Merl.*
 –head down on pillow, a heavy weight—*Merc. i. f.*
 –downward through head, blunt instrument were—*Calc. c.*

Pressed—*Continued*

–into head, eyes would be—*Bapt.*

–out of head, both eyes would be—*Bry., Ham.*

–like an elastic ball in head and spine—*Benz. ac.*

–upon by a hand on left parietal bone, head were—*Kali ar.*

–into forehead and root of nose on stooping, contents of head were—*Zing.*

–asunder, brain would be—*Nux v., Sil.*

–against skull, brain would be—*Mez.*

–against upper part of skull, brain—*Laur.*

–against forehead, brain were—*Chin., Mag. m.*

–against forehead, brain fell forward and—*Coff.*

–against skull, brain were being—*Calc. p., Kali c., Rhod.*

–against frontal bones, brain were—*Hydr.*

–sharp corners, brain were—*Saba.*

–asunder, brain were—*Hyper., Saba.*

–backward, brain were—*Tab.*

–down in middle of brain—*Cina*

–forward, brain were—*Senec.*

–into a ball, brain were—*Chin.*

–into brain, nail were—*Nux v.*

–inward, brain were—*Ther.*

–out, brain were—*Acon., Bry.*

–out at forehead, brain were—*Am. c., Berb., Bry., Cupr., Hell., Kreos., Rat.*

–out on nodding head, brain were—*Thuj.*

–outward, brain were too full and—*Bry.*

–outward in temples, brain would be—*Thuj.*

–to all sides, brain—*Laur.*

–to forehead, brain were—*Bell., Cupr. ar.*

–together, brain would be—*Calc. c., Cocc.*

–together from both sides and forehead, brain were—*Chin.*

–together in one lump, brain were—*Ant. t.*

–together and lying loose in skull, brain were—*Staph.*

–together against sharp corner, brain were—*Saba.*

–upon brain, heavy substance—*Still.*

–upon brain at every step, a weight were—*Meny.*

–upward, brain were—*Fl. ac.*

–forehead were—*Laur.*

–asunder in temples and especially in forehead—*Op.*

–or strapped to forehead, board were—*Dulc., Plat., Rhus t.*

Pressed—*Continued*

    –by a tight hat, forehead were—*Alumn.*

    –flat, forehead were—*Cor. r.*

    –as in measles, forehead were—*Nat. m.*

    –in, forehead would be—*Bapt.*

    –in, forehead were—*Nux v., Stann.*

    –inward, forehead would be—*Stann.*

    –into forehead, a nail were—*Puls. n.*

    –out, forehead were as large again and—*Nux m.*

    –out at forehead, something would be—*Chin.*

    –against right frontal eminence, sharp point were—*Par.*

    –firmly, right side of head were—*Phyt.*

    –together in sides of head—*Glon.*

    –on left parietal bone which was sore, a hand—*Kali ar.*

    –asunder in temporal eminence—*Sabin.*

    –in by thumbs, temples were—*Bapt.*

    –down as far as temples, tight cap were—*Phys.*

    –in, temples and malar bones were—*Pip. n.*

    –out, temples would be—*Ign., Saponin., Spong.*

    –out, temples and eyes were—*Par.*

    –together in temples—*Op.*

    –together, temples were—*Sang.*

    –out, bones in left temple would be—*Staph.*

    –against wall, top of head—*Sulph.*

    –asunder on vertex—*Ran. b.*

    –asunder in vertex and must hold it together, head were—*Carb. an.*

    –together, vertex and sides of head were—*Glon.*

    –into right side of head near vertex, nail were—*Euon.*

    –on vertex, dull instrument—*Ran. s.*

    –asunder in back of head—*Lach.*

    –out, occiput were—*Bry., Carb. o., Chin., Fago., Stront.*

    –out, occiput were being—*Eriod.*

    –in occiput and point pierced brain, a nail were —*Mosch.*

    –in occiput, wedge would be—*Bov.*

    –near occiput, wound were—*Saba.*

    –at point where head and neck unite, a finger were—*Rheum*

    –against skull, brain were expanded and—*Cupr. ar.*

    –skull asunder, something—*Bry., Nux v.*

    –inward, skull were—*Hell.*

    –out of skull, everything would be—*Sil.*

Pressed—*Continued*
 –out, bones would be—*Staph.*
 –outward and raised upward, bones were—*Laur.*
 –outward by sharp plug, skull would be—*Prun.*
Pressing down in head, blood were—*Con.*
 –down in head, load were—*Con.*
 –through whole head, board were—*Zing.*
 –on left head, convex button were—*Thuj.*
 –above ears, band tied around head were—*Am. br., Gels.*
 –down, cast were fitted over head and—*Lyss.*
 –in root of nose, over and around ears, a band were—*Ther.*
 –on back of head, fingers were—*Meph.*
 –head, someone were forcibly—*Nit. ac.*
 –against head, something were—*Cast. eq.*
 –upon head, something were—*Sars.*
 –on head from above downward, weight were—*Phos. ac.*
 –head down on pillow, heavy weight were—*Merc. i. f.*
 –head, wobbling body were—*Asar.*
 –inward, dull instrument were—*Olnd., Asaf.*
 –head forward, pain in brain were—*Olnd.*
 –brain forward, a hundred weight were—*Olnd.*
 –in one-half of brain, nail or plug were—*Hep.*
 –into brain, nail were—*Nux v.*
 –brain inward, weight were—*Thuj.*
 –on brain, something were—*Coff.*
 –against bone, brain were—*Mez.*
 –on brain in frontal region, hard substance were—*Still.*
 –out of brain, something heavy were—*Phys.*
 –together, brain were—*Agar.*
 –brain, weight on vertex were—*Peti.*
 –against forehead, board were—*Dulc., Plat.*
 –in forehead, dull point were—*Rhus t.*
 –in forehead, stone were—*Bell., Cham., Elect.*
 –upward in forehead, a fullness were—*Meph.*
 –on brows, something were—*Carb. an., Linum*
 –against each temple, something were—*Iodof., Phaseo.*
 –asunder in right eminence of temporal bone—*Sabi.*
 –inward in temple, pointed plug were—*Asaf.*
 –from temple to temple and screwed, a bolt were—*Ham.*
 –temples would be broken from—*Pip. n.*
 –in vertex, nail were—*Form., Hell., Thuj.*

Pressing—*Continued*
  –in vertex, temples and eyes, thumbs were—*Nit. ac.*
  –against occiput, something firm were—*Cast. eq.*
  –skull in, stone on vertex were—*Nux v.*
  –on skull, hard substance were—*Staph.*
  –within skull, a tumor were—*Helod.*
Pressure in head were caused by congestion—*Dig.*
  –head would fall forward because of—*Agn.*
  –from fingertips on head—*Pall.*
  –in head, there were great—*Oxyt.*
  –on head, hot—*Carb. v.*
  –in head, sweat would follow—*Camph.*
  –brain were constricted on all sides by—*Tarax.*
  –of fingers on forehead—*Cham.*
  –in bones of frontal sinuses—*Nux v.*
  –forehead were flattened by—*Cor. r.*
  –in temples—*Ang., Nux v.*
  –of finger in left temple—*Staph.*
  –outward in right temple—*Spong.*
  –of weight in vertex—*Sulph.*
  –of hat, icy cold in vertex from—*Valer.*
  –two fingers into it at occiput, head were in a cushion and
      someone were—*Sil.*
  –in occiput would force brain out at forehead—*Caps.*
  –from head-rest in occiput—*Nat. a.*
Pricked into temple, sharp substance inside which—*Raph.*
Pricking in head and other parts, nail were—*Asc. t.*
  –into brain, a thousand needles were—*Tarent.*
  –in forehead, pins were—*Aur. m., Calad.*
Prickling sweat on bald vertex—*All. c.*
Pried apart, atlas and axis had been—*Cur.*
Prolapse from forehead, all would—*Berb.*
Protrude through forehead, everything would—*Psor.*
Puffed up, head were—*Par.*
Puffy, head were—*Berb.*
Pulled up with half of brain, upper part of skull were being—
      Cund.
  –skin on forehead were—*Bapt.*
  –by hair of vertex—*Acon., Indg., Kali n., Mag. c., Mag. m.,
      Mur. ac., Sulph.*

Pulled—*Continued*
  —from vertex, a bunch of hair were—*Indg.*
  —out in occiput, hair were—*Arn.*
  —backward toward occiput, skin of forehead were—*Bapt.*
  —back by a weight in occiput, head were—*Syph.*
  —down tight, scalp of occiput were—*Hell.*
  —occiput were being—*Dios., Fer. g.*
  —hair had been—*Acon., Æth., Alum., Eupi., Kali p., Mag. c., Phos., Psor., Rhus t., Sec., Sel., Stry., Vib.*
  —single hairs were being—*Acet. ac.*
  —hair had been severely—*Sol. n.*
  —upward, roots of hair were—*Arg. n.*
  —out, hair were being—*Caps., Prun.*
  —it out by roots, hand struck left side of head, grasped hair and—*Sep.*
  —a lock of hair were—*Laur.*
Pulling in forehead—*Ang., Kreos., Lepi.*
  —at occipital region, heavy weight were—*Oxyt.*
  —lock of hair upward on vertex, someone were—*Canth.*
  —hair on back of head, someone were—*Kali p.*
Pulsating, vessels in head were—*Nux m.*
Pulsation would arise in head—*Fl. ac.*
Pulses were beating in head, all—*Paraf.*
Pumped into brain, something were—*Glon.*
Pumping in vertex, something were—*Glon.*
Pus under scalp—*Cinch. s.*
Push through top of head from throbbing deep in, brain would—*Parth.*
  —out forehead, everything would—*Acon.*
Pushed forward, head were—*Ferr. p., Gymn.*
  —out, forehead were—*Nux m.*
  —through orbit into brain, needles were—*Ign.*
  —out in left frontal eminence, bone were being—*Calc. c.*
  —from occiput to forehead at each respiration, wedge were—*Pall.*
  —it forward, something stuck behind ear and (when brushing hair on occiput)—*Ars. s. f.*
  —from occiput to forehead on each expiration, load were—*Pall.*
  —upward, skull were—*Ferr.*
Pushing in right forehead, something were—*Arg. n.*

Pushing—*Continued*

  –two fingers in at occiput, head were in a cushion and some-
      one were—*Sil.*

  –skull open, membranes were tense and were—*Meny.*

Putty, head were made of—*Nit. ac.*

Queer feeling in whole head with painless throbbing—*Ap. g.*

Quivering in head, a nerve were—*Ferr.*

  –in brain—*Xanth.*

Racked and shaken, brain were—*Rhod.*

Railroad train were going through brain—*Chin. s.*

Raise head after stooping, he could not—*Spig.*

Raised about five inches and brain were coming out, top of head
      were lifted or—*Lac d.*

  –upward, bones were pressed outward and—*Laur.*

  –brain were—*Acon., Rhod., Thuj.*

  –brain were moved or—*Acon., Agar., Rheum*

  –from pillow, occiput could not be—*Chel.*

  –by pulling, hair were—*Mag. m.*

Raising up, occiput were—*Dign.*

Ran over whole head, something cold—*Carl.*

Raw, head were—*Sulph.*

  –in occipital protuberance—*Elaps*

Relaxed and contracted alternately, inner head—*Calc. c., Lac c.,
      Med.*

Remained lying held firmly by neck, head moved forward while
      occiput—*Chel.*

Remove vertex, she would like to—*Ther.*

Removed, calvaria were—*Arum t., Cann. i.*

Rent asunder, brain were—*Ferr.*

Rested on lower jaws, bones of face and cranium—*Pip. n.*

  –on brain, skull—*Cur.*

Reunited, skin of scalp were cut and—*Ol. an.*

Revolving on an axis, brain were—*Nux v., Rob.*

  –over forehead, ring were—*Hura*

Ring, hot iron, were binding head—*Acon.*

  –were tightened about head—*Spire.*

  –head were being squeezed tighter and tighter by an iron—
      Tub.

  –forehead were compressed by—*Fuc. ves.*

  –were revolving over forehead—*Hura*

Ringing in head—*Kali i., Kreos., Sulph.*

Rise, top of head would—*Lac. ac.*
Rising in head, foam were—*Myric.*
   –in head, something were—*Glon., Nat. c., Nux v., Rhus t., Tab.*
   –from throat to brain, ball were—*Plb.*
   –from vertex, something were—*Glon.*
   –up on left occiput, hair were—*Cocc.*
   –from occiput to vertex, something were—*Glon.*
   –of scalp, a sudden—*Polyg.*
Roaring in forehead—*Verat. a.*
   –in head—*Aur., Chin. s., Cinnb., Ferr., Graph., Hura, Hyper., Kali bi., Kreos., Lach., Mur. ac., Narcot., Nat. c., Nat. m., Nit. ac., Petr., Phos. ac., Phos., Sep., Sil., Tab., Thuj., Verat. a., Zinc.*
Rocked and swayed in brain, something—*Bell.*
Rocket had passed through head—*Kali p.*
Rod or bolt, iron, from temple to temple and screwed tighter and tighter—*Phos.*
   –iron, were thrust from right eyebrow to lower part of occiput—*Syph.*
Rolled about in skull, brain—*Chin., Phys.*
   –over, brain—*Lob. e.*
   –up in a lump, brain were—*Ant. t., Arn., Cocc.*
   –up against frontal bone, waves of pain—*Sep.*
Rolling about in head, something were—*Eug., Sep.*
   –from side to side, brain were loose and—*Tub.*
   –in brain, small leaden balls were—*Lyss.*
   –and surging in forehead, waves were—*Sep.*
   –in left forehead, something were—*Berb.*
Room in head, there were not enough—*Daph. o.*
   –enough in forehead, brain had not—*Psor.*
   –enough in skull, there were not—*Helod.*
Rose and fell at every step, brain—*Bell.*
   –into brain, smoke—*Op.*
Rope around head drawn tighter and tighter—*Nat. m.*
Rough, forehead were—*Alumn., Fl. ac., Kali bi., Pall., Rhus v., Sars., Sep.*
Rubber band around forehead—*Carb. ac., Plat., Sulph.*
   –cap on head, tight—*Stel.*
Run through head above tips of ears, bolt were—*Dulc.*
Running upward from nape of neck, hot water were—*Glon.*
   –needles into brain—*Lyss.*

Running—*Continued*

    –down temple, drop of water were (not cool)—*Verat. a.*

    –over scalp, lice were—*Caps., Pedi.*

    –and crawling in hair, something were—*Cast. eq.*

Rushed through head, a current of cold air—*Aur.*

    –to head, blood—*Calc. c., Cinch., Ferr., Glon., Meli., Phos., Sal. ac., Sulph., Upas, Valer., Verat. a.*

    –to heart then head, blood—*Nux m.*

    –to brain vanishing thought, blood—*Ran. b.*

    –to forehead and temples, blood—*Phys.*

    –like lightning through brain down neck, something—*Chin. a.*

    –upward in vertex, something—*Aml. n.*

    –to occiput, all blood—*Ol. an.*

Rushing through head from right to left, fluid were—*Lil. t.*

    –in head, something were—*Acon., Chlor., Indg., Pimp.*

    –into head and ears, all blood were—*Aml. n., Mill.*

    –into head and face, all blood were—*Cur., Ferr. s.*

    –across head, blood were—*Eup. per.*

    –through brain, blood were—*Con.*

    –of boiling water in occiput—*Indg., Pimp.*

Salt, brain were sprinkled with—*Zinc. ac.*

Saw were tearing in head—*Sulph.*

Scalded, brain were—*Helod.*

Scalding, vertex were—*Sol*

Scraped, head were being—*X-ray*

    –bones of head were—*Phos. ac.*

    –off from back of head, scalp were—*Acon.*

    –scalp were contracted and bones—*Par.*

Screw were being driven into right temple—*Nat. s.*

    –behind each ear compressing head--*Ox. ac.*

Screwed asunder, head were—*Thuj.*

    –together, head were—*Æth., Alumn., Atro., Bell., Castor., Caust., Cina, Clem., Cocc., Coloc., Daph., Graph., Ind., Indg., Kali i., Mag. c., Mag. s., Merc., Mill., Nicc., Petr., Plat., Rat., Saba., Sars., Stann., Sulph., Zinc.*

    –up, head were—*Atro., Glon.*

    –in, whole brain were—*Euph.*

    –together, brain were—*Clem.*

    –together, brain and zygoma were—*Euph.*

    –together and over forehead, board were—*Sulph.*

    –forehead were—*Chel., Grat., Hyos., Merc. s.*

Screwed—*Continued*

–in, forehead were—*Plat.*

–together, forehead were—*Sulph.*

–apart at temples, head were being—*Cast. eq.*

–in, temples were—*Plat.*

–together, temples were—*Lyc.*

–a bolt were pressing from temple to temple and were tightly —*Ham.*

–tighter and tighter, bolt or iron rod through from temple to temple and—*Phos.*

–together, both sides of head were being—*Zinc.*

–together above ears—*Sul. ac.*

–together, right side of head were—*Mill.*

–up in a vise, vertex were—*Daph., Daph. o.*

–together in vertex—*Grat.*

–in, occiput were—*Am. m.*

–inward frequently, head were—*Stann.*

–together from below upward, head were—*Daph. o.*

–together from both sides of head in morning—*Kali i.*

–together in occiput—*Grat., Mag. c., Merc.*

–together in muscles of back part of head, parts were—*Rhus t.*

Screwing from behind forward, something were working in top of head and—*Plb.*

Screws, head were between—*Puls.*

Seething in head—*Euph., Pæon.*

–in occiput extending to loins—*Euph. amyg.*

Seized, head were—*Lith.*

–with incipient apoplexy—*Ran. g.*

–with pincers, parts over zygomatic arch were—*Puls.*

–by something in occiput extending around back of ears, eyes and forehead with rush of blood to head and electric shocks —*Ricin.*

Senseless, head were—*Lyc.*

Sensitive, brain were very—*Genist.*

Separate, head would—*Dol.*

Separated from body, head were—*Cann. i., Daph., Psor.*

–or forced apart in pieces, head were—*Arg. n., Bufo, Glon., Kali bi., Lyc., Mez.*

–from rest of head or she could lift it off, vertex were—*Ther.*

–from bone on touch, flesh were—*Caust.*

–bones of skull were—*Arg. n.*

Set in, catarrh would—*Rhod.*
Settled down on head, a cloud—*Samars.*
Shaken, brain were—*Pall., Mez.*
  –and racked, brain were—*Rhod.*
  –by electric shocks, brain were—*Aster.*
  –in skull, brain were—*Bell.*
  –brain were (with nausea)—*Elaps*
  –brain were rudely—*Upas*
  –when walking, brain were—*Cic.*
  –from side to side when walking, brain were—*Rhod.*
Shaking head, brain were crushed on—*Squill.*
  –in morning, something in head were—*Tab.*
  –in forehead on motion—*Spig.*
  –in skull, brain were—*Spig.*
  –about in skull on moving head, brain were—*Sol. n.*
Sharp corner, brain were pressed against a—*Saba.*
  –corner were placed against top of head—*Prun.*
  –point were pressed against right frontal eminence—*Par.*
Shattered at a blow, brain were made of glass and—*Dig.*
  –head were—*Æth., Calc. c., Euph., Kali c., Lact., Rhus t.,*
    Stront., Stry., Sul. ac., Verat. a.
  –by toothache, head were—*Euph.*
  –in morning on waking—*Sul. ac.*
  –forehead were—*Stann.*
Shattering, head were—*Stry.*
  –in brain when stepping hard—*Sil.*
  –so as to hold on to temples, coughing causes—*Cur.*
Sheet-lightning, crisping of blood in brain like—*Cann. i.*
Shivering in forehead > touch—*Castor.*
  –of skin under hair, slight—*Verat. a.*
Shock, electric, in head—*Carb. v.*
  –strong, of electricity from head extending to all parts of body
    —*Mag. p.*
  –from right temple to left occiput, electric—*Iris*
  –in occiput from a blow—*Arg. m.*
  –electric, in occiput—*Arn.*
  –in scalp, gentle electric—*Cench.*
  –passed through head, a strong electric—*Zinc. s.*
  –of electricity passed through head—*All. c., Graph., Hell.,*
    Laur., Nat. s., Ricin.

Shocks, electric, in head—*Cic.*

  –shooting rapidly from one part of head to another—*Sang.*

  –of electricity pass through brain—*Hell.*

  –at night, brain were shaken by—*Aster.*

  –fine electric, in vertex—*Carb. ac.*

  –in brain as when sitting down suddenly—*Raph.*

Shook from behind forward from hiccough, brain—*Bry.*

  –from noise, brain—*Mag. p. Arct.*

Shooting rapidly from one part of head to another, electric shocks
  —*Sang.*

Short and head would be drawn backward, tendons were too—
  Laur.

Shot down to abdomen on swallowing, head opened and pain—
  Lyc.

  –through head like lightning, something—*Morph.*

Shrunken, brain were—*Morph.*

  –left side of head were—*Cinnm.*

Shut and calvarium were lifted, top of head opened and—*Cann. i.*

  –top of head opened and—*Cann. i., Cimic., Cocc.*

  –like a door, occiput opened and—*Bell., Cann. i., Cimic., Cocc.,*
   Sep.

Shutting and opening in left parietal region—*Vib.*

  –and opening in right temple and vertex—*Cann. s.*

Sick in head—*Ars., Zinc.*

Sink down, head would—*Sulph.*

  –to right side, head would—*Prun. p.*

Sinking backward when turning in bed, head were—*Tub.*

  –down in head, something heavy were—*Nux v.*

  –transversely across frontal eminence, weight were—*Thuj.*

  –vertex were—*Sep.*

  –from occiput on stooping, something were—*Kali c.*

Sleep, brain had gone to—*Apis, Con.*

  –in vertex, head were going to—*Cupr. s.*

  –occiput had gone to—*Cast. eq.*

Small, head were too—*Coff.*

  –for brain, skull were too—*Clem., Glon.*

  –skull were too—*Morph.*

Smaller, head were—*Acon., Grat., Ign., Pic. ac.*

  –left side of head were—*Cinnm.*

Smashed, forehead were—*Hyper.*

Smoke passing through brain—*Anthr.*

   —rose into brain—*Op.*

   —one side of head were filled with—*Sul. ac.*

Snap, right temple were drawn so tight it would—*Am. c.*

Snapped off, melody were ground on an organ in head and after a few turns it—*Merc.*

Snapping in head were nearly driving him crazy—*Antip.*

   —of a piano string in head—*Lyc.*

   —in occiput, an electric machine were—*Calc. c.*

Soft, head were—*Sulph.*

   —and spongy, whole side of head were—*Paraf.*

Soldered together, head and teeth were—*Lyss.*

Solid head, there were no—*Cot.*

Someone else, head belonged to—*Ther.*

Sore, brain were—*Arn., Bapt., Camph., Chin., Zinc. ac.*

   —and collided with skull, brain were—*Sil.*

   —spot on right side of head if hair is touched—*Ambr.*

Sound came through forehead and brain—*Sulph.*

   —hurt brain—*Kali p.*

Sounds of a swarm of bees in head—*Sal. ac.*

   —in brain of striking a piece of silver—*Phel.*

Space enough in forehead, brain had not—*Psor.*

Sparks, electric, in forehead—*Ol. an.*

   —electric, in temples—*Spig.*

   —fine electric, in vertex (changing to prickling)—*Carb. ac.*

Splashing in left side of brain—*Carb. an.*

Splinters in scalp—*Nit. ac.*

Split, head would—*Am. m., Asar., Aster., Calc. ar., Calc. c., Caps., Coc. c., Coch., Helod., Lyss., Nat. s., Nux v., Ol. j., Peti., Sarr., Sol. n.*

   —open, head were being—*Podo.*

   —when coughing, head would—*Calc. c.*

   —in two, head would be—*Nat. ntrs.*

   —head, pain would—*Calc. ar.*

   —open with a wedge, head were—*Lachn.*

   —in two, brain were—*Nux v.*

   —brain would—*Aster.*

   —open, frontal bones would—*Pic. ac.*

   —forehead would—*Æth., Olnd., Thuj., Vacc., Vario.*

   —in two in median line, forehead would—*Vacc., Vario.*

   —on going into cold, forehead would—*Lac c.*

Split—*Continued*

　　–in two, vertex were—*Zinc.*

　　–top of head would—*Nat. s.*

　　–skull would—*Bar. c., Caps., Mez., Peti.*

　　–skull had been—*Carb. ac., Carb. an.*

Splitting, head were—*Am. m.*

Sprinkled with salt, brain were—*Zinc. ac.*

Spongy and soft when touched, whole side of head were—*Paraf.*

Spoon, brain were stirred with a—*Arg. n., Iod.*

Spot in head opposite center of forehead, cold were in—*Bell.*

　　–in forehead, someone touched him with cold thumb in small—*Arn.*

Sprained, back of head were—*Psor.*

Squeezed between two beams, head had been—*Sal. ac.*

　　–flat, head were—*Manc.*

　　–after breakfast, head were—*Dios.*

　　–in a vise, head were—*Sars., Sul. i.*

　　–brain were—*Rhus v.*

　　–together by an iron ring, brain were being—*Tub.*

　　–and relaxed alternately, brain were—*Calc. c.*

　　–in vertex—*Con.*

　　–forehead were—*Acon., Eupi.*

　　–above nose—*Acon.*

Squeezing together, head were—*Bar. c.*

Stabbed in forehead, eyes and ears with knife—*Thuj.*

Stabbing from temple to temple, knife were—*Bell.*

　　–under right temporal bone, knife were—*Paraf.*

　　–in right frontal eminence—*Saba.*

Stand on end, hair would—*Am. c.*

Standing on end, hair were—*Acon., Lachn., Spong.*

　　–on end on vertex, hair were—*Spong.*

Start out through eye, whole brain would—*Acon.*

Step were felt in head, every—*Calc. p., Lyc., Nat. m., Rhus t., Stann., Sulph.*

　　–had an echo in head, every—*Calc. ar.*

Stick in temple, dull—*Asaf.*

　　–large, thrust through head from left to right—*Apis*

Sticking into head until head was turned toward side, a number of needles were (associated with chest symptoms)—*Pip. n.*

　　–in brain, a pin were—*Nux v.*

　　–in forehead, knife were—*Ter.*

7

Sticking—*Continued*
  –in left side of forehead, needle were—*Verb.*
  –with a penknife in temples—*Ferr.*
  –in left temple, needles were—*Staph.*
  –in right temple, plug were—*Plat.*
  –into her head, hairpins were—*Kali p.*
  –in vertex, nail were—*Nicc.*
  –in middle of vertex, needles were—*Cic.*
Stirred with a spoon, brain were—*Arg. n., Iod.*
Stitch of needle in left temple—*Tarax.*
Stitches were thrust into occiput—*Stront.*
Stitching in vertex, fine needles were—*Staph.*
  –in forehead, knife were—*Ferr., Lact.*
  –in occiput, knives were—*Nat. m.*
  –just above right temple, knife-like—*Verb.*
Stolid, head were—*Merc. i. r.*
Stone in forehead—*Cham., Kali c.*
  –pressing in forehead—*Bell., Cham., Elect.*
  –on upper forehead—*Con.*
  –in parietes, lying upon a—*Plat.*
  –or lump on top of head—*Ang., Nux v., Phel.*
  –on vertex pressing skull in—*Nux v.*
  –upon vertex—*Cann. s.*
  –in vertex—*Kali c.*
Stood still, blood collected in head and—*Elaps*
  –on end, hair—*Acon., Bar. c., Carb. v., Cham., Chel., Dulc., Mur. ac., Sal. ac., Spong.*
  –on end with itching, hair—*Sal. ac.*
  –on end, hairs on forehead—*Calc. c., Ran. b.*
  –on end, a hair in sinciput—*Ran. b.*
  –on end, hair on vertex—*Sulph.*
Stooping, brain were cut in pieces on—*Nicc.*
Stopped up, head were—*Ham., Nat. c.*
Strained in forehead—*Hyper., Op.*
  –head were—*Calc. s., Phys.*
Strange, head were—*Thea*
Strap were drawn tightly across forehead—*Carb. v.*
Strapped or pressed to forehead, board were—*Calc. c., Dulc., Plat., Rhus t.*
Stream of wind from chest to head—*Mill.*
Streamed from head into body, all blood—*Elaps*

Street car were running through brain—*Chin. s.*
Stretched, brain were—*Plat.*
   —over forehead, a band of ribbon were—*Lil. t.*
   —over forehead, a rubber band were—*Carb. ac., Coca*
   —from above, skin above eyes were—*Stach.*
   —left side of head were—*Cupr. ac.*
   —skull were—*Samb.*
   —over skull, skin of forehead were tightly—*Cann. i.*
Striking of a large bell in head, with buzzing—*Sars.*
   —head from within outward, hammers were—*Psor.*
   —wedge in head, every beat of heart were—*Calc. ar.*
   —a piece of silver, sounds in brain as if—*Phel.*
   —each other over ear when walking, two marbles were—*Ars.*
   —on back of head, invisible hammers were—*Lyss.*
String snapped in head with a clang—*Lyc.*
Stroke, he might have an apoplectic—*Arg. m.*
Struck, head had been—*Med.*
   —head had been covered by a leaden cap and then—*Paull.*
   —by apoplexy—*Kali cy.*
   —when walking, head were—*Naja*
   —by apoplexy, he would be—*Fl. ac., Tarent.*
   —in head, a large bell had been; causing buzzing—*Sars.*
   —against skull on moving, brain—*Rob.*
   —against side of head, brain wobbled and—*Nux m.*
   —with hammer on right side of head—*Tab.*
   —with hammer on vertex—*Sal. ac.*
   —with hammer, occiput were—*Tarent.*
Stuck into forehead, needles were—*All. c., Caul.*
   —into vertex, a red-hot iron were—*Crot. c.*
   —behind ear and pushed it forward when brushing hair on
      occiput, something—*Ars. s. f.*
Stuffed, head were—*Acon., Glon., Graph., Sep., Sulph., Ust.*
   —forehead were—*Glon.*
Stung her on left temple, bee had—*Apis*
Stunned in forehead—*Agar., Fl. ac., Thuj.*
   —in head—*Sarr.*
Stupid in left half of occiput—*Dig.*
Substance, foreign, in brain—*Iod.*
  —heavy, pressed upon brain—*Still.*
  —sharp, inside which pricked into temple—*Raph.*

Substance—*Continued*
 –light, were rolling from above eyes to vertex—*Tub.*
 –hard, pressing on skull—*Staph.*
Sun, head had been exposed to the—*Manc.*
 –without dinner, he had been in hot—*Glon.*
Support head, muscles were too weak to—*Crot. h.*
Suppurate, a spot on occiput would—*Rhus t.*
Suppurating on head, < when touched—*Agar., Graph.*
 –head were—*Mez., Petr.*
 –on left side of head—*Sulph.*
 –in brain—*Nux v.*
 –under right side of scalp—*Cinch. s.*
 –vertex were—*Castor.*
 –on touch, skin of vertex were—*Paraf.*
 –in occiput—*Puls.*
Surcharged with electricity, head were—*Kalm.*
Surging in head—*Alumn., Fago., Ox. ac.*
 –of waves rolling in forehead—*Sep.*
 –from occiput to forehead—*Cann. i.*
Surrounded head, a tight band—*Xanth.*
 –with band, head were—*Chel.*
 –by hot air, head were—*Aster.*
Suspended, head were—*Cere. b.*
Swashed about in vertex, brain—*Carb. ac.*
Swashing in head—*Hep., Plect., Squill.*
 –in head, water were—*Hyos.*
 –around in head with each step, brain were—*Rhus t.*
 –of brain when walking—*Spig.*
 –about in forehead, brain were—*Cina*
 –about in top of head, brain were—*Carb. ac.*
Swayed and rocked in brain, something—*Bell.*
Swaying in head—*Daph.*
 –in a jerking manner in head, rocking and—*Bell.*
 –brain were—*Meli.*
 –to one side while sitting, occiput were—*Gins.*
Sweat would follow pressure in head—*Camph.*
 –ice-cold, on forehead, but none there—*Glon.*
 –prickling on bald vertex—*All. c.*
Swelled up, head were—*Par.*
 –over eyes suddenly, with horrid pain—*Tub.*

Swelling, head were—*Bapt., Berb., Rhus t.*
  –right side of head were—*Par.*
  –of head and hands—*Aran.*
Swinging, head were—*Thuj.*
Swollen, head were—*Æth., All. c., Ars. m., Cedr., Gels.*
  –to an enormous size, head were—*Bov.*
  –head were greatly—*Aran.*
  –head, face and hands were swollen, < washing—*Æth.*
  –head above eyes were—*Tub.*
  –and heavy on crown of head—*All. c.*
  –bones of head were—*Ant. c., Cedr.*
  –back of head were—*Crat. ox.*
  –brain were (in fever)—*Pop.*
  –skin of forehead were—*Stann.*
  –scalp were—*Coc. c.*
Sword were jagging in and out—*Carb. ac.*
Swung backward and forward, head were—*Pall.*
Taken off by flashes of throb-like pain, top of head would be—*Xanth.*
  –by straining at stool, head would be—*Ind.*
Tape around head—*Gels., Graph., Iod., Nit. ac., Plat., Sulph.*
  –head were constricted by—*Gels., Nit. ac., Sulph.*
  –drawn tightly from ear to ear—*Anac.*
Tea, brain were excited after—*Hyper.*
Tear head asunder, sticking in vertex would—*Nit. ac.*
Tearing around in brain—*Thuj.*
  –brain to pieces, cats were—*Ars.*
Teeming with live things whirling around it, head were—*Sil.*
Tense and pushing skull open, membranes were—*Meny.*
  –membrane of brain were—*Par.*
  –scalp were—*Thuj.*
Tension in head and large cords were drawn to each other, there were three points of—*Med.*
Thick as natural, head were twice as—*Nux m.*
  –head were—*Ail., Clem., Colch., Nat. m., Nicc., Petr., Ran. s., Thea*
  –head were too—*Daph. o.*
  –it were a strange head, head were so—*Ther.*
  –in forehead—*Calc. c., Mag. s., Ruta, Spong.*
  –heavy atmosphere, one were staying in a room with—*Agn.*

Thick—*Continued*

—feeling extending from right frontal eminence to right side of vertex—*Sac. lac.*

—and could not be wrinkled, skin in occiput were—*Par.*

Thin, frontal bones were too—*Puls.*

—head were a bushel and walls were too—*Par.*

—skull were quite—*Bell., Par.*

Thread were drawn tightly through eyes to middle of head—*Par.*

—had been drawn from middle of forehead to occiput—*Saba.*

Threads were being drawn through head and trunk—*Meph.*

—deep within head extended to ears—*All. c.*

Throb-like pain, top of head would be taken off by flashes of—*Xanth.*

Throbbing internally and externally would burst head—*Sil.*

—a vein in head were too full and—*Ferr.*

—deep in, brain would push through top of head from—*Parth.*

—in arteries of brain—*Hyos.*

—in cerebellum from hammer—*Camph.*

—would come out at forehead—*Zinc. ac.*

—in vertex—*Ferr.*

Thrust from right eyebrow to lower part of occiput, iron rod or bolt were—*Syph.*

—quickly by increasingly severe blows into head, plug were—*Sul. ac.*

—through head from left to right, a large stick were—*Apis*

—into right side of head, nail were—*Agar., Lycpr.*

—through brain to forehead, something were—*Saba.*

—into brow, knives were being—*Lach.*

—in right temple, gimlet were—*Puls.*

—in temples, pointed irons were—*Anan.*

—into temple, nail were—*Arn.*

—from temple to temple, some sharp instrument were—*Asc. c.*

—from side to side in head, a sharp knife were—*Arg. m.*

—from occiput to forehead, knife were—*Gels.*

—into occiput, stitches were—*Stront.*

Thrusts from behind forward in occiput—*Coloc.*

Thumb in small spot on forehead, someone touched him with cold—*Arn.*

Thumbs, temples were pressed in by—*Bapt.*

—were pressing in vertex, temples and eyes—*Nit. ac.*

Ticking in forehead, clock were—*Mag. s.*
  –in temples, watch were—*Chel.*
  –in vertex, watch were—*Graph.*
Tickling in right forehead, something were—*Brom.*
Tied up, head were—*Colch., Pimp.*
  –with a band, head were—*Dios., Merc.*
  –around head above ears pressing, band were—*Am. br., Gels*
  –about head, handkerchief were—*Carb. v.*
  –tightly around forehead, band were—*Sulph.*
  –together close to occiput, parts were—*Plat.*
Tight, head were too—*Kali c.*
  –on head, skin were too—*Sulph.*
  –band surrounded head—*Xanth.*
  –iron hoop around head—*Tub.*
  –cord, head were bound by—*Cocc., Merc. i. r.*
  –large cover over head were drawn very—*Helod.*
  –around head and forehead, band of hat were too—*Sars.*
  –rubber cap on head—*Stel.*
  –brain were too—*Kali br.*
  –over brain and occiput, dura mater were drawn—*Par.*
  –in brain just beneath scalp, it were heavy and—*Merc.*
  –skin of forehead were too—*Anag., Equis., Med., Phos.*
  –to forehead, skin had grown—*Sabi.*
  –cord in frontal region, bound by—*Merc. i. f., Tub.*
  –hat pressed forehead—*Alumn.*
  –cap were pressed down as far as temples—*Phys.*
  –over vertex, scalp were—*Tarax.*
  –hair on occiput were too—*Lach.*
  –over occiput, scalp were—*Hell.*
  –left occiput were held (in confusion)—*Crot. t.*
  –scalp were drawn—*Arg. n.*
  –scalp were too—*Arg. n., Brach., Merc., Stict., Stront.*
  –over skull, scalp were drawn—*Helod.*
Tightened to cut head in two, cord were frequently drawn and—*Mosch.*
  –about head, ring were—*Spire.*
  –around forehead, rubber band were—*Samars.*
  –up and remained so, scalp were wrinkled up and—*Zinc.*
Tightening in head, something were—*Med.*
  –in brain, something were—*Sabal*

Tighter and tighter, rope around head were drawn—*Nat. m.*
　　–and tighter, iron band around head just above ears and growing—*Berb. a.*
　　–and tighter by an iron ring, head were being squeezed—*Tub.*
　　–and smaller, head were—*Grat.*
Tightly, brain were wound up—*Morph.*
　　–compressed, head were—*Cocc.*
　　–bound, head were—*Colch., Nit. ac., Spig., Verat. v.*
　　–about forehead, strap were drawn—*Carb. v.*
　　–bound, temples were too—*Plat.*
　　–from ear to ear tape were drawn—*Anac.*
　　–bound to occiput, something hard were—*Phys.*
　　–stretched over skull, skin of forehead were—*Cann. i.*
　　–over skull, something were drawn down—*Arg. n.*
Tingling from pins and needles in forehead—*Stram.*
Tired and gone to sleep, brain were—*Apis*
Tore loose in brain when coughing, something—*Sep.*
Torn asunder, head were—*Sil.*
　　–asunder, head would be—*Cupr.*
　　–after vertigo, head were—*Plat.*
　　–on coughing or moving, head were—*Cur.*
　　–and bruised on coughing, head were—*Sulph.*
　　–off when sneezing, head would be—*Bell.*
　　–to pieces, head would be—*Chin. s., Lil. t.*
　　–brain were—*Am. m., Canth., Coff., Con., Ferr., Mur. ac., Rhus t., Staph., Verat. a.*
　　–brain were being—*Op.*
　　–or crushed, brain were—*Coff.*
　　–in morning, brain in vertex were—*Caust.*
　　–to pieces, brain were—*Am. m., Ars., Mur. ac., Puls., Staph.*
　　–to pieces, brain would be—*Hyper.*
　　–in left side of brain, a nerve were being—*Arg. m.*
　　–out with fine instruments, nerves on right side of forehead and temple were being—*Spig.*
　　–asunder, forehead would be—*Sil.*
　　–out, forehead would be—*Hep.*
　　–to pieces, forehead were—*Puls.*
　　–asunder, temples would be—*Puls.*
　　–from head, pieces of parietal bone were—*Ant. t.*
　　–out, mastoid process would be—*Canth.*
　　–asunder, skull had been—*Carb. an.*

Torn—*Continued*
  —open, skull would be—*Sulph.*
  —open, sutures of skull were being—*Bell.*
  —out, hair would be—*Sulph.*
  —out on vertex, hair would be—*Sol. t. æ., Sulph.*
Tornado in head—*Carb. an.*
Torpor in vertex—*Arist. m.*
  —awful, in brain—*Senec. j.*
Touch, skin of vertex were suppurating on—*Paraf.*
Touched or pierced head, sharp points of ice or ice-cold needles
      —*Agar.*
  —suppurating on head only when—*Graph.*
  —hole were in head and brain were—*Stram.*
  —by an icy cold hand on forehead—*Hyper.*
  —him with cold thumb in small spot on forehead, someone—
      Arn.
Transfixed with lance, head were—*Op.*
Transparent, skull were—*Bell.*
Trickling from forehead to back of head, blood were—*Lac. ac.*
Tube went through head from one ear to other—*Med.*
Tumble about on rising, head would—*Bar. c.*
Tumor were pressing within skull—*Helod.*
Turned around in head, something—*Anan.*
  —wrong side out on raising up, head would be—*Bar. c.*
  —around when walking, something in head—*Rhus t.*
Turning around, brain were—*Bry.*
  —in a circle, anterior half of brain were—*Bism.*
  —and twisting toward forehead, something were loose in head
      and—*Kali c.*
  —around in forehead, something were—*Æth., Merc., Mosch.*
  —around, occiput were—*Iber.*
Twisted, brain were clasped by a hand and were being—*Mur. ac.*
  —about in head, everything were alive and—*Sil.*
Twisting toward forehead, something were loose in head and
      turning and—*Kali c.*
  —in forehead, something were—*Nicc.*
  —in vertex—*Bell., Merl.*
Two heads, he has—*Mosch.*
Twitched toward forehead, scalp of occiput—*Aml. n.*
Ulcer in brain—*Nux v.*

Ulcerated, head were—*Eupi.*
   –in vertex—*Spig.*
   –occiput were hollow and—*Sep.*
   –scalp were—*Kali i.*
   –roots of hair were—*Chel.*
Ulceration, subcutaneous, of scalp—*Sul. ac.*
Uncovered, upper part of head were opened and—*Arum t.*
Undulating in head—*Sol*
   –in whole head—*Indg.*
   –in brain—*Hyos.*
   –frontal part of head were—*Cocc.*
Upward and outward, blood in head were coursing—*Ox. ac.*
Up and down, brain went—*Cob.*
Vacillating to and fro, brain were—*Lyc.*
Vapor ascended from throat through head—*Aml. n.*
   –were going through head on swallowing—*Form.*
   –ascended from occiput—*Atham.*
Vermin, scalp were full of—*Lyc.*
   –on scalp—*Arg. n.*
Vessels in head were pulsating—*Nux m.*
Vibration in forehead, there were—*Merc.*
Vise, head were in a—*Æth., Alum., Arg. n., Bry., Cocc., Merc.*
     Nat. m., Op., Parth., Puls., Ran. s., Rat.
   –around head—*Cinnb.*
   –front of head were in—*Alet.*
   –head were compressed in a—*Bar. c., Cact., Rat., Zinc. s.*
   –contents of head were in a—*Alum.*
   –head were held in a—*Coca*
   –head were seized in—*Cocc.*
   –head were squeezed in a—*Sars., Sul. i.*
   –base of brain were crushed in a—*Nat. s.*
   –forehead were in a—*Puls.*
   –temples were in a—*Daph., Dios., Nux m., Plb.*
   –from ear to ear over vertex, head were in—*Nit. ac.*
   –occiput were held in a—*Coca*
   –vertex were screwed in a—*Daph., Daph. o.*
Walking inside of head in a circle, something alive were—*Crot. c.*
   –backward when walking forward (felt in head)—*Sil.*
Wall, top of head were pressed against—*Sulph.*
Wanted to get out of skull, brain moved and—*Prim.*

Watch were ticking in temples—*Chel.*
  –were ticking in vertex—*Graph.*
Water during headache, head were wrapped in warm—*All. c.*
  –were drawn tightly over head, cap filled with—*Phys.*
  –in head—*Anan., Plat., Samb.*
  –warm, in head—*Am. c., Peti., Sant.*
  –head were full of boiling—*Rob.*
  –were dropping on head, drops of cold—*Cann. s.*
  –dropping in cranium—*Chin. s.*
  –head were filled with—*Samb.*
  –gushing forward in head on stooping—*Ars. m.*
  –in head, humming of boiling—*Bar. c.*
  –cold, were poured on head—*Cupr., Saba.*
  –were poured on head, a large quantity of—*Tarent.*
  –splashing in head, water were—*Sol. t. æ.*
  –splashing in left hemisphere on walking—*Carb. ac.*
  –were swashing in head—*Hyos.*
  –swashing, head were full of—*Acon., Asaf., Bell., Hep., Hyos., Samb.*
  –swashing and running to side as if in a large wash basin; no pain; (always came on when taking Hood's Sarsaparilla)
  –trickling down left brain, cold—*Kali c.*
  –were undulating in head—*Samb.*
  –boiling, whizzing in side of head on which he lies—*Mag. m.*
  –brain were agitated with boiling—*Acon.*
  –were falling on brain, drops of—*Cann. s.*
  –brain were moved by boiling—*Acon.*
  –hot, on scalp penetrating brain—*Peti.*
  –pipes bursting in brain—*Sil.*
  –wobbling in brain—*Hep.*
  –in forehead—*Plat.*
  –cold, were poured over forehead—*Tarent.*
  –(not cool) running down temple, a drop of—*Verat. a.*
  –had fallen on right frontal bone, drop of cold—*Croc.*
  –gurgling behind upper portion of frontal bones—*Asaf.*
  –warm, were pouring down inside of forehead—*Glon.*
  –had fallen on left parietal bone, a drop of cold—*Croc.*
  –were in vertex—*Daph. o.*
  –cold, on vertex—*Tarent.*
  –from occiput over vertex to forehead, waves of—*Sil.*
  –boiling, were rushing in occiput—*Indg., Pimp.*

Water—*Continued*
   –hot, were running upward from nape of neck—*Glon.*
   –beating on skull, waves of—*Dig.*
   –had been injected into sinuses—*Lach.*
Wave were beating on right side of head—*Zinc.*
   –from occiput to sinciput—*Senec.*
Waves with hunger, brain moved in—*Sep.*
   –to brain, something moved in—*Glon.*
   –against skull, brain were beating in—*Chin., Glon.*
   –of pain rolling up and beating against frontal bone—*Sep.*
   –of water from occiput over vertex to forehead—*Sil.*
   –from right to left side of occiput—*Zinc.*
   –of water were beating on skull—*Dig.*
Weak to support head, muscles were too—*Crot. h.*
Weariness at junction of atlas and head on arising in morning—*Maland.*
Wedge from outside, head were split open with—*Lachn.*
   –in head, every beat of heart were striking—*Calc. ar.*
   –of wood or ball were in forehead—*Staph.*
   –were driven into temple—*Thuj.*
   –would be pressed into occiput—*Bov.*
   –pushed from occiput to forehead at each respiration—*Pall.*
Weep with sudden headache, patient were going to—*Ferr. ma.*
Weight in head, there were no—*Trom.*
   –heavy, were in head—*Arn., Mosch., Phos. ac., Ran. g., Sars.*
   –moved to and fro in head on raising it—*Op.*
   –head were pressed down with—*Merl.*
   –pressing on head from above downward—*Phos. ac.*
   –heavy, were pressing head down on pillow—*Merc. i. f.*
   –whole contents of head had greatly diminished in—*Momor.*
   –on top of head—*Amyg., Laur., Mag. p. Arct., Phel.*
   –a hundred, were pressing brain forward—*Olnd.*
   –were lying on brain—*Pall., Sulph.*
   –pressed upon brain at every step—*Meny.*
   –were pressing brain inward—*Thuj.*
   –above eyes—*Cist.*
   –fell toward forehead when leaning forward—*Paraf.*
   –fell forward into forehead dragging head down on stooping *Rhus t.*
   –were sinking transversely across frontal eminence—*Thuj.*
   –in forehead were falling out—*Chel.*

Weight—*Continued*

--in head from too much blood—*Sep.*

--on head, a heavy—*Prim.*

--on vertex pressing brain—*Peti.*

--on vertex—*Cact., Med., Naja, Sulph.*

--great, on vertex—*Med., Zinc.*

--heavy, were lying on vertex—*Plat.*

--tremendous, falling on vertex—*Bry., Sil.*

--in occiput would draw head backward and neck had not
    enough strength to prevent it—*Alet.*

--of an iron band from ear to ear through occiput—*Ferr.*

--in occiput—*Bell., Carb. v., Luna, Sil., Sulph., Syph.*

--heavy, were pulling at occipital region—*Oxyt.*

--on nape of neck, head would be drawn backward by—*Phel.*

--in occiput, head were pulled back by a—*Syph.*

--jolting in occiput at every step—*Bell.*

Whirled from chest to brain, something—*Cact.*

--round and round, brain—*Saba.*

Whirling in head like a millwheel—*Chin. s.*

--around it, head were teeming with live things—*Sil.*

Whirring in head—*Lact., Puls.*

Whizzing in head and sounds as in an empty barrel—*Pimp.*

Widened, head were—*Aloe*

Wind during headache, head were in a hot—*Puls.*

--in head—*Alco., Petr., Puls., Verat. a.*

--in head extending to abdomen—*Aloe*

--cold, blowing on head—*Laur., Meny., Petr.*

--from chest to head, stream of—*Mill.*

--passed through it, head were open and—*Sanic.*

--blowing through head on shaking it—*Cor. r.*

--cold, blowing through head—*Nat. m., Verat. a.*

--through brain, a sharp—*Puls.*

--cold, in forehead from—*Phos. ac.*

--cold in right frontal eminence were from—*Arg. n.*

--cutting, from behind caused coldness in occiput—*Pimp.*

--sharp, penetrated left occiput—*Sabin.*

Wobbled and struck against side of head, brain—*Nux m.*

--when walking, brain—*Cyc.*

Wobbling of water in brain—*Hep.*

Wood, head were made of—*Petr.*

    --lying across back of head, piece of—*Psor.*

Wood—*Continued*

 —and could not think, back of brain were made of—*Staph.*

 —or ball were in forehead, wedge of—*Staph.*

Working in top of head and screwing from behind forward, something were—*Plb.*

Worm were crawling through forehead—*Sulph.*

Wound up tightly, brain were—*Morph.*

 —pain in head were caused by a—*Mag. p. Ambo*

 —on parietal bone, there were—*Kali ar.*

 —were pressed near occiput—*Saba.*

Wounded or bruised, hair were—*Sulph.*

Wrapped up in warm water during headache, head were—*All. c.*

 —in fog, brain were—*Petr.*

Wrinkle his forehead, he must—*Viol. o.*

Wrinkled up and kept tightening, scalp were—*Zinc.*

Writhing above eyes, something were—*Lach.*

Wrong in head, something were—*Epiph.*

EYES AND VISION

Abscess would form in right eye—*Anan.*
Acid were biting in eyes—*Graph., Rhus t.*
  —fumes in eye—*Sang.*
Adhered to lids, eyes had—*Zinc.*
Affected, eyes were being—*Irid.*
Agglutinated, eyelid were—*Caust., Plat.*
Air, eyelids were distended with—*Ars.*
  —cold, blew in left eye—*Croc.*
  —were blowing on eyes, stream of cold—*Mez.*
  —were blowing out through eyes when uncovered, cold stream of—*Thuj.*
  —cold, blew under lids—*Fl. ac.*
  —cold, blowing on exposed eyes, lids were wide open and—*Syph.*
  —cold, blowing on right eye, lids were open and—*Sulph.*
  —cold, were rushing through eyes—*Croc.*
  —cool, blowing on left eye—*Mag. p. Arct.*
  —hot, streamed out of eyes—*Kreos.*
  —hot, streamed out of eyes, passing over face—*Dios.*
Albumen, eyes were covered with—*Verat. a.*
Animals and birds, smoke were in form of—*Ammc.*
  —moving in cup—*Hyos.*
  —black, before vision on lying down to sleep—*Nat. a.*
Appear a long way off, objects—*Anac.*
  —larger than normal, objects—*Laur.*
Approach and recede, objects—*Cic.*
Attached to posterior parts of eyes, weights were—*Sep.*
Back into head, eyes extended—*Lac f.*
Ball of fire, eyes were—*Merc., Ruta, Sep.*
  —hard, were moving around when moving eye—*Rhus t.*
Balls floating before eyes—*Kali c.*
  —before eyes, two large black—*Cund.*
  —of fire rolling about—*Stram.*
  —luminous, before vision—*Cyc.*
Band around eyeball—*Laur.*
  —narrow, drawn tightly across eyeball—*Lac d.*

103

Bandage, white, obscured vision—*Lepi.*

Bars, vertical and of various colors, moving with eyes—*Stram.*

Bathed in hot water, right eye were—*Am. br.*

Bathing eyes, hot tears were—*Cor. r.*

Beaten, eyes were—*Tarax.*

–in right canthus—*Verat. a.*

–eyeballs were (renewed if talking about it)—*Calc. p.*

Bifurcated bodies before eyes—*Carl.*

Big for orbits, eyeballs were too—*Chin. m.*

Bird, little, were flying from left to right when reading—*Calc. p.*

Birds and animals, smoke were in form of—*Ammc.*

Biting in eyes, acid were—*Graph., Rhus t.*

–in eyes, something corrosive were—*Phel.*

–in eyes, dust were—*Ambr.*

–in eyes, horseradish were—*Merc., Phyt.*

–in eyes, foreign substance were—*Rheum*

–in eyes, salt were—*Caust., Chin., Rhus t.*

–in eyes as from rubbing with woolen cloth—*Stann.*

–in eyes, soap were—*Alum.*

–in eyes, smoke were—*Croc., Mosch., Petr.*

–in left eye, sweat were—*Viol. t.*

–in eye as from being in wind—*Merc.*

Black—*Acon., Agar., Ambr., Am. m., Anac., Arn., Ars., Asaf., Bell., Calc. c., Carb. v., Caust., Cham., Chin., Cic., Cocc., Con., Cupr., Dig., Dros., Euphr., Ferr., Hep., Kali c., Laur., Lyc., Mag. c., Mang., Meny., Merc., Mosch., Mur. ac., Nat. c., Nat. m., Nit. ac., Nux v., Olnd., Op., Petr., Phos., Phos. ac., Plb., Ruta, Saba., Sec., Sep., Sil., Squill., Staph., Stram., Sulph., Thuj., Verat. a., Verb.*

–animals before vision on lying down—*Nat. a.*

–balls before right eye—*Cund.*

–balls floating before eyes—*Kali c.*

–bug below doorknob—*Atro.*

–disk before left eye when walking—*Elaps*

–dots filled visual field—*Tab.*

–figures—*Petr.*

–flickerings—*Lach.*

–flies floating before eyes—*Sulph.*

–two black horns with large black balls on upper ends and a mound of crystals between them, their tops tapering off and tipped with—*Cund.*

Black—*Continued*

  –lightnings—*Staph.*

  –objects—*Sol. n.*, *Stram.*

  –objects which turn as one turns—*Cocc.*

  –plate—*Kali bi.*

  –point before right eye—*Elect.*

  –points before eyes—*Bell.*, *Calc. c.*, *Carb. an.*, *Cic.*, *Con.*, *Der.*, *Elaps*, *Jatr.*, *Kali c.*, *Merc.*, *Mez.*, *Mosch.*, *Nux v.*, *Sol. n.*, *Tab.*, *Thuj.*

  –points, letters change to—*Calc. p.*

  –points flickering before eyes—*Coca*

  –points floating before eyes—*Chin.*, *Chlf.*, *Cop.*, *Daph.*, *Gins.*, *Led.*, *Phos.*, *Ter.*

  –points move downward—*Merc.*

  –rings—*Dig.*, *Dign.*, *Nit. s. d.*, *Sol. n.*

  –rings float before eyes—*Dign.*

  –serpents jumping before eyes—*Cund.*

  –sparks before eyes—*Stry.*

  –spots—*Asc. t.*, *Bar. c.*, *Calc. c.*, *Camph.*, *Chlf.*, *Cimic.*, *Cupr. ar.*, *Dulc.*, *Elaps*, *Hell.*, *Lyc.*, *Nit. ac.*, *Nit. s. d.*, *Petr.*, *Scroph.*, *Sep.*, *Stram.*, *Tab.*, *Verat. a.*

  –spots floating—*Acon.*, *Agar.*, *Alco.*, *Am. c.*, *Ant. t.*, *Asaf.*, *Bell.*, *Calc. c.*, *Carb. v.*, *Carl.*, *Chlol.*, *Cob.*, *Coff. t.*, *Dign.*, *Hyos.*, *Itu*, *Kiss.*, *Lact.*, *Lil. t.*, *Lyc.*, *Macrot.*, *Mez.*, *Morph.*, *Nit. s. d.*, *Phos.*, *Phys.*, *Sil.*, *Sol. n.*, *Stram.*, *Tab.*, *Thuj.*

  –spots floating when eyes are closed—*Elaps*

  –spots moving with eyes—*Chin. s.*

  –stripes—*Bell.*, *Con.*, *Phos. ac.*, *Sol. n.*

  –tadpoles floating in a mist—*Sep.*

  –woolen thread floating before left eye—*Thuj.*

  –veil before eyes—*Aur.*, *Paraf.*, *Phos.*

Blew in eyes, cold air—*Croc.*

  –under lids, cold air—*Fl. ac.*

  –out of socket, eyes were gone and cold wind—*Sulph.*

  –out of socket, eyes were gone and cool wind—*Sep.*

  –in eyes, hot air—*Dios.*

Blood in eyes, there were too much—*Mill.*

  –would burst out of forehead or eyes—*Lac. ac.*, *Meïi.*

  –ran into eyes upon stooping, all—*Ferr. p.*

  –went to right inner canthus and could go no farther—*Syph.*

  –globules passing with every beat of pulse, he saw—*Glon.*

Blow on eyes—*Sulph.*
  –on right eye, he had been struck a—*Agn.*
  –pain in eyeballs were from a—*Urt. u.*
Blowing across eyes, cold wind were—*Berb., Croc.*
  –on eye, stream of cold air were—*Mez.*
  –under eyelids, cold wind were—*Fl. ac.*
  –on left eye, cool air were—*Mag. p. Arct.*
  –on right eye, lids were open and cold air were—*Sulph.*
  –into sore eyes from ears, cold wind were—*Alum.*
  –in eyes, cold wind were—*Med., Paraf., Syph.*
  –on exposed eyes, lids were wide open and cold air were—*Syph.*
  –in them, eyes were opened by force and fresh wind were—
    Fl. ac.
  –out of eyes, cold stream of air were—*Thuj.*
Blown in eye suddenly, something had been—*Homar.*
Blue—*Acon., Act. sp., Am. br., Bell., Crot. c., Cyc., Dig., Hipp.
    Kreos., Lach., Lyc., Stram., Stront., Sulph., Tril., Zinc.*
  –when eyes are closed—*Thuj.*
  –circles—*Zinc.*
  –circles around light—*Lach.*
  –sparks—*Ars.*
  –spots—*Acon., Hipp., Kali c., Thuj., Stram.*
Blur before eyes—*Crot. c., Lac v., Nux v.*
  –before left eye—*Cund.*
  –before eyes suddenly—*Podo.*
Blurred, eyes were—*Fago.*
  –from winking mucus over pupils—*Pic. ac.*
Body, foreign, in eye—*Bor., Calc. c., Calc. p., Calc. s., Caps.,
    Carl., Cinnb., Cist., Dios., Dros., Gels., Hyos., Kali bi.,
    Lach., Meph., Nat. m., Par., Phos., Puls., Sulph., Sumb.,
    Thuj., Upas*
  –foreign, in eye, caused aching—*Caps., Carl., Lyc.*
  –foreign, in eyes (burning)—*Chel.*
  –foreign, in left eye—*Apis, Am. m., Stram.*
  –foreign, in right eye—*Bov., Sulph.*
  –foreign, between lid and ball—*Coc. c.*
  –foreign, in left eye between lid and ball—*Ammc.*
  –foreign, under lids—*Caul., Coc. c., Merc., Plb., Psor., Upas*
  –foreign, under right upper lid—*Lob. s., Paraf.*
  –foreign, in rim of canthus—*Berb.*
  –foreign, in right outer canthus—*Sul. ac.*

Body—*Continued*
 --foreign, near outer canthus when closing eyes—*Sulph.*
 --foreign, in conjunctiva—*Tab.*
 --foreign, caused pain in eyes—*Nat. m.*
 --foreign, scraping in left eye—*Lycps.*
 --rose before left eye impeding sight—*Am. m.*
 --hard, were between upper lid and eyeball—*Viol. t.*
 --hard, behind right eyelid—*Stann.*
 --sharp, were cutting under lids—*Merc.*
Boil would form on eyebrow—*Kali c.*
Bound, eyes were—*Lith.*
 --by a cloth, eyes were tightly—*Puls.*
 --with strings which held them together and snapped when
     opened, lids were—*Cob.*
Bows, bright—*Con.*
Brain would start out through eyes—*Acon.*
Breadcrumbs in eyes—*Hura*
Breaking glass on opening lids—*Meph.*
Breathed upon cornea so as to dim its luster—*Plb.*
Breeze in eyes when in house—*Cinnb.*
Bright—*Calc. c., Camph., Carb. an., Chin. s., Chel., Cic., Con.,
     Eug., Hyos., Mill., Phys., Sol. n., Stry.*
 --and glittering, all objects were too—*Camph.*
 --circles—*Ammc., Camph., Carb. v., Fl. ac., Tax.*
 --colors—*Kali c.*
 --glow around letters—*Atro.*
 --spots—*Acon., Atro., Chlf., Cic., Con., Dign., Hell., Jatr.,
     Stram., Thuj.*
 --stripes—*Chlf., Cic.*
Bristle of hairbrush stuck in eyes—*Agar.*
Brown spot before left eye—*Agar.*
 --worm on brown carpet—*Atro.*
Bruise over eye, he had received a—*Nux v.*
Bruised, eyes were—*Lyc., Nat. p., Sep., Rhus t.*
 -in right eye—*Iodof.*
 --eyebrow were—*Plan.*
Bubble were bursting in eyes—*Puls.*
Bubbling in eyes—*Berb.*
 -in margins of lids—*Berb.*
Bug, black, below black door-knob—*Atro.*
Bulging, right eye were—*X-ray*

Bullets, eyes were two cold—*Stry.*
Burned, eyelids were—*Merc. c.*
Burning in eyes, a foreign body were—*Chel.*
   –horseradish were—*Merc.*
   –ring around each eye—*Chlol.*
   –sand were—*Psor., Ter.*
   –smoke were—*Æth., Nat. a.*
Burst, eyes would—*Nux v., Prun., Stach.*
   –eyeballs would—*Staph., Sulph.*
   –from pressure, eyeballs would—*Lycpr.*
   –out of forehead or eyes, blood would—*Lac. ac., Meli.*
Bursting, eyeballs were—*Samars.*
   –in eyes—*Daph., Lac. ac., Juni., Stram.*
   –from their sockets, eyes were—*Juni.*
   –in eyes, bubble were—*Puls.*
Chalk, middle of wood were marked with—*Ign.*
Cinders, sharp, in left eye—*Dulc.*
Ciphers before eyes—*Phos. ac.*
Circle, green, around light which on closing eyes turns red—*Verat. v.*
   –of colors when looking at light, a zigzag—*Sep.*
Circles—*Carb. v., Cyc., Dign., Hell., Kali c., Plb.*
   –colored—*Hyos.*
   –half, during headache—*Viol. o.*
   –quivering—*Carl.*
   –objects move in—*Cic., Hep.*
   –oval—*Ferr. ma.*
   –zigzag—*Ign., Sep.*
Clogged, eye were—*Stram.*
Close, eyes were about to—*Cyc.*
   –eyes would—*Sabin.*
   –eyes would not—*Phos.*
   –with heaviness, eyes would—*Plb.*
   –lids, unable to—*Meli., Par.*
Closed eye, something forcibly—*Cocc.*
   –too tightly, eyes had been—*Ambr.*
   –to protect eyes, lids must be—*Nat. a.*
Cloud before eyes—*Cahin., Corn., Corn. f., Ether., Euon., Lac d., Lachn.*
   –before left eye—*Tarent.*
   –over outer half of left eye—*Gels.*

Cloud—*Continued*
  —continually before left eye, in twilight—*Arg. n.*
  —dark, before eyes—*Coca*
  —upper part of field of vision were covered with a dark—*Dig.*
  —of dust before eyes—*Ammc.*
  —thick, before eyes—*Caust., Zinc.*
  —white, passed over eyes—*Sanic.*
Clouds floating before eyes—*Hydr. ac.*
  —moving up and down with vision—*Carl.*
  —were rising behind eyes—*Sabin.*
Clutched and pulled backward for a moment, eyes were—*Sanic.*
Coals of fire on lids—*Phyt.*
  —glowing, in small spots in eyes—*Caust.*
Cobwebs before eyes—*Agar., Lyc., Merl., Nit. ac., Tarent.*
Cold, eyes were—*Alumn., Con., Mez., Stry., Thuj.*
  —behind eye—*Calc. p.*
Colors, Illusions of, and **Color-Blindness,** see the GENERAL
    REPERTORIES
Colors, outlines of objects were shaded by—*Gels.*
Coming out, eyes were—*Acon.*
Commingled, all objects—*Camph.*
Compressed, eyeballs were—*Viol. o.*
  —in a vise, eyes were—*Rat.*
  —from all sides, eyeballs were—*Cham.*
Confusion and tumult, everything in street appears (when look-
    ing through window)—*Camph.*
Congested, left eye were—*Sarr.*
Constricted, eyes were—*Chlol.*
  —left upper lid were—*Gins.*
Contracted, eyeball were much—*Lycpr.*
  —in sockets, eyes were—*Verb.*
  —ciliary muscles were irregularly—*Phys.*
Contracting, right upper lid were—*Bor.*
Cord, eyes were drawing together by a—*Zinc.*
  —right eye were strung together with a—*Amph.*
Cords, eyes were being pushed out yet at same time held back
    by—*Fago.*
Corroded, eyelids were—*Hep.*
Corrosive were biting in eye—*Phel.*
Corrugated, eyebrow were—*Dirc.*
Coryza were beginning—*Jug. r., Naja, Nat. m., Ox. ac., Psor.*

Cotton in eyes—*Rad.*
Cover balls, eyelids would not—*Meli.*
 –he were looking through a gray—*Sil.*
Covered with a cobweb, eyes were—*Agar.*
 –with a dark body, half of object were—*Aur.*
 –by a dark cloud, upper part of field of vision were—*Dig.*
 –with a veil, eyes were—*Gent. c.*
 –with a film, eye were—*Sulph.*
 –with a bluish-gray film—*Bell.*
 –with much mucus, cornea were—*Euphr.*
 –with a gray veil, objects were—*Phos.*
 –with a thin veil, objects were—*Nat. m.*
Crawling in eyes, something were—*Nat. s.*
Creeping about ciliary region, something were—*Phys.*
Cried much, he had—*Eupi., Verat. v.*
Crooked, objects were—*Bell., Bufo*
Crossed, eyes were—*Bell., Calc. c., Con., Op., Puls.*
Crumbs in eyes- -*Hura*
Crushed, eyeballs were—*Aster., Prun.*
Crying hard, eyes were—*Kali p.*
 –she had been—*Nux m.*
 –a long time, he had been—*Pyrus*
Curled hair before right eye and a blur before left, causing
    letters to run together—*Cund.*
Curtain, dark, were slowly let down before eyes—*Ferr.*
Cut had been made around eye—*Crot. h.*
 –out of head, eyes would be—*Samb.*
Cutting in lower lid, something were—*Nux v.*
 –under lids, sharp body were pressing and—*Merc.*
 –around eyeball as if it were being taken out with a pen-knife—
    Crot. c.
Dance, objects were moving in a confused—*Olnd.*
 –objects seemed to totter and—*Sant.*
Danced before eyes, tadpoles—*Cimic.*
 –before eyes, bright stars—*Croc.*
Dancing before vision, objects were—*Glon., Sant.*
 –before vision, letters were—*Calc. c.*
Darting out of eyes when walking in sun, fire were—*Dulc.*
Dazzling before eyes, snow were—*Olnd.*
 –like lightning before eyes—*Nat. m.*
Dead, eyes were—*Cich.*

Deep in head, eyes were—*Elect.*
  –in head, eyes lay—*Zinc.*
  –in sockets, eyes were lying—*Gent. c.*
Denuded, margins of upper lid were—*Plat.*
Develop, a corneal ulcer might—*Plb.*
Difficult to move lids (stiffness)—*Rhus t.*
Dim—see also GENERAL REPERTORIES and special rubrics such
    as VEIL, VISION, OBSCURED, *etc.*
Dim, edges of objects were—*Bell.*
  –its luster, one breathed on cornea so as to—*Plb.*
Dimness of eyes as if tears were in them—*Ign.*
  –before eyes—*Doryph., Gels., Lac v., Morph., Viol. o.*
  –of vision were caused by film—*Aml. n.*
Displaced, focus of right eye were suddenly—*Glon.*
Distance, everything were at a great—*Magnol.*
Distant, objects were—*All. c., Anac., Atro., Bell., Calc. c., Merc.
    c., Nux m., Stram., Sulph.*
Distended, eyeballs were—*Calc. p.*
  –them, fluid pressed into eyeballs and—*Seneg.*
  –with air, eyeballs were—*Ars.*
Distorted, objects were—*Bell., Benz. n., Card. b., Dig., Morph.,
    Nux v.*
Divided horizontally, objects were—*Aur.*
Dolls, people were as small as—*Plb.*
Doorway were not wide enough—*Samars.*
Dots, black, filled visual field—*Tab.*
Double, objects were—*Atro., Eug., Camph., Phys.*
Draft of air, light flickers from a—*Hell. f.*
Dragged back into head by a string, both eyes were being—*Par.,
    Sil.*
Draw within themselves, eyes would—*Sep.*
Drawing into head, eyes were—*Ars.*
  –together by cord, eyes were—*Zinc.*
  –together in left upper lid—*Bry.*
Drawn tightly across eyeball, narrow band were—*Lac d.*
  –back, eyes were—*Aster., Bov., Graph., Hep., Lach., Mez., Plb.,
    Puls., Rhod., Sil., Sulph.*
  –tightly backward, eyeball were—*Cham.*
  –back a moment, eyeball were clutched and—*Sanic.*
  –from behind eye to eye, a thread were—*Lach.*
  –tightly through eyeball to middle of head, thread were—*Par.*

Drawn—*Continued*

–deep into head, eyes were—*Ars., Aur. m.*

–out, eyes were being—*Sil.*

–out of their sockets, eyes were—*Glon.*

–together from sleep, eyelids must be—*Viol. o.*

–upward causing him to wink, supraorbital muscles would be—
    Tus. p.

–together, eyes were—*Zinc.*

–toward temple, left eye were—*Crot. c.*

–backward and forward, left eye were—*Spig.*

–out, right eyeball were—*Crot. c.*

–back, eyes were suddenly stiffened and—*Stry.*

–before eyes, veil were—*Arum t.*

–down, right upper lid were—*Carb. an.*

–over eyes, skin were—*Apis*

–up and down through globe of left eye, a saw were—*Maland.*

Dried to ball, left lid were—*Cedr.*

Drill-point pressed downward in eyeball—*Ran. b.*

Drooping, upper lids were—*Alum., Bell., Dulc., Euph., Gins.,
    Nat. m., Op., Plb., Squill., Stram., Zinc.*

Dropping out, eyes were—*Acet. ac., Hell.*

–out during menses, eyes were—*Brom.*

Drowsiness, irresistible, in eyes—*Ferr. p., Upas*

Dry, eyes were—*Lyc.*

–and hot in eyes—*Cor. r.*

–internally, eyes were too—*Crot. h.*

–eyes were very—*Staph.*

–from long weeping, eyes were—*Nat. c.*

–lids were too—*Ign., Laur.*

–after reading, lids were—*Lith.*

–and sore, lids were—*Arn.*

–upper lid were too—*Ign.*

–edges of lids were—*Ars.*

–from inflammation, lids were—*Mez.*

–inner surfaces of lids were too—*Verat. a.*

Dryness in eyes—*Rumx., Sil.*

–in eyes, can move lids only with difficulty—*Nux m.*

Dull looking and weak, eyes were—*Rheum*

Dust in eyes—*Cocc., Dios., Lachn., Lyc., Op., Rhus t., Ruta,
    Sulph.*

–in right eye—*Lac f., Phos., Zinc.*

Dust—*Continued*
   –were biting in eyes—*Ambr.*
   –before eyes, waving cloud of—*Ammc.*
   –acrid, in eyes—*Aur.*
   –were tickling in eye—*Zinc.*
   –eyes were covered with a fine—*Sulph.*
   –cornea were covered with—*Hell.*
   –on cornea, vision perceived through—*Cocc.*
   –under lower lid—*Phos.*

Eclipse of sun were taking place—*Phys.*

Electric lights, eyes were long exposed to—*Oxyt.*
   –sparks flashing before eyes in daytime—*Croc.*

Elevation on bulb of eye, upper lid passed over an—*Symph.*

Elongated, lashes were—*Mez.*
   –objects were—*Atro., Zinc.*

Encircled by a cloud, objects were—*Camph.*

Enlarged, eyeballs were—*Cimic., Macrot., Pulx., Stram.*

Enveloped in a mist or halo, objects were—*Merc. c.*
   –in a yellow mist, objects were—*Kali bi.*
   –in smoke, eyes were—*Phos., Sulph.*

Excoriated, eyeballs were—*Arn.*

Exposed to electric lights, eyes were long—*Oxyt.*

Expanded, eyeballs were being—*Seneg.*

Expansion of eyes—*Acon., Agar., Ambr., Benz. n., Card. b., Chel., Chr. ac., Colch., Macrot., Nat. a., Nat. m., Onos., Par., Plb., Seneg., Stram., Tril.*

Extended back into head, eyes—*Lac f.*

Eyelash in eyes—*Dios.*

Fade if one used eye longer than a minute, objects—*Chlol.*
   –and reappear, objects would—*Gels.*

Fall out of head, eyes would—*All. c., Carb. an., Cham., Coloc., Glon., Ign., Lyc., Puls., Sep., Tril.*
   –out on stooping, eyes would—*Brom., Coloc.*
   –near objects seem to—*Hyos.*

Fallen in, eyes were—*Chin.*

Falling from a height and resting on eyes, stone were—*Cocaine*
   –straight down before eyes, snowflakes were—*Camph. br.*
   –over eyes, fringe were—*Con.*
   –on conjunctiva and burning it, snowflakes were—*Form.*

Far off, all objects were too—*Stann.*

Farther apart, objects were—*Carb. an.*

Fat were in eyes—*Calc. c., Paraf.*

Fatty matter under lids—*Vesp.*

Feathers before eyes—*Alum., Calc. c., Kreos., Mag. c., Nat. c., Sulph.*

  —on eyelashes—*Spig.*

  —came from corner of eye—*Merc.*

  —looking through—*Nat. m.*

  —sight were obscured with—*Lyc.*

Fell from sockets, eyes were too large and—*Tril.*

Fiery points burning lids—*Merc.*

  —stars passed before left eye—*Card. b.*

  —objects were—*Dig., Iod., Stram., Verat. a., Viol. o.*

  —body before eyes in dark—*Arg. n.*

  —circles—*Calc. p., Ip., Puls.*

  —half-circles—*Viol. o.*

  —flakes floating in circles—*Zinc.*

  —lines radiating outward—*Iod., Thea*

  —points—*Ammc., Coca, Elaps*

  —rays about light—*Lach.*

  —showers—*Plb.*

  —sparks—*Merc.*

  —stripes—*Card. b.*

  —wheels—*Camph., Spire.*

  —zigzags—*Con., Graph., Nat. m., Sep.*

Figure, black, floats before eyes—*Cocc.*

Figures, zigzag, before eyes—*Lach.*

  —from floor rise to her face—*Atro.*

  —hovering before eyes—*Tarent.*

Filled with dirty fluid, vessels of eye were—*Stram.*

  —with sharp salt, eyes were—*Nat. m.*

  —with smoke, eyes were—*Chin., Croc., Nat. a., Valer.*

Film before eyes—*Aml. n., Lact., Phys., Scroph.*

  —eyes were covered with a—*Sulph.*

  —eye were covered with a bluish-gray—*Bell.*

  —dimness of vision were caused by a—*Aml. n.*

  —he were looking through a—*Lac c.*

  —of mucus over eye—*Croc., Sang. n.*

Fingers before eyes, one were playing with his—*Psor.*

Fire, eyes were a ball of—*Merc., Ruta, Sep.*

  —came out of eyes—*Eug.*

  —coming out of eyes, sparks of—*Merc.*

Fire—*Continued*

—even when eyes are closed, looking into a sea of—*Phos.*

—were darting out of eyes when walking in sun—*Dulc.*

—when in dark night, eyes were a pillar of—*Staph.*

—were rolling about, balls of—*Stram.*

—before eyes as if he had been slapped in face (following dimness of vision) flashes of—*Puls.*

—rushing from stomach to eye, spark of—*Stram.*

—were streaming from eyes—*Clem.*

—were before eyes on closing them, wheels of—*Spira.*

—on lids, coals of—*Phyt.*

Firefly were hovering before eyes—*Thuj.*

Fistula would form, a lachrymal—*Puls.*

Flame before eyes—*Bell., Coca, Canth., Myric., Staph., Ther. Viol. o.*

Flames, everything were enveloped in—*Spong.*

Flashes—*Alco., Arg. n., Atro., Bell., Benz. n., Chlf., Dig., Dign., Iber., Ment., Op., Puls., Sec., Stram., Tab., Tarent.*

—sudden, like electric sparks, were before eyes—*Croc.*

—of fire before eyes as if he had been slapped in face (following dimness of vision)—*Puls.*

Flea-bites caused itching in eyes—*Myric.*

Flickering before eyes—*Chin. m., Cyc., Vinc.*

—as from threads or rays of sun before eyes—*Lach.*

Flickers from draft of air, light—*Hell. f.*

Flies were before eyes—*Cocc., Dig.*

—black, were floating before eyes—*Sulph.*

—little black, were before eyes—*Paraf.*

Flitted before eyes, shadow—*Ruta*

Floated before eyes, black objects like tadpoles in mist—*Sep.*

Floating in field of vision, red spot were—*Dub.*

—about, balls were—*Kali c.*

—before eyes obliging to wipe constantly, something were—*Kreos.*

—before eyes, objects were—*Camph., Dig., Hell., Kali c., Nux m., Petr.*

Floats before eyes, a black figure—*Cocc.*

Flow but they do not, tears would—*Spire.*

Flowing over right to left and from eyes, warm water—*Nit. ac.*

Fluid. vessels of eye were filled with dirty—*Stram.*

—pressed into eyeballs and distended them—*Seneg.*

Flutters, eyeball—*Dub.*

Fluttering before vision—*Carb. o., Petr., Sil., Thuj.*

Fly into pieces, eye would—*Spig.*

Flying from left to right when reading, a little bird were—*Calc. p.*

Focus of right eye were suddenly displaced—*Glon.*

Fog before eyes—*Aur., Bism., Camph., Carb. s., Coff. t., Cyc., Kali c., Lach., Lonic., Med., Merc., Morph., Sal. ac., Sil., Sulph., Vinc.*

–objects were seen through a—*Alum., Camph., Euphr., Ign., Lach., Lyc., Merc., Morph., Sars., Sol, Sulph., Tab., Verb., Vinc., Zinc.*

–or smoke before right eye—*Kali c.*

–before left eye—*Crot. t.*

–before eyes when closing them—*Bar. c.*

–before eyes on attempting to read—*Arn.*

–he were looking through a dense—*Cund.*

–gray, before eyes—*Sulph.*

–thick, before eyes—*Caust., Zinc.*

–eyes were wrapped in—*Petr.*

Force eyes out of sockets, swelling of eyes would—*Sol*

Forced forward, brain and eyes were—*Sil.*

–deep into eye, something pointed were being—*Fl. ac.*

–out, eyes were being—*Bell., Berb., Carb. v., Card. b., Caust., Iber., Ign., Laur., Led., Lyc., Mag. c., Phos. ac., Ran. b., Seneg., Thuj.*

–out of head, both eyes would be—*Hom.*

–out, eyeballs would be—*Led., Med., Merc. c., Stram.*

–out when throat is pressed, eyes would be—*Lach.*

–out, upper part of eyeball would be—*Acon.*

–out of eyes, blood were being—*Lac. ac.*

–open, lids were—*Fl. ac.*

Forehead, he must look out under—*Phos. ac.*

Form in right eye, abscess would—*Anan.*

–lachrymal fistula would—*Puls.*

Forming on inside of lid, pimples were—*Hura*

Forward, eyes were pushed—*Gymn.*

Fringe falling down over eyes—*Con.*

Full of sleep, eyes were—*Ferr., Staph.*

–of smoke, eyes had been—*Kali p.*

Full—*Continued*
  –of water, left eye were—*Sil.*
  –of water, eyes were—*Staph.*
Fumes of acid in eye—*Sang.*
Gauze before eyes—*Alum., Bar. c., Caust., Cina, Clem., Croc., Dulc., Gamb., Kali bi., Kreos., Nat. m., Nitro. o., Rhod., Rhus t., Stram., Sulph., Til.*
  –black, before eyes—*Sulph.*
  –before eyes in morning—*Bar. c.*
  –looking through a—*Calc. c., Caust., Cina, Dulc., Hydr. ac., Kreos., Lact., Lepi., Nat. m., Plb., Sang. n.*
  –looking through white—*Ars.*
  –pearly, before right eye—*Elaps*
  –spread over left eye—*Sars.*
Gazing at some distant object—*Lyss.*
Glare before right eye so she could hardly read—*Chel.*
Glass were in eye, piece of—*Rhus t.*
  –breaking on opening lids—*Meph.*
  –eyeball rubbed against spiculæ of—*Sulph.*
  –looking through a dark blue—*Cyc.*
Glasses, she had been looking through too strong—*Croc.*
Glimmering—*Aran. s., Bar. c., Bell., Calc. p., Cann. i., Gels., Kalm., Zing.*
  –before eyes—*Gels.*
Glistening bodies moved back and forth—*Ol. an.*
  –objects—*Kali c., Nux v., Dros.*
Glittering objects—*Calc. p., Camph., Chel., Con., Cyc., Ign., Nat. s.*
Globules were floating in air, endless strings of white—*Upas*
Glued up, outer canthus were—*Colch.*
  –together, eyelids were—*Lyss.*
Glutinous, right eye were—*Euph.*
  –on closing, lids were—*Merl.*
  –mass were lying between lid and ball—*Bell.*
Goiter and could not see over it, she had a large—*Zinc.*
Golden, everything were—*Acon., Atro., Bell., Hyos.*
Gnats, many, came before sight—*Tab.*
Gone into bright sunlight, she had—*Sep.*
  –and cool wind blew out of socket, eyes were—*Sep., Sulph.*
Grain of sand in eye—*Agar., Alum., Caust., Con., Ferr., Ign., Iod., Mag. m., Merc., Sars.*

Grain—*Continued*
 –of sand in right eye—*Sep., Zing.*
 –of sand on inner margin of lids—*Sel.*
 –of sand in upper lids—*Calc. c., Pæon.*
 –of sand under lids—*Calc. c.*
 –of sand in outer canthus of eye—*Con., Euphr.*
Grains, little, in eyes—*Lith.*
Granular, blood-vessels on inner side of lid were—*Nat. a.*
Granulated, edges of lids were—*Phyt.*
Gravel, first in left and then in right eye—*Med.*
Gray, objects were—*Arg. n., Brom., Calc. p., Card. b., Carl.,
  Chlf., Cic., Elaps, Guare., Gins., Lachn., Nit. ac., Nux v.,
  Phal., Phos., Sep., Sil., Stram.*
 –reddish-gray—*Stram.*
Green—*Cann. i., Canth., Carb. s., Cina, Cot., Cyc., Dig., Mag.
  m., Merc., Osm., Phos., Ruta, Sant., Sep., Sil., Stram., Stry.,
  Tab., Zinc.*
 –about light—*Verat. v.*
 –bluish-green about light—*Osm.*
 –pea-green about light—*Cann. i.*
 –halo about light—*Mag. m., Phos., Sep., Sil.*
 –spots—*Hipp., Kali c., Nit. ac., Stram., Stront.*
 –yellow-green—*Sant.*
Hair were in eyes—*Plan., Puls., Ran. b., Sang., Tab.*
 –in right eye—*Lappa a.*
 –in left eye—*Tarent.*
 –were under lids—*Coc. c.*
 –were between eyeballs and lids—*Coc. c.*
 –curled, in front of right eye—*Cund.*
 –hung over eyes—*Euphr.*
Hairs before eyes—*Dig.*
 –were on lashes—*Spig.*
Halo about light—*Alum., Anac., Bell., Calc. c., Cham., Coff. t.,
  Dign., Kali c., Nat. p., Nit. ac., Staph., Sulph., Tub.*
 –yellow before eyes even when closed—*Aml. n.*
 –green around light—*Caust.*
 –red and green about light—*Sil.*
 –variegated, around light—*Ferr. ma.*
 –objects were enveloped in—*Merc. c.*
Hammering in left eye—*Ham.*

Hanging down over eyes, skin were—*Ol. an.*
   –before eyes, obscuring sight, mucus that could not be wiped away were—*Puls.*
   –before eyes, threads were—*Seneg.*
   –by a string, eyes were torn or—*All. c.*
   –over eyes, veil were—*Hep.*
Hard and immovable, upper lids were—*Spig.*
   –as marble, eye were—*Cann. i.*
   –lids were—*Franc.*
   –substance behind right eyelid—*Stann.*
   –substance under right upper lid—*Spig.*
Haze of light, objects were in a yellow—*Sant.*
Heavy as lead, eyes were—*Par.*
   –eyelids were—*Daph. o.*
   –eyelids were too—*Sep.*
Held back by cords, eyes were being pushed out yet at same time—*Fago.*
Holding lids together and snapping when opening them, strings were—*Cob.*
Horns, two black, before eyes—*Cund.*
Horseradish in eyes—*Merc. sul., Phyt.*
   –he had been near someone scraping—*Iris t.*
Hot, eyeball were—*Nat. s.*
   –something in left eye were—*Lac d.*
Hung over eyes, hair—*Euphr.*
   –before eyes, something—*Cast.*
   –down over eyes, something—*Eupi.*
   –down preventing vision, skin of eyebrow—*Ol. an.*
Ice, eyeballs were—*Lyc.*
   –lay in orbit, lump of—*Mag. p. Arct.*
Illuminated, white objects were strongly—*Sant.*
   –objects were—*Hyos.*
Immovable, upper lids were hard and—*Spig.*
Impeding sight, a body rose before left eye—*Am. m.*
Inflamed, eyes were—*Chr. ac., Nat. m.*
   –lids would become—*Sulph.*
Inflammation would arise—*Saba.*
Insects, black floating—*Merc.*
Inverted, lines were—*Kali c.*
   –objects were—*Bell., Guare.*

Iron, even when eyes are closed, looking into a vessel of molten
—*Phos.*

—pierced through right eye with a piece of cold—*Til.*

Issue from forehead and eyes, everything would—*Sep.*

Jumping, objects were—*Bell., Meny., Plb.*

—out of his head, eyes were—*Gels.*

—in eyes—*Tarent.*

—before right eye, black serpents were—*Cund.*

Knife, cutting around eyeball as if it were being taken out with
a pen—*Crot. c.*

—were stabbing in ears and eyes—*Vib.*

—were thrust between ball and socket and turned about—*Chin.*

Knives, eyes were pierced with—*Chel.*

—were sticking in eyes—*Lach., Vib.*

—were sticking in right eyeball—*Coloc., Sulph.*

Lachrymation were present but is not—*Spig.*

—would set in—*Ars. i., Merc. i. f.*

Large, eyes were too—*Cean., Chlol., Com., Daph. o., Laur., Lyc.,
Nat. m., Mez., Phos., Phos. ac., Par., Phyt., Plb., Spig.*

—for orbit, eyes were too—*Carl., Daph. o., Op., Meli., Seneg.*

—on closing eyes, eyes were—*Am. br.*

—and fell from sockets, eyes were too—*Tril.*

—objects were—*Æth., Atro., Berb., Cann. i., Cann. s., Carb. s.,
Coniin., Dig., Hyos., Laur., Mand., Nicc., Nitro. o., Nux m.,
Op., Osm., Ox. ac., Phys., Staph., Verb.*

—smooth substance lying beneath left upper lid—*Staph.*

—smooth substance in eyes—*Dios.*

—for socket, eyeball were swollen too—*Spig.*

—upper lid would not cover it, left eyeball were so—*Chel.*

—everything were too—*Laur., Tub.*

—distant objects look—*Onos.*

—substance in eye—*Caust.*

—as natural, objects were twice as—*Berb.*

Larger than it is, everything appears—*Euph.*

—than usual, eyes were—*Com.*

—and more protruded than left, right eyeball were—*Com.*

—and starting from orbits, eyes were becoming—*Dign.*

Lashes in eyes—*Dios., Iod., Tarent.*

Lattice, one were looking through a fine—*Lyc.*

Lay deep in head, eyes—*Zinc.*
–in orbit, lump of ice—*Mag. p. Arct.*
–above eyes, something—*Carb. an.*
Lead, lids were of—*Nat. s.*
–eyebrows and lids were of—*Lac f.*
Leaf, white, before right eye—*Nat. s.*
Letters were written in red ink—*Phos.*
–expand and contract—*Atro.*
–placed irregularly on line—*Stram.*
Light were surrounded by halo—*Coff. t., Sulph., Tub.*
–were at end of room—*Oxyt.*
–pupil admitted too much—*Helon.*
–points—*Nat. m.*
–spots—*Con., Dig.*
–snakes or worms—*Phys.*
Lightning were dazzling before eyes—*Nat. m.*
Lightnings—*Brom., Cyc., Dig., Glon., Olnd., Nat. c., Sulph.*
–distant sheet—*Coca*
Lights before eyes—*Ammc., Calc. c., Chin. s., Dig., Fl. ac., Valer.*
Lilac—*Acon., Stram.*
Line or thread horizontally before right eye—*Con.*
Linen, one were looking through coarse—*Stram.*
Look at objects far away, she wanted to—*Onos.*
Looked too long and too intently at an object, one had—*Ruta*
–at sun a few minutes before, objects appear as if one had—
    Podo.
Looking through coarse linen, one were—*Stram.*
–through concave glasses, one were—*Mez.*
–down, he were—*Phos.*
–at sun, one had been—*Nit. ac.*
–through white bandage, he were—*Lepi.*
–through feathers—*Nat. m.*
–through film—*Lac c.*
–through a lace veil—*Xanth.*
–through a gauze—*Calc. c., Cina, Caust., Dulc., Hydr. ac.,
    Kreos., Lact., Lepi., Nat. m., Plb., Sang. n.*
–through glass when in open air—*Nat. m.*
–through clear water which produced prismatic colors, one
    were—*Oxyt.*
–through white gauze—*Ars.*
–through a dark blue glass—*Cyc.*

9

Looking—*Continued*
  –through a fine lattice, one were—*Lyc.*
  –too long and too intently at an object—*Ruta*
  –through too strong glasses, she had been—*Croc.*
  –through mist—see MIST
  –through rain—*Nat. m.*
  –through a sieve—*Puls.*
  –through a gray veil—*Phos.*
  –through a veil—*Cocc., Lyc., Verb.*
  –upon the ground, one were—*Verat. a.*
  –into a vessel of molten iron, even when eyes are closed—*Phos.*
Loose, eyes were lying in sockets—*Carb. an.*
  –in socket, left eyeball were too small and—*Croc.*
Lubricating so lid would not stick, eyeball wanted—*Sac. lac.*
Luminous—*Arund., Cann. i., Cyc., Dig., Nitro. o., Stram.,*
    Sulph., Thuj.
Lump in right outer canthus—*Sul. ac.*
  –of ice lay in orbit—*Mag. p. Arct.*
Lying deep in sockets, eyes were—*Gent. c.*
  –beneath left upper lid, large smooth substance were—*Staph.*
  –loose in sockets, eyes were—*Carb. an.*
  –between lid and ball, glutinous mass were—*Bell.*
Marble, eye were as hard as—*Cann. i.*
Mass of hypertrophied tissue, cornea were a—*Sil.*
Melting away, eye were—*Ham.*
Membrane extended across eye—*Daph.*
  –over eyes—*Caust.*
Mist before eyes—*Agar., Am. m., Aran., Arg. m., Bism., Calc.*
    ar., Cahin., Caust., Croc., Cyc., Dub., Ether., Form., Gels.,
    Glon., Graph., Grat., Kali m., Lact., Mill., Merl., Momor.,
    Myric., Paraf., Podo., Sulph., Thuj., Zinc.
  –before eyes in morning—*Merl.*
  –distant objects enveloped in a—*Phos. ac.*
  –before eyes but at a distance—*Mill.*
  –about light—*Sil.*
  –before eyes when looking keenly at objects—*Calc. c.*
  –before eyes in which black objects like tadpoles floated—*Sep.*
  –everything were enveloped in a—*Eupi., Phos.*
  –looking through a—*Ambr., Arn., Lact., Zinc.*
  –thick, before eyes—*Ammc.*

Mist—*Continued*

--white, before right eye—*Lac f.*

--objects were enveloped in—*Merc. c.*

--objects were enveloped in yellow—*Kali bi.*

Moist in eyes—*Paraf.*

Moisture, eye were dim from glutinous—*Lyc.*

Molten iron, even when eyes are closed, looking into vessel of—
Phos.

Motion, every object were in—*Sep.*

Mounted to eyes, something hot—*Spire.*

Move eyes, she could not—*Rat.*

--eyes, it were difficult to—*Seneg.*

--lids, it were difficult to—*Rhus t.*

--objects at a distance—*Spira.*

Moved involuntary, eye—*Calc. c.*

--in eyes, > rubbing, something—*Carb. an.*

--to and fro before eyes, something—*Lyss.*

--up and down, objects—*Cocc.*

Moves before eyes, everything—*Eug.*

Moving in eye, something were—*Caust.*

--about while lying on left side, right eye were—*Lac f.*

--in a confused dance, objects were—*Olnd.*

--in ball, something were—*Calc. p.*

--letters were—*Agar., Am. c., Merc., Phys.*

--around when moving eye, hard ball were—*Rhus t.*

--up and down, lines of print were—*Con.*

--objects were—*Carb. ac., Con., Euphr., Hydr. ac., Ign., Nitro.
o., Petr., Spire., Wies.*

--to and fro, objects were—*Cic., Elaps*

--before eyes, something were—*Lyss., Psor.*

Mucus over eye, a film of—*Croc., Sang. n.*

--were over eyes; must wink and wipe eyes—*Croc.*

--were in left eye—*Apis*

--that could be wiped away were hanging over eyes, obscuring
sight—*Puls.*

--cornea were covered with much—*Euphr.*

Multiplied, objects were—*Bell., Iod., Phys., Phyt., Stram.*

Muscles of eye inferior and internal were too short on looking
up—*Sabin.*

Nail in margin of orbit—*Ars., Hell.*

Nearer, objects were—*Phys., Rhus t.*
  —to each other, objects—*Nux m.*
Needle under lid, a prick of—*Paraf.*
  —lens had been punctured by a—*Sulph.*
  —were sticking in eye—*Sulph.*
  —stitched in eyebrow—*All. c.*
  —thrust into right eyeball—*Spig.*
  —red-hot, were stitching in right eye—*Rhod.*
  —points suddenly thrust into lid, a hundred—*Verat. a.*
Needles in eyes—*Meph.*
  —were run into eyeball through cornea—*Cimic.*
  —were sticking into eyes from washing in cold water—*Sac. lac.*
  —fine, sticking in right lower and left upper lids—*Zinc.*
  —stinging in eye—*Calc. c., Caust.*
  —were thrust into eyeball—*Spig.*
Net before eyes—*Chin. s., Hyos.*
  —were swimming before eyes—*Carb. an.*
Nose a shapeless mass, he sees his—*Coniin.*
Obscuration before eyes—*Sulph.*
Obscured, objects were—*Cact., Sil.*
  —cornea were—*Ang.*
  —with feathers, sight were—*Lyc.*
  —vision, something—*Sil.*
  —vision, white paper—*Bell.*
  —vision, white bandage—*Lepi.*
Obscuring sight, scales were before eyes—*Kali bi.*
Obstructed by thin secretion—*Fago.*
  —by something before axis—*Nat. c.*
Obstruction, pear-shaped, before eye with large end up, on
      waking in morning—*Cund.*
Occur, strabismus would—*Podo.*
Open, eyes were wide—*Onos., Fl. ac.*
  —enough, not—*Chin. m.*
  —than usual, lids were wider—*Fl. ac.*
  —and cold air were blowing on right eye, lids were—*Sulph.*
  —and cold air were blowing on exposed eyes, lids were wide—
      Syph.
  —eyes, he could not—*Par.*
  —eyelids again, he would not be able to—*Spig.*
  —eyes could not be kept—*Ars., Lachn.*
  —eyes wide and press on them, he wanted to—*Adren.*

Opened wider so field of vision becomes enlarged—*Fl. ac.*

  –by force and fresh wind were blowing in them, eyes were—*Fl. ac.*

Oppressed with sleep, eyes were—*Stram.*

Orange spots—*Cere. b.*

Out of their sockets, eyes were coming—*Acon., Bell.*

Outlines of objects were shaded by colors—*Gels.*

Overcome with sleep, in eyelids—*Asaf.*

Pain were situated between eyeballs and orbital plate of parietal bone—*Cimic.*

  –in eye would drive him crazy—*Spig.*

  –surrounded eyeball deep in left socket—*Æsc.*

  –pressed down into eyes by a weight—*Phos.*

Pale, objects were—*Agar., Cop., Dig., Eupi., Ind., Rhus t., Sil.*

Paper, white, obscured vision—*Bell.*

Paralyzed, eyeballs were—*Cocc.*

  –right eye were—*Caust.*

  –lids were—*Cocc., Op., Plb., Sep.*

  –upper lid were—*Alum., Dulc., Morph., Spig., Zinc.*

Particle in left external canthus—*Ign.*

Pass before eyes, a dark veil would—*Nat. m.*

  –out of eye, something were seeking to—*Elect.*

Passed over an elevation on bulb of eye, lid—*Symph.*

  –over eyes, a white cloud—*Sanic.*

  –before left eye, fiery stars—*Card. b.*

  –from eyes to light, rays of light—*Cham.*

Passing around in eye with stitches, something were—*Cist.*

Pear-shaped obstruction before eyes—*Cund.*

Pepper had been thrown into eyes causing lachrymation and spasms of lids—*Zinc.*

  –had been thrown into right eye and on upper lid—*Eug.*

Phosphorescence on closing eyes, clouds of—*Dig.*

Pieces, left eye would fly to—*Spig.*

Pierced in eyes with knives—*Chel.*

  –through right eye with piece of cold iron—*Til.*

Pin were sticking in eyeball if pressed upon—*Sin.*

Pinched upper lid, something—*Chin. m.*

Playing with his fingers before eyes, one were—*Psor.*

Pleasant sensation in eye—*Fl. ac.*

Plug were pressing on upper border of sight—*Anac.*

Point, black, before right eye—*Elect.*

  —of drill pressed downward in eyeball—*Ran. b.*

  —from within outward, pressure with a dull—*Asar.*

Pointed were being forced deep into eye, something—*Fl. ac.*

Points in lids, fiery—*Merc.*

  —suddenly thrust into lid, a hundred needle—*Verat. a.*

Press eyes, she should—*Calc. c.*

  —on them, he wanted to open eyes wide and—*Adren.*

Pressed into eyeballs and distended them, fluid—*Seneg.*

  —against sides of orbits, eyeballs were—*Card. m.*

  —asunder, eye were—*Led., Prun.*

  —asunder, eye would be—*Asar., Prun.*

  —asunder, then out of orbit, left eye were—*Led.*

  —from above downward, eyeballs—*Coloc., Sin.*

  —down, eyeballs were—*Coloc., Corn.*

  —down from vertex, eyes would be—*Sulph.*

  —down, lids and eyes were—*Hell.*

  —down, lids were—*Chin. s., Hell.*

  —around something, a stick were—*Form.*

  —down into eyes, weight—*Phos.*

  —down by a heavy weight, upper lids were—*Con.*

  —downward in eyeball, a drill point—*Ran. b.*

  —forward, eyes—*Gymn.*

  —from behind, right eye were—*Fl. ac.*

  —in on reading, eyes were—*Kali c.*

  —into head, eye would be—*Bapt., Bell., Calc. c., Caust., Cocc., Daph. o., Kali c., Puls., Zinc.*

  —into orbits, eyes were—*Cor. r.*

  —inward with waning sight, eyeball were—*Thlaspi*

  —off from pressure in left cheek, eye would be—*Lachn.*

  —open from above, eyeballs were—*Bry., Camph., Guare., Iber., Ign., Med., Merc. c., Nux v., Phos., Psor., Puls., Sabin., Sang., Seneg., Spig., Stram., Thuj.*

  —out, eyes would be—*Bry., Card. b., Cimic., Eupi., Laur., Nux v., Ovi g. p., Pip. m., Phos., Rhus t., Sabin., Sang., Scut., Thuj., Valer.*

  —out from above—*Com.*

  —out of eyes, water would be—*Laur.*

  —out of orbit, eye were—*Led.*

  —out, right eye would be—*Apoc., Camph., Ign.*

  —out, eyes were forcibly—*Daph. o.*

Pressed—*Continued*

  –out when hair was combed, eye were—*Nux v.*

  –out, temples and eyes were—*Par.*

  –out, eyes were being—*Con., Meli.*

  –out of head, eyes were swollen and—*Thuj.*

  –or squeezed tightly together, lids were—*Kali i.*

  –together, eyes would be—*Op.*

  –an ulcer were being—*Nit. ac.*

  –upward, eyes were—*Meli.*

  –upward, lids were—*Rat.*

  –by a weight, eyelids and balls were—*Corn.*

Pressing and cutting under lids, a sharp body—*Merc.*

  –on top of eyeballs, something were—*Com.*

  –on upper border of sight, dull plug were—*Anac.*

  –out, right eye were—*Zing.*

  –upon eyes, someone were—*Euphr.*

Pressure in frontal bone at inner left canthus—*Sac. lac.*

  –with a dull point from within outward—*Asar.*

  –behind right eyeball—*Fl. ac.*

  –on eyelids—*Lac d.*

Prick of needle under lid—*Paraf.*

Pricking in eye, something were—*Caust.*

  –in lower lid, splinter were—*Sep.*

Printed upon, paper were not (by artificial light)—*Aur. m.*

Projected, eyes—*Bell., Guai.*

  –from forehead so that he could not see over it, something were—*Phel.*

Projecting, eyes were—*Bell., Guai., Par.*

Protrude, eyes would—*Ferr., Hep.*

Protruded, eyes—*Acon., Bell., Med.*

  –and she stared at everything, eyes—*Med.*

  –right eyeball—*Com.*

  –eyes swelled and—*Guai., Phos., Sol, Thlaspi*

Protruding, eyes were—*Ars. s. f., Con., Glon., Scut.*

Pulled backward into head, eyes were—*Hep.*

  –toward temple by a thread, eyes were—*Crot. c.*

  –backward for a moment, eyes were clutched and—*Sanic.*

  –out of head, eyes were being—*Med.*

  –outward from nose, eyes were—*Con.*

  –into head, eyes were—*Crot. t., Par.*

  –tight over eyes, something were—*Phos.*

Pulled—*Continued*

  —out, eyes were—*Nat. c.*

  —inward when pressing on spot near ears, eyes were—*Raph.*

  —eyes were being—*Crot. c., Mur. ac., Raph., Sep.*

Pulling eyes from within outward, somebody were—*Glon.*

  —eyeball back into head, string were—*Crot. t., Par., Ruta, Sil.*

Punctured by a needle, lens had been—*Sulph.*

Purple vertical bar before eyes—*Stram.*

  —obstruction before right eye—*Cund.*

Pushed forward, eyes were—*Gymn.*

  —back into orbits, eyes were—*Puls.*

  —into orbit, whole eyeball were—*Acon.*

  —out, eyes were—*Aur., Com., Ephed., Passi., Peti., Rhus v.*

  —out, eye would be—*Spig.*

  —out, eyeball were being—*Guare.*

  —out of head, enormously enlarged eye were—*Spig.*

  —out yet at same time held back by cords, eyes were being—*Fago.*

  —out of sockets, eyes were swelled and—*Phos.*

  —upon, eyes were—*Rhus v.*

Rainbow—*Bar. c., Bell., Bry., Cic., Con., Dig., Dign., Euph., Ferr. ma., Ip., Kali c., Kali n., Mim., Osm., Phos. ac., Phos., Stann., Stram., Sulph.*

Raise eyelids, weight and heaviness on upper lids so she could not—*Sep.*

  —upper lids, he could not—*Caust.*

Raised, eyelids cannot be—*Arn.*

Ran into eyes on stooping, all blood—*Ferr. p.*

Raw in eyes—*Clem.*

  —edges of lids were—*Phyt.*

Rays of light passed from eyes to light—*Cham.*

Reading, eyes were strained by—*Ruta*

Receding, objects were—*Bell., Cic., Sep.*

Red—*Atro., Bell., Cact., Cann. s., Cedr., Chin., Con., Croc., Cund., Dig., Elaps, Fl. ac., Hep., Hyos., Iodof., Mag. m., Nux m., Osm., Plat., Phos., Saba., Sars., Spig., Stram., Stront., Sulph.*

  —at night, objects were—*Cedr.*

  —objects look cherry—*Phos.*

  —ink, letters were written in—*Phos.*

  —circles—*Cact., Stront., Sulph., Verat. v.*

Red—*Continued*

  –disk or bar—*Elaps*

  –halo—*Bell., Sil.*

  –masses—*Spig.*

  –sparks—*Fl. ac., Stry.*

  –spots—*Cot., Hipp.*

Reflected from a bright copper plate at left side, a light were—*Oxyt.*

Rested on eyes, a heavy weight—*Carb. v.*

Resting on eyes, stone falling from a height and—*Cocaine*

  –on right eye, a round weight were—*Lepi.*

Ring, burning, around each eye—*Chlol.*

  –around light, a bluish-gray—*Lach.*

  –about eye, pain were from a heavy—*Sep.*

Rise, inflammation would—*Saba.*

Rising behind eyes, clouds were—*Sabin.*

Riveted in their sockets, eyes were—*Cupr. ac.*

Rocket rushed out of eyes—*Pana.*

Rolling around beneath lids, sand were—*Ign., Med.*

Room, brightly lighted in dark—*Elect.*

  –in orbits, eyes had no—*Ars.*

Rose before left eye impeding sight, a body—*Am. m.*

Rotated, eyes were spasmodically—*Sec.*

Rotating, objects were—*Atro., Bell.*

Rough, eyeball were—*Elaps*

  –from sand, eye were—*Asaf.*

  –skin of right lower lid were—*Nat. m.*

  –inner surface of lids were—*Conv.*

Round objects passing before eyes—*Caust.*

  –with a whirling sensation, eyes went—*Saba.*

Rub lids, he must—*Ars.*

Rubbed against lids, eyeballs—*Sulph.*

  –between lid and ball, something—*Anac.*

  –by lids, eyes were—*Ars.*

  –margins of lids were—*Nux v.*

  –sore, eyelids were—*Verat. a.*

Rubbing with a woolen cloth, biting in eyes as from—*Stann.*

Run into eyeball through cornea, needles were—*Cimic.*

Rushed out of eyes, a rocket—*Pana.*

Rushing through eyes, cold air were—*Croc.*

  –from stomach to eye, spark of fire were—*Stram.*

Saffron-colored—*Ind.*

Salt in eye—*Canth., Chin., Nat. m., Nux v., Sulph., Verat. a., Zinc.*

　–between lids and eyes—*Verat. a.*

　–were biting in eyes—*Caust., Chin., Rhus t.*

　–eyes were filled with sharp—*Nat. m.*

　–in margin of lids—*Canth.*

Sand in eyes—*Am. br., Am. m., Ang., Ars., Apis, Apoc., Asc. t., Aur., Bar. c., Bell., Berb., Bry., Cann. s., Carb. v., Caust., Chel., Chin., Chin. m., Chlol., Cob., Con., Cor. r., Dig., Elaps, Euph., Euphr., Fago., Ferr., Fl. ac., Form., Gas., Grat., Hæm., Hep., Hura, Ign., Jac., Kali bi., Kali m., Kali p., Lach., Led., Lith., Luna, Lyc., Med., Merc., Myric., Nat. m., Nat. p., Nit. ac., Op., Ox. ac., Pæon., Peti., Petr., Phos. ac., Phos., Phyt., Pic. ac., Plat., Psor., Puls., Rad., Rhod., Rhus t., Rhus v., Sep., Sil., Sol. n., Spig., Stram., Sulph., Syph., Tarent., Thuj., Upas, Urt. u., Vib., Xanth., Zinc., Zing.*

　–in eye, grain of—*Alum., Ferr., Sars.*

　–in right internal canthus, pressure as from—*Tarax.*

　–in left eye—*Hura, Phos., Rhus t., Zing.*

　–in right eye—*Amph., Bry., Cann. s., Sulph.*

　–in right eye, grain of—*Sep., Zing.*

　–in eyes with tears—*Chel.*

　–caused itching in right eye—*Arg.*

　–in eyes made them rough—*Asaf.*

　–had got in eyes on reading—*Cina*

　–were thrown into eye—*Psor.*

　–were thrown violently into eye—*Ter.*

　–under lids—*Cob., Ign., Med.*

　–under lids, grain of—*Calc. c.*

　–at outer angles of eye, grain of—*Con., Euphr.*

　–in inner left canthus—*Acon.*

　–in inner right canthus—*Thuj.*

　–in lids—*Berb., Cob., Chel., Phyt., Seneg., Sulph., Tarent.*

　–in upper lid—*Cob.*

　–in upper lids, grain of—*Calc. c., Pæon.*

　–on inner margin of lids, grain of—*Sel.*

　–fine, in eyes under eyelids—*Thuj.*

Saw were drawn up and down through globe of left eye—*Maland.*

Scalded and raw, edges of lid were—*Phyt.*

Scales were before eyes obscuring sight—*Kali bi.*
  —were before eyes—*Verat. v.*
Scraped with a knife, eyes were—*Puls.*
Scraping in left eye, foreign body were—*Lycps.*
Scratching ball, there were a stick under lids—*Zinc.*
Screwed in and immovable, eyes were—*Rat.*
Sea of fire even when eyes are closed, looking into—*Phos.*
Separated itself, something in eye—*Lachn.*
Serrated, objects were—*Hyos.*
Serpents—*Arg. n., Cund., Ign., Phys.*
Shadow flitted before eyes—*Ruta*
Shears into her eyes, someone would stick—*Bov.*
Shining shooting bodies before eyes—*Aloe*
  —particles floating before eyes when closed—*Ars.*
  —white points—*Cann. s.*
  —spots—*Seneg., Verat. a.*
Short and unable to cover eyes, lids were—*Guai.*
  —when looking up, muscles of lids were too—*Cinnb.*
  —when looking up, inferior and internal muscles were too—*Sabin.*
Sieve, one were looking through a—*Puls.*
Silvery clouds—*Bell.*
Skin were drawn over eyes—*Apis*
  —before eyes—*Rat.*
  —came half-way down over right eye—*Caust.*
  —were hanging down over eyes—*Ol. an.*
  —were on cornea—*Kali bi.*
Sleep, eyes were full of—*Ferr., Staph.*
  —had been long deprived of—*Merc.*
  —heavy with—*Ind.*
  —eyes were oppressed with—*Stram.*
  —in eyelids, overcome with—*Asaf.*
Sleepy in lids—*Equis., Verat. v.*
Slept enough, he had not—*Bapt., Benz. ac., Colch., Ferr., Lac. ac., Nux v., Onos., Ran. b., Thuj.*
Small, eyes were—*Bry., Croc., Euphr., Grat., Kreos., Morph.*
  —eye were—*Aloe, Cinnb., Croc., Dig., Grat., Hura, Merc., Nat. m., Squill., Tab.*
  —for socket, eyes were too—*Morph.*
  —left eye were—*Euphr.*
  —right eye were—*Eupi.*

Small—*Continued*

—and loose in socket, left eyeball were too—*Croc.*

—as dolls, people were—*Plb.*

—lids were—*Euphr.*

—letters were—*All. c., Glon., Phys.*

—objects were—*Hyos., Merc. c., Op., Stram.*

Smaller than usual, eyes were—*Croc.*

—and swayed to and fro, eyes were—*Acon.*

—left eye were—*Cinnm.*

—than right eye, left eye were—*Rhod.*

Smarting from wood smoke—*Nat. a., Ran. b.*

—from a hair in eye—*Coc. c.*

—from soap—*Seneg.*

—from weeping—*Pedi.*

—in left eye—*Zinc.*

Smeared over, upper half of left eye were—*Coloc.*

Smoke before eyes—*Aur., Cyc., Gels., Kali m.*

—were burning in eyes—*Æth., Nat. a.*

—eyes were enveloped in—*Phos., Sulph.*

—eyes were filled with—*Chin., Croc., Nat. a., Nit. ac., Valer.*

—in air—*Stram.*

—were in eyes—*All. c., Ran. b., Valer.*

—biting, in eyes—*Croc., Mosch., Petr.*

—in room—*Crot. t.*

—after using eyes a few moments, room were filled with—*Croc.*

—eyes had been full of—*Kali p.*

—sees through—*Kali c.*

—in form of birds, animals and circles—*Ammc.*

Smoky before eyes—*Bell., Crot. t., Cyc., Gels., Mag. p. Ambo, Osm., Phos., Pic. ac., Plat., Stram., Sulph., Til.*

—room were—*Lac. ac., Osm., Thuj.*

Smooth substance, large, lying beneath left upper lid—*Staph.*

—large substance in eyes—*Dios.*

Snake were before vision—*Gels.*

—or worm before vision—*Phys.*

Snapping when opening them, little strings holding eyelids together and—*Cob.*

Snow were dazzling before eyes—*Olnd.*

—blind in afternoon, he were—*Sang.*

—objects were covered with—*Dig.*

Snowflakes were falling on conjunctiva and burning—*Form.*
   –were falling—*Bell., Jab., Plb.*
   –were falling straight down before eyes—*Camph. br.*
Soap in eyes—*Seneg.*
   –were biting in left eye—*Alum.*
Sockets, eyes were too small for—*Morph.*
   –eyes were gone and wind blew out of—*Sep., Sulph.*
Something were under lids—*Caul.*
   –were under upper lid—*Cob.*
   –would come out of eyeballs—*Elect.*
   –were in eye < if others speak of it—*Calc. p.*
   –in eye that could be rubbed out—*Fl. ac.*
   –lay above eyes, preventing looking up—*Carb. ac.*
Sore, eyelids were rubbed—*Verat. a.*
Spark of fire rushing from stomach to eyes—*Stram.*
   –caused pain in eye—*Tarent.*
Sparks—see the GENERAL REPERTORIES
Sparks, electric, flashing before eyes in daytime—*Croc.*
   –of fire coming from eyes—*Merc.*
Speck, white, before eyes—*Rat.*
Specks, black, before eyes—*Gels.*
Spider-web over objects—*Carb. s.*
Splinter in eye—*Calc. s.*
   –in upper lid—*Sil.*
   –in left eye—*Elat.*
   –under lids—*Ham.*
   –were sticking in eye—*Sulph.*
   –pricking in lower lid—*Sep.*
Splinters of glass rubbed in eye—*Sulph.*
Split, eyes would—*Vacc., Vario.*
Spots—*Act. sp., Cyc., Dig., Kali bi., Kali c., Hipp., Sil., Sol. n.,*
      Sulph.
   –black, before eyes—*Cocc., Glon., Sep., Syph.*
   –bright, before eyes—*Gels.*
   –dark, before eyes—*Dig.*
   –dancing to and fro—*Ust.*
   –floating—*Cann. i., Dig., Hell., Phos.*
   –red, floating in field of vision—*Dub.*
Spread over left eye, gauze were—*Sars.*
Spring out of head when pressing on throat, eyes would—*Lach.*

Squeezed, upper part of eyeballs were—*Chel.*
  —together, lids were pressed or tightly—*Kali i.*
  —and put back again, eyes had been taken out—*Lach.*
  —in a vise, eyes were—*Spig.*
  —left eyeball were—*Coloc.*
Squinting—*Calc. c., Con., Coniin.*
  —inward, eyes were—*Coca*
Stab in left eye—*Cinch. b.*
Stabbed in eyes—*Thuj.*
Stabbing in ears and eyes, knife were—*Vib.*
Staring, eyes were—*Med.*
Stars—*Ammc., Atro., Cast., Croc., Hyos., Sec., Puls., Tarent.*
  —bright, danced before eyes—*Croc.*
  —fiery, passed before left eye—*Card. b.*
Start from its socket, right eye would—*Mag. s.*
Starting, eyes were—*Amyg., Chlor., Dign., Kali i., Stry.*
  —from their sockets, eyes were—*Bell., Chlol.*
  —from orbits, eyes were becoming larger and—*Dign.*
Stick shears into her eyes, someone would—*Bov.*
  —in eyes—*Caust., Dios., Kali p., Med., Pic. ac.*
  —were pressed around something in eyes—*Form.*
  —under lids, scratching ball—*Zinc.*
Sticks in eyes, lids and inner canthus—*Med.*
  —eyes full of small—*Naph.*
  —in eyes—*Dios.*
Sticking in eyes from washing in cold water, needles were—*Sac. lac.*
  —in right lower and left upper lids, fine needles were—*Zinc.*
  —in eyeball if pressed upon, a pin were—*Sin.*
  —in eyes, splinter were—*Sulph.*
  —in right eyeball, knives were—*Coloc., Sulph.*
  —in eyes, knives were—*Lach., Vib.*
  —in eye, needle were—*Sulph.*
  —to lids because of dryness, eyeballs were—*Sanic.*
Stiff as from tonic spasm, eyelids were—*Meny.*
  —eyes were—*Ars., Bar. m., Bell., Caust., Cupr. s., Lach., Merc., Mosch., Nat. h., Op., Phos., Stry.*
Stiffened and drawn back, eyes were suddenly—*Stry.*
Stiffness: difficult to move lids—*Rhus t.*
Stinging in eye, needles were—*Calc. c., Caust.*
Stitched with needle in eyebrow—*All. c.*

Stitches, something were passing around in eye with—*Cist.*
  —from knives in eyes—*Lach.*
  —with red-hot needle in right eye—*Rhod.*
Stone were falling from a height and resting on eyes—*Cocaine*
Stones, eyes were full of little—*Lac d.*
Strained by reading, eyes were—*Ruta*
  —eyes were—*Adren.*
Straining by reading, tension in eyes as from—*Onos.*
Straw hanging before each eye—*Merc.*
Stream of cold air were blowing on eye—*Mez.*
  —of cold air were blowing out or through eyes—*Thuj.*
Streamed out of eyes, hot air—*Dios., Kreos.*
Streaming from eyes, fire were—*Clem.*
Stretching eyes open—*Onos.*
String, eyes were torn or hanging by a—*All. c.*
  —were pulling eyeball back into head—*Crot. t., Par., Sil., Ruta*
  —little, holding eyelids together and snapping when opening
    them—*Cob.*
Striped—*Am. c., Am. m., Bell., Cham., Cic., Con., Dig., Iod.,
    Kali c., Nat. m., Phos., Puls., Sep.*
Struck by blow in right eye—*Agn.*
  —in eye, he had been—*Eup. per.*
Strung together with a cord, right eye were—*Amph.*
Stuck together, eyelids were—*Agar.*
  —in eyes, bristle of hairbrush were—*Agar.*
  —fast to ball, lid were—*Verat. a.*
Stung in right eye by some insect—*Luna*
Stupefied, eye were—*Hell., Op.*
Sty would form in eye—*Meph., Thuj.*
  —were in eye when holding it still—*Meny.*
  —would begin—*Carb. s.*
Substance, foreign, were in eye—*Asim.*
  —foreign, biting in eyes—*Rheum*
  —foreign, in right eye then left—*Med.*
  —hard, under right upper lid—*Spig.*
  —hard, behind right eye—*Stann.*
  —large, in eyes—*Caust.*
  —large, smooth, lying beneath left upper lid—*Staph.*
  —large, smooth, in eyes—*Dios.*
Sun were flickering before eyes—*Lach.*
  —were taking place, eclipse of—*Phys.*

Sun—*Continued*
  —a few minutes before, objects appear as if one had looked at—*Podo.*
  —one had been looking at—*Nit. ac.*
Sunlight, she had gone out into bright—*Sep.*
Sunken into head, eyes were—*Calc. s., Gent. c., Sulph.*
  —lower lids were—*Glon.*
Surrounded by halo, light were—*Coff. t., Sulph., Tub.*
  —by a hot vapor—*Bell.*
  —by a white vapor—*Bell.*
  —by pain, eyeball deep in left socket—*Æsc.*
Spasm, eyelids were stiff as from tonic—*Meny.*
Suppurating when pressed, left eyeball were—*Dros.*
Swayed to and fro, eyes were smaller and—*Acon.*
Sweat were biting in left eye—*Viol. t.*
Swelled and pushed out of sockets, eyes were—*Phos.*
  —and protruded, eyes were—*Guai., Phos., Sol, Thlaspi*
Swelling, eyes were—*Coloc.*
  —and would force themselves out of sockets, eyes were—*Sol*
  —in left inner canthus—*Helio.*
  —lids were—*Carb. s., Caust., Chel., Cimic., Croc., Cyc., Euphr., Fago., Meny., Tarax., Thuj.*
  —inner surface of lids were—*Ammc.*
  —lower lids were—*Coloc., Nat. a.*
Swimming before eyes, net were—*Carb. an.*
  —in cold water, eyes were—*Chin., Sil., Squill.*
  —in tears, eyes were—*Cor. r.*
  —before eyes, letters were—*Bell., Coca*
  —before eyes, objects were—*Amyg., Carb. ac., Carl., Digit., Gins., Inul., Jab., Mez., Par., Sumb., Thuj., Til., Zinc.*
Swollen, eyeballs were—*Calc. c., Calc. p., Cann. i., Caust., Con., Ham., Mag. c., Phys., Thuj.*
  —eyes were—*Ant. t., Dign., Op.*
  —during one-sided headaches, eyes were—*Arg. n.*
  —eyes were enormously—*Bell.*
  —left eye were—*Rhus t.*
  —and too large for socket, eyeball were—*Spig.*
  —and pressed out of head, eyes were—*Thuj.*
  —eyelids were—*Arum t., Croc., Cyc., Lact., Stram., Sumb., Tarax., Thuj.*

Swollen—*Continued*

    –but they were not, eyelids were—*Carb. s.*, *Sac. lac.*

    –lower lids were—*Arum t.*

Tadpoles floated in mist before eyes—*Sep.*

    –danced before eyes—*Cimic.*

Tearing in bones above left eye—*Merc. c.*

Tears would flow but they do not—*Spire.*

    –were in it, dimness of eye as if—*Ign.*

    –came out of eyes in a stream—*Eug.*

    –eyes were swimming in—*Cor. r.*

    –hot, were bathing eyes—*Cor. r.*

    –were in eyes—*Berb.*, *Cor. r.*, *Eupi.*, *Fago.*, *Glon.*, *Hyos.*, *Lil. t.*, *Merc.*, *Nit. ac.*, *Pyrus*, *Spire.*

    –were in one eye—*Ign.*, *Paraf.*

    –were in left eye—*Sep.*

Tense, eyeballs were too—*Stach.*

Tension in eyes as from straining—*Onos.*

Thick, upper lid were—*Caj.*

Thickened, inner surface of lids were—*Kali bi.*, *Nat. a.*

Thorn in left eye on rising—*Calc. c.*

Thread before left eye, black woolen—*Thuj.*

Threads before eyes she could not wipe away—*Sulph.*

    –were hanging before eyes—*Seneg.*

    –in eye—*Tab.*

    –before eyes on looking up—*Kali c.*

    –drawn from behind eye to eye—*Lach.*

    –were drawn tightly through eye to middle of head—*Par.*

    –or line horizontally before right eye—*Con.*

    –white, moving before eyes—*Elaps*

    –were flickering before eye—*Lach.*

    –were hovering before eye—*Coca*

    –were swimming before eye—*Con.*

Thrown into eyes, pepper had been—*Eug.*, *Zinc.*

    -into eyes, sand were—*Psor.*

    –violently into eye, sand were—*Ter.*

Thrust between ball and socket and turned about, knife were—*Chin.*

    –suddenly into lid, hundred needle points were—*Verat. a.*

    –into right eyeball, needle were—*Spig.*

Tickling in eye, dust were—*Zinc.*

    –in eye—*Agar.*, *Aspar.*, *Card. b.*, *Hep.*, *Lyss.*

Tight and did not cover ball, lids were too—*Sep.*
Tightly backward, eyeball were drawn—*Cham.*
  –bound by a cloth, eyes were—*Puls.*
Tired of reading, eyes were—*Lappa a.*
Torn open, inner canthus were—*Nat. m.*
  –eyes were—*All. c.*
  –out, eyes were being—*All. c., Carb. v., Chel., Cocc.*
  –out, eyes had been—*Bell.*
  –out, inner portion of right eyeball would be—*Prun.*
Tossed up from below in every direction, eyes were—*Lac d.*
Totter and dance, objects seem to—*Sant.*
Trembling, vision tremulous as if eyes were—*Con.*
Transparency, cornea had lost its—*Sulph.*
Triple, objects were—*Con., Sec.*
Tumult and confusion, everything in street appears (when looking through window)—*Camph.*
Turn in head, eyeballs seem to—*Gels.*
Turned in, eyelashes were—*Tell.*
  –about, knife were thrust between ball and socket and—*Chin.*
  –in, lashes of lower lid were—*Tell.*
  –up and light came only from above, pupil were—*Cahin.*
Twisted around, eyes were—*Sang., Spong.*
  –eyes would become—*Petr.*
  –left eye were—*Pop.*
Twisting in eye—*Phys.*
Twitched about in eyes, water were—*Stram.*
Ulcer were being pressed—*Nit. ac.*
  –corneal, might develop—*Plb.*
Vapor, white, before eyes—*Bell.*
  –eye were surrounded by hot—*Bell.*
Veil before eyes—*Acon., Agar., Am. c., Ant. t., Arum t., Arund
  Asaf., Bell., Bov., Bry., Bufo, Calc. c., Calc. p., Carb. s
  Carl., Caust., Clem., Croc., Crot. t., Cupr., Dig., Dros., Dulc
  Euph., Euphr., Eupi., Gels., Hæm., Hep., Hyos., Ign., Iod
  Laur., Lil. t., Lith., Lyc., Merl., Nat. m., Nat. p., Nit. ac
  Op., Paraf., Petr., Phos., Pic. ac., Pin. s., Plat., Puls., Rat
  Rhus t., Sec., Sil., Stram., Sulph., Syph., Tarent., Ther
  Thuj., Til.*
  –between light and eyes—*Croc.*
  –eyes were covered by—*Gent. c.*
  –were drawn before eyes—*Arum t.*

Veil—*Continued*
  –were hanging over eyes—*Hep.*
  –looking through a—*Berb., Bufo, Cocc., Lyc., Tab., Verb.*
  –black, before eyes—*Aur., Paraf., Phos.*
  –dark, will pass before eyes—*Nat. m.*
  –objects were covered with a gray—*Elaps, Phos.*
  –seen through a green—*Carb. s.*
  –looking through a lace—*Xanth.*
  –thick, before eyes—*Ant. t.*
  –thin, before eyes—*Eupi.*
  –objects were covered with a thin—*Nat. m.*
  –white, over objects—*Staph.*

Vessel of molten iron, even when eyes are closed, looking into
    a—*Phos.*

Violet—*Cann. i., Elaps, Sant.*

Vise, eyes were compressed in a—*Rat.*
  –eyes were squeezed in a—*Spig.*

Vision:
  –animals and birds, smoke were in form of—*Ammc.*
      black, before vision on lying down to sleep—*Nat. a.*
      moving in cup—*Hyos.*
  –approach and recede, objects seem to—*Cic.*
  –bandage, white, obscured vision—*Lepi.*
  –balls floating before eyes—*Kali c.*
      before eyes, two large black—*Cund.*
      of fire rolling about—*Stram.*
      luminous, before vision—*Cyc.*
  –bandage, white, obscured vision—*Lepi.*
  –bars, vertical and of various colors, moving with eyes—*Stram.*
  –bifurcated bodies in axis—*Carl.*
  –bird, little, were flying from left to right when reading—*Calc.
    p.*
  –birds and animals, smoke were in form of—*Ammc.*
  –black—*Acon., Agar., Ambr., Am. m., Anac., Arn., Ars., Asaf.,
    Bell., Calc. c., Carb. v., Caust., Cham., Chin., Cic., Cocc.,
    Con., Cupr., Dig., Dros., Euphr., Ferr., Hep., Kali c., Laur.,
    Lyc., Mag. c., Mang., Meny., Merc., Mosch., Mur. ac., Nat.
    c., Nat. m., Nit. ac., Nux v., Olnd., Op., Petr., Phos., Phos.
    ac., Plb., Ruta, Saba., Sec., Sep., Sil., Squill., Staph., Stram.,
    Sulph., Thuj., Verat. a., Verb.*
      animals on lying down—*Nat. a.*

Vision—*Continued*

  balls before right eye—*Cund.*

  balls floating before eyes—*Kali c.*

  balls were before eyes, two large—*Cund.*

  bug below a black door-knob—*Atro.*

  disk before left eye when walking—*Elaps*

  dots filled visual field—*Tab.*

  figures—*Petr.*

  flickerings—*Lach.*

  flies floating before eyes—*Sulph.*

  two black horns, with large black balls on upper ends and
   a mound of crystals between them, their tops tapering
   off and tipped with—*Cund.*

  lightnings—*Staph.*

  objects—*Sol. n., Stram.*

  objects which turn as one turns—*Cocc.*

  plate—*Kali bi.*

  point before right eye—*Elect.*

  points before eyes—*Bell., Calc. c., Carb. an., Cic., Con.,
   Der., Elaps, Jatr., Kali c., Merc., Mez., Mosch., Nux v.,
   Sol. n., Tab., Thuj.*

  points, letters change to—*Calc. p.*

  points flickering before eyes—*Coca*

  points floating before eyes—*Chin., Chlf., Cop., Daph., Gins.,
   Led., Phos., Ter.*

  points move downward—*Merc.*

  rings—*Dig., Dign., Nit. s. d., Sol. n.*

  rings float before eyes—*Dign.*

  serpents jumping before eyes—*Cund.*

  sparks before eyes—*Stry.*

  spots—*Asc. t., Bar. c., Calc. c., Camph., Chlf., Cimic., Cupr.
   ar., Dulc., Elaps, Hell., Lyc., Nit. ac., Nit. s. d., Petr.,
   Scroph., Sep., Stram., Tab., Verat. a.*

  spots floating—*Acon., Agar., Alco., Am. c., Ant. t., Asaf.,
   Bell., Calc. c., Carb. v., Carl., Chlol., Cob., Coff. t., Dign.,
   Hyos., Itu, Kiss., Lact., Lil. t., Lyc., Macrot., Mez.,
   Morph., Nit. s. d., Phos., Phys., Sil., Sol. n., Stram., Tab.,
   Thuj.*

  spots floating when eyes are closed—*Elaps*

  spots moving with eyes—*Chin. s.*

  stripes—*Bell., Con., Phos. ac., Sol. n.*

Vision—*Continued*

    tadpoles floating in a mist—*Sep.*

    woolen thread floating before left eye—*Thuj.*

    veil before eyes—*Aur., Paraf., Phos.*

–blood globules passing with every beat of pulse, he saw—*Glon.*

–blue—*Acon., Act. sp., Am. br., Bell., Crot. c., Cyc., Dig., Hipp., Kreos., Lach., Lyc., Stram., Stront., Sulph., Tril., Zinc.*

    when eyes are closed—*Thuj.*

    circles—*Zinc.*

    circles around light—*Lach.*

    sparks—*Ars.*

    spots—*Acon., Hipp., Kali c., Thuj., Stram.*

–blur before eyes—*Crot. c., Lac v., Nux v.*

    before left eye—*Cund.*

    before eyes suddenly—*Podo.*

–blurred, eyes were—*Fago.*

    from winking mucus over pupil—*Pic. ac.*

–bows, bright—*Con.*

–bright—*Calc. c., Camph., Carb. an., Chin. s., Chel., Cic., Con., Eug., Hyos., Mill., Phys., Sol. n., Stry.*

    and glittering, all objects were too—*Camph.*

    circles—*Ammc., Camph., Carb. v., Fl. ac., Tax.*

    colors—*Kali c.*

    glow around letters—*Atro.*

    spots—*Acon., Atro., Chlf., Cic., Con., Dign., Hell., Jatr., Stram., Thuj.*

    stripes—*Chlf., Cic.*

–brown spot before left eye—*Agar.*

    worm on brown carpet—*Atro.*

–bug, black, below door-knob—*Atro.*

–chalk, middle of wood were marked with—*Ign.*

–ciphers before eyes—*Phos. ac.*

–circle, green, around light which on closing eyes turns red—*Verat. v.*

    of colors when looking at light, a zigzag—*Sep.*

–circles—*Carb. v., Cyc., Dign., Hell., Kali c., Plb.*

    colored—*Hyos.*

    half, during headache—*Viol. o.*

    quivering—*Carl.*

    objects move in—*Cic., Hep.*

Vision—*Continued*

    oval—*Ferr. ma.*

    zigzag—*Ign., Sep.*

—cloud before eyes—*Cahin., Corn., Corn. f., Ether., Euon., Lac d., Lachn.*

    before left eye—*Tarent.*

    over outer half of left eye—*Gels.*

    continually before left eye, in twilight—*Arg. n.*

    dark, before eyes—*Coca*

    upper part of field of vision were covered with a dark—*Dig.*

    of dust before eyes—*Ammc.*

    thick, before eyes—*Caust., Zinc.*

    white, passed over eyes—*Sanic.*

—clouds floating before eyes—*Hydr. ac.*

    moving up and down with vision—*Carl.*

    were rising behind eyes—*Sabin.*

—cobwebs before eyes—*Agar., Lyc., Merl., Nit. ac., Tarent.*

—colors, illusions of, and color-blindness—see the GENERAL REPERTORIES

—colors, outlines of colors were shaded by—*Gels.*

—commingled, all objects were—*Camph.*

—confusion and tumult, everything in street appears in (when looking through window)—*Camph.*

—cover, he were looking through a gray—*Sil.*

—covered with a cobweb, eyes were—*Agar.*

    with a dark body, half of object were—*Aur.*

    by a dark cloud, upper part of vision were—*Dig.*

    with a veil, eyes were—*Gent. c.*

    with a film, eye were—*Sulph.*

    with a bluish-gray film—*Bell.*

    with a gray veil, objects were—*Phos.*

    with a thin veil, objects were—*Nat. m.*

—crooked, objects were—*Bell., Bufo*

—curled hair before right eye and a blur before left causing letters to run together—*Cund.*

—curtain, dark, were slowly let down before eyes—*Ferr.*

—dance, objects were moving in a confused—*Olnd.*

    objects seemed to totter and—*Sant.*

—danced before eyes, tadpoles—*Cimic.*

    before vision, bright stars—*Croc.*

Vision—*Continued*

　–dancing before vision, objects were—*Glon., Sant.*
　　before vision, letters were—*Calc. c.*
　–dazzling before eyes, snow were—*Olnd.*
　　like lightning before eyes—*Nat. m.*
　–dim—see also GENERAL REPERTORIES and special rubrics such
　　as VEIL, OBSCURED, *etc.*
　–dim, edges of objects were—*Bell.*
　–dimness of vision were caused by film—*Aml. n.*
　　before eyes—*Doryph., Gels., Lac v., Morph., Viol. o.*
　　of eyes as if tears were in them—*Ign.*
　–displaced, focus of right eye were suddenly—*Glon.*
　–distance, everything were at a great—*Magnol.*
　–distant, objects were—*All. c., Anac., Atro., Bell., Calc. c.,
　　Merc. c., Nux m., Stram., Sulph.*
　–distorted, objects were—*Bell., Benz. n., Card. b., Dig., Morph.,
　　Nux v.*
　–divided horizontally, objects were—*Aur.*
　–dolls, people were as small as—*Plb.*
　–doorway were not wide enough—*Samars.*
　–dots, black, filled visual field—*Tab.*
　–double, objects were—*Atro., Eug., Camph., Phys.*
　–draft of air, light flickers from—*Hell. f.*
　–dust before eyes, waving cloud of—*Ammc.*
　–eclipse of sun were taking place—*Phys.*
　–electric sparks flashing before eyes in daytime—*Croc.*
　–elongated, objects were—*Atro., Zinc.*
　–encircled by a cloud, objects were—*Camph.*
　–enveloped in a mist or halo, objects were—*Merc. c.*
　　in a yellow mist, objects were—*Kali bi.*
　　in smoke, eyes were—*Phos., Sulph.*
　–fade and reappear, objects would—*Gels.*
　　if one used eye longer than a minute, objects—*Chlol.*
　–fall, near objects seem to—*Hyos.*
　–falling straight down before eyes, snowflakes were—*Camph.
　　br.*
　　over eyes, fringe were—*Con.*
　–far off, all objects were too—*Stann.*
　–farther apart, objects were—*Carb. an.*
　–feathers before eyes—*Alum., Calc. c., Kreos., Mag. c., Nat.
　　c., Sulph.*

Vision—*Continued*

        on eyelashes—*Spig.*

        came from corner of eye—*Merc.*

        looking through—*Nat. m.*

        sight were obscured with—*Lyc.*

—fiery stars passed before left eye—*Card. b.*

        objects were—*Dig., Iod., Stram., Verat. a., Viol. o.*

        body before eyes in dark—*Arg. n.*

        circles—*Calc. p., Ip., Puls.*

        half-circles—*Viol. o.*

        flakes floating in circles—*Zinc.*

        lines radiating outward—*Iod., Thea*

        points—*Ammc., Coca, Elaps*

        rays about light—*Lach.*

        showers—*Plb.*

        sparks—*Merc.*

        stripes—*Card. b.*

        wheels—*Camph., Spire.*

        zigzags—*Con., Graph., Nat. m., Sep.*

—figure, black, floats before eyes—*Cocc.*

—figures, zigzag, before eyes—*Lach.*

        from floor rise to her face—*Atro.*

        hovering before eyes—*Tarent.*

—film before eyes—*Aml. n., Lact., Phys., Scroph.*

        eyes were covered with a—*Sulph.*

        eye were covered with a bluish-gray—*Bell.*

        dimness of vision were caused by a—*Aml. n.ˢ*

        he were looking through a—*Lac c.*

—fingers before eyes, one were playing with his—*Psor.*

—fire, even when eyes are closed, looking into a sea of—*Phos.*

        when in dark night, eyes were a pillar of—*Staph.*

        were rolling about, balls of—*Stram.*

        before eyes as if he had been slapped in face (following dimness of vision) flashes of—*Puls.*

        were before eyes on closing them, wheels of—*Spira.*

—firefly were hovering before eyes—*Thuj.*

—flame before eyes—*Bell., Coca, Canth., Myric., Staph., Ther., Viol. o.*

—flames, everything were enveloped in—*Spong.*

—flashes—*Alco., Arg. n., Atro., Bell., Benz. n., Chlf., Dig., Dign., Iber., Ment., Op., Puls., Sec., Stram., Tab., Tarent.*

Vision—*Continued*

    sudden, like electric sparks, were before eyes—*Croc.*

    of fire before eyes as if he had been slapped in face (following dimness of vision)—*Puls.*

—flickering before eyes—*Chin. m., Cyc., Vinc.*

    as from threads or rays of sun before eyes—*Lach.*

—flickers from draft of air, light—*Hell. f.*

—flies were before eyes—*Cocc., Dig.*

    black, were floating before eyes—*Sulph.*

    little black, were before eyes—*Paraf.*

—flitted before eyes, shadow—*Ruta*

—floated before eyes, black objects like tadpoles in mist—*Sep.*

—floating in field of vision, red spot were—*Dub.*

    about, balls were—*Kali c.*

    before eyes obliging to wipe constantly, something were—*Kreos.*

    before eyes, objects were—*Camph., Dig., Hell., Kali c., Nux m., Petr.*

—floats before eyes, a black figure—*Cocc.*

—fluttering before vision—*Carb. o., Petr., Sil., Thuj.*

—flying from left to right when reading, a little bird were—*Calc. p.*

—focus of right eye were suddenly displaced—*Glon.*

—fog before eyes—*Aur., Bism., Camph., Carb. s., Coff. t., Cyc., Kali c., Lach., Lonic., Med., Merc., Morph., Sal. ac., Sil., Sulph., Vinc.*

    objects were seen through a—*Alum., Camph., Euphr., Ign., Lach., Lyc., Merc., Morph., Sars., Sol, Sulph., Tab., Verb., Vinc., Zinc.*

    or smoke before right eye—*Kali c.*

    before left eye—*Crot. t.*

    before eyes when closing them—*Bar. c.*

    before eyes on attempting to read—*Arn.*

    he were looking through a dense—*Cund.*

    gray, before eyes—*Sulph.*

    thick, before eyes—*Caust., Zinc.*

—forehead, he must look out under—*Phos. ac.*

—fringe falling down over eyes—*Con.*

—gauze before eyes—*Alum., Bar. c., Caust., Cina, Clem., Croc., Dulc., Gamb., Kali bi., Kreos., Nat. m., Nitro. o., Rhod., Rhus t., Stram., Sulph., Til.*

Vision—*Continued*

> black, before eyes—*Sulph.*
> before eyes in morning—*Bar. c.*
> looking through a—*Calc. c., Caust., Cina, Dulc., Hydr. ac., Kreos., Lact., Lepi., Nat. m., Plb., Sang. n.*
> looking through white—*Ars.*
> pearly, before right eye—*Elaps*
> spread over left eye—*Sars.*

—gazing at some distant object—*Lyss.*

—glare before right eye so she could hardly read—*Chel.*

—glass, looking through a dark blue—*Cyc.*

—glimmering—*Aran. s., Bar. c., Bell., Calc. p., Cann. i., Gels., Kalm., Zing.*
> before eyes—*Gels.*

—glistening bodies moved back and forth—*Ol. an.*
> objects—*Kali c., Nux v., Dros.*

—glittering objects—*Calc. p., Camph., Chel., Con., Cyc., Ign., Nat. s.*

—globules were floating in air, endless strings of white—*Upas*

—goiter and could not see over it, she had a large—*Zinc.*

—golden, everything were—*Acon., Atro., Bell., Hyos.*

—gnats, many, came before sight—*Tab.*

—gone into bright sunlight, she had—*Sep.*

—gray, objects were—*Arg. n., Brom., Calc. p., Card. b., Carl., Chlf., Cic., Elaps, Guare., Gins., Lachn., Nit. ac., Nux v., Phal., Phos., Sep., Sil., Stram.*
> reddish-gray—*Stram.*

—green—*Cann. i., Canth., Carb. s., Cina, Cot., Cyc., Dig., Mag. m., Merc., Osm., Phos., Ruta, Sant., Sep., Sil., Stram., Stry., Tab., Zinc.*
> about light—*Verat. v.*
> bluish-green about light—*Osm.*
> pea-green about light—*Cann. i.*
> halo about light—*Mag. m., Phos., Sep., Sil.*
> spots—*Hipp., Kali c., Nit. ac., Stram., Stront.*
> yellow-green—*Sant.*

—hair, curled, in front of right eye—*Cund.*
> hung over eyes—*Euphr.*

—hairs before eyes—*Dig.*
> were on lashes—*Spig.*

Vision—*Continued*

　　–halo about light—*Alum., Anac., Bell., Calc. c., Cham., Coff. t., Dign., Kali c., Nat. p., Nit. ac., Staph., Sulph., Tub.*

　　　　yellow before eyes even when closed—*Aml. n.*

　　　　green around light—*Caust.*

　　　　red and green about light—*Sil.*

　　　　variegated, around light—*Ferr. ma.*

　　　　objects were enveloped in—*Merc. c.*

　　–hanging down over eyes, skin were—*Ol. an.*

　　　　before eyes, obscuring sight, mucus that could not be wiped away were—*Puls.*

　　　　before eyes, threads were—*Seneg.*

　　　　over eyes, veil were—*Hep.*

　　–haze of light, objects were in a yellow—*Sant.*

　　–horns, two black, before eyes—*Cund.*

　　–hung over eyes, hair—*Euphr.*

　　　　before eyes, something—*Cast.*

　　　　down over eyes, something—*Eupi.*

　　　　down preventing vision, skin of eyebrow—*Ol. an.*

　　–illuminated, white objects were strongly—*Sant.*

　　　　objects were—*Hyos.*

　　–impeding sight, a body rose before left eye—*Am. m.*

　　–insects, black floating—*Merc.*

　　–inverted, lines were—*Kali c.*

　　　　objects were—*Bell., Guare.*

　　–iron even when eyes are closed, looking into a vessel of molten —*Phos.*

　　–jumping, objects were—*Bell., Meny., Plb.*

　　　　before right eye, black serpents were—*Cund.*

　　–large, objects were—see EYES, LARGE

　　–large, distant objects look—*Onos.*

　　　　everything were too—*Laur., Tub.*

　　　　as natural, objects were twice as—*Berb.*

　　–larger than it is, everything appears—*Euph.*

　　–lattice, one were looking through a fine—*Lyc.*

　　–leaf, white, before right eye—*Nat. s.*

　　–letters were written in red ink—*Phos.*

　　　　expand and contract—*Atro.*

　　　　placed irregularly on line—*Stram.*

　　–light were surrounded by halo—*Coff. t., Sulph., Tub.*

　　　　were at end of room—*Oxyt.*

Vision—*Continued*

    points—*Nat. m.*

    spots—*Con., Dig.*

    snakes or worms—*Phys.*

—lightning were dazzling before eyes—*Nat. m.*

—lightnings—*Brom., Coca, Cyc., Dig., Glon., Olnd., Nat. c., Sulph.*

—lights before eyes—*Ammc., Calc. c., Chin. s., Dig., Fl. ac., Valer.*

—lilac—*Acon., Stram.*

—line or thread horizontally before right eye—*Con.*

—linen, one were looking through coarse—*Stram.*

—looked at sun a few minutes before, objects appear as if one had—*Podo.*

—looking through coarse linen, one were—*Stram.*

    through concave glasses, one were—*Mez.*

    down, he were—*Phos.*

    at sun, one had been—*Nit. ac.*

    through white bandage, he were—*Lepi.*

    through feathers—*Nat. m.*

    through film—*Lac c.*

    through a lace veil—*Xanth.*

    through a gauze—*Calc. c., Cina, Caust., Dulc., Hydr. ac., Kreos., Lact., Lepi., Nat. m., Plb., Sang. n.*

    through glass when in open air—*Nat. m.*

    through clear water which produced prismatic colors, one were—*Oxyt.*

    through white gauze—*Ars.*

    through a dark blue glass—*Cyc.*

    through a fine lattice, one were—*Lyc.*

    too long and too intently at an object—*Ruta*

    through too strong glasses, she had been—*Croc.*

    through mist—see Mist

    through rain—*Nat. m.*

    through a sieve—*Puls.*

    through a gray veil—*Phos.*

    through a veil—*Cocc., Lyc., Verb.*

    upon the ground, one were—*Verat. a.*

    into a vessel of molten iron, even when eyes are closed—*Phos.*

Vision—*Continued*

　—luminous—*Arund., Cann. i., Cyc., Dig., Nitro. o., Stram., Sulph., Thuj.*

　—mist before eyes—*Agar., Aran., Am. m., Arg. m., Bism., Calc. ar., Cahin., Caust., Croc., Cyc., Dub., Ether., Form., Gels., Glon., Graph., Grat., Kali m., Lact., Mill., Merl., Momor., Myric., Paraf., Podo., Sulph., Thuj., Zinc.*

　　before eyes in morning—*Merl.*

　　distant objects enveloped in—*Phos. ac.*

　　before eyes but at a distance—*Mill.*

　　about light—*Sil.*

　　before eyes when looking keenly at objects—*Calc. c.*

　　before eyes in which black objects like tadpoles floated—*Sep.*

　　everything were enveloped in a—*Eupi., Phos.*

　　looking through a—*Ambr., Arn., Lact., Zinc.*

　　thick, before eyes—*Ammc.*

　　white, before right eye—*Lac f.*

　　objects were enveloped in—*Merc. c.*

　　objects were enveloped in a yellow—*Kali bi.*

　—molten iron, even when eyes are closed looking into a vessel of—*Phos.*

　—motion, every object in—*Sep.*

　—move, objects at a distance—*Spira.*

　—moved to and fro before eyes, something—*Lyss.*

　　up and down, objects—*Cocc.*

　—moves before eyes, everything—*Eug.*

　—moving in a confused dance, objects were—*Olnd.*

　　letters were—*Agar., Am. c., Merc., Phys.*

　　up and down, lines of print were—*Con.*

　　objects were—*Carb. ac., Con., Euphr., Hydr. ac., Ign., Nitro. o., Petr., Spire., Wies.*

　　to and fro, objects were—*Cic., Elaps*

　　before eyes, something were—*Lyss., Psor.*

　—mucus that could be wiped away were hanging over eyes, obscuring sight—*Puls.*

　—multiplied, objects were—*Bell., Iod., Phys., Phyt., Stram.*

　—nearer, objects were—*Phys., Rhus t.*

　　to each other, objects—*Nux m.*

　—net before eyes—*Chin. s., Hyos.*

　　were swimming before eyes—*Carb. an.*

Vision—*Continued*

  –nose a shapeless mass, he sees his—*Coniin.*

  –obscuration before eyes—*Sulph.*

  –obscured, objects were—*Cact., Sil.*

    with feathers, sight were—*Lyc.*

    vision, something—*Sil.*

    vision, white paper—*Bell.*

    vision, white bandage—*Lepi.*

  –obscuring sight, scales were before eyes—*Kali bi.*

  –obstruction, pear-shaped, before eye with large end up, on waking in morning—*Cund.*

  –opened wider so field of vision becomes enlarged—*Fl. ac.*

  –orange spots—*Cere. b.*

  –outlines of objects were shaded by colors—*Gels.*

  –pale, objects were—*Agar., Cop., Dig., Eupi., Ind., Rhus t., Sil.*

  –paper, white, obscured vision—*Bell.*

  –pass before eyes, a dark veil would—*Nat. m.*

  –passed over eyes, a white cloud—*Sanic.*

    before left eye, fiery stars—*Card. b.*

    from eyes to light, rays of light—*Cham.*

  –pear-shaped obstruction before eyes—*Cund.*

  –phosphorescence on closing eyes, clouds of—*Dig.*

  –playing with his fingers before eyes, one were—*Psor.*

  –point, black, before right eye—*Elect.*

  –printed upon, paper were not (by artificial light)—*Aur. m.*

  –projected from forehead so that he could not see over it something were—*Phel.*

  –purple vertical bar before eyes—*Stram.*

    obstruction before right eye—*Cund.*

  –rainbow—*Bar. c., Bell., Bry., Cic., Con., Dig., Dign., Euph. Ferr. ma., Ip., Kali c., Kali n., Mim., Osm., Phos. ac., Phos. Stann., Stram., Sulph.*

  –rays of light passed from eyes to light—*Cham.*

  –receding, objects were—*Bell., Cic., Sep.*

  –red—*Atro., Bell., Cact., Cann. s., Cedr., Chin., Con., Croc. Cund., Dig., Elaps, Fl. ac., Hep., Hyos., Iodof., Mag. m. Nux m., Osm., Plat., Phos., Saba., Sars., Spig., Stram. Stront., Sulph.*

    at night, objects were—*Cedr.*

    objects look cherry—*Phos.*

Vision—*Continued*

    ink, letters were written in—*Phos.*

    circles—*Cact., Stront., Sulph., Verat. v.*

    disk or bar—*Elaps*

    halo—*Bell., Sil.*

    masses—*Spig.*

    sparks—*Fl. ac., Stry.*

    spots—*Cot., Hipp.*

—reflected from a bright copper plate at left side, a light were
    —*Oxyt.*

—room, brightly lighted in dark—*Elect.*

—rose before left eye impeding sight, a body—*Am. m.*

—rotating, objects were—*Atro., Bell.*

—round objects passing before eyes—*Caust.*

—saffron-colored—*Ind.*

—scales were before eyes obscuring sight—*Kali bi.*

    were before eyes—*Verat. v.*

—sea of fire even when eyes are closed, looking into a—*Phos.*

—serpents—*Arg. n., Cund., Ign., Phys.*

—serrated, objects were—*Hyos.*

—shadow flitted before eyes—*Ruta*

—shining shooting bodies before eyes—*Aloe*

    particles floating before eyes when closed—*Ars.*

    white points—*Cann. s.*

    spots—*Seneg., Verat. a.*

—sieve, one were looking through a—*Puls.*

—silvery clouds—*Bell.*

—small as dolls, people were—*Plb.*

    letters were—*All. c., Glon., Phys.*

    objects were—*Hyos., Merc. c., Op., Stram.*

—smoke before eyes—*Aur., Cyc., Gels., Kali m., Lach.*

    in air—*Stram.*

    in room—*Crot. t.*

    after using eyes a few moments, room were filled with—
      Croc.

    sees through—*Kali c.*

    in form of birds, animals and circles—*Ammc.*

—smoky before eyes—*Bell., Crot. t., Cyc., Gels., Mag. p. Ambo,
    Osm., Phos., Pic. ac., Plat., Stram., Sulph., Til.*

    room were—*Lac. ac., Osm., Thuj.*

Vision—*Continued*

 —snake were before vision—*Gels.*
  or worm before vision—*Phys.*
 —snow were dazzling before eyes—*Olnd.*
  objects were covered with—*Dig.*
 —snowflakes were falling—*Bell., Jab., Plb.*
  were falling straight down before eyes—*Camph. br.*
 —sparks—see the GENERAL REPERTORIES
 —sparks, electric, flashing before eyes in daytime—*Croc.*
 —speck, white, before eyes—*Rat.*
 —specks, black, before eyes—*Gels.*
 —spider-web over objects—*Carb. s.*
 —spots—*Act. sp., Cyc., Dig., Kali bi., Kali c., Hipp., Sil., Sol. n., Sulph.*
  black, before eyes—*Cocc., Glon., Sep., Syph.*
  bright, before eyes—*Gels.*
  dark, before eyes—*Dig.*
  dancing to and fro—*Ust.*
  floating—*Cann. i., Dig., Hell., Phos.*
  red, floating in field of vision—*Dub.*
 —spread over left eye, gauze were—*Sars.*
 —squinting—*Calc. c., Con., Coniin.*
  inward, eyes were—*Coca*
 —staring, eyes were—*Med.*
 —stars—*Ammc., Atro., Cast., Croc., Hyos., Sec., Puls., Tarent.*
  bright, danced before eyes—*Croc.*
  fiery, passed before left eye—*Card. b.*
 —straw hanging before each eye—*Merc.*
 —striped—*Am. c., Am. m., Bell., Cham., Cic., Con., Dig., Iod., Kali c., Nat. m., Phos., Puls., Sep.*
 —sun were flickering before eyes—*Lach.*
  were taking place, eclipse of—*Phys.*
  a few minutes before, objects appear as if one had looked at—*Podo.*
  one had been looking at—*Nit. ac.*
 —sunlight, she had gone out into bright—*Sep.*
 —surrounded by halo, light were—*Coff. t., Sulph., Tub.*
  by a hot vapor—*Bell.*
  by a white vapor—*Bell.*
 —swimming before eyes, net were—*Carb. an.*
  before eyes, letters were—*Bell., Coca*

Vision—*Continued*

before eyes, objects were—*Amyg., Carb. ac., Carl., Digit., Gins., Inul., Jab., Mez., Par., Sumb., Thuj., Til., Zinc.*

—tadpoles floated in mist before eyes—*Sep.*

danced before eyes—*Cimic.*

—tears were in it, dimness of eyes as if—*Ign.*

—thread before left eye, black woolen—*Thuj.*

—threads before eyes, she could not wipe away—*Sulph.*

were hanging before eyes—*Seneg.*

before eye on looking up—*Kali c.*

or line horizontally before right eye—*Con.*

white, moving before eyes—*Elaps*

were flickering before eye—*Lach.*

were hovering before eye—*Coca*

were swimming before eye—*Con.*

—totter and dance, objects seem to—*Sant.*

—trembling, vision tremulous as if eyes were—*Con.*

—triple, objects were—*Con., Sec.*

—tumult and confusion, everything in street appears (when looking through window)—*Camph.*

—vapor, white, before eyes—*Bell.*

—veil before eyes—*Acon., Agar., Am. c., Ant. t., Arum t., Arund., Asaf., Bell., Bov., Bry., Bufo, Calc. c., Calc. p., Carb. s., Carl., Caust., Clem., Croc., Crot. t., Cupr., Dig., Dros., Dulc., Euph., Euphr., Eupi., Gels., Hæm., Hep., Hyos., Ign., Iod., Laur., Lil. t., Lith., Lyc., Merl., Nat. m., Nat. p., Nit. ac., Op., Paraf., Petr., Phos., Pic. ac., Pin. s., Plat., Puls., Rat., Rhus t., Sec., Sil., Stram., Sulph., Syph., Tarent., Ther., Thuj., Til.*

between light and eyes—*Croc.*

eyes were covered by a—*Gent. c.*

were drawn before eyes—*Arum t.*

were hanging over eyes—*Hep.*

looking through a—*Berb., Bufo, Cocc., Lyc., Tab., Verb.*

black, before eyes—*Aur., Paraf., Phos.*

dark, will pass before eyes—*Nat. m.*

objects were covered with a gray—*Elaps, Phos.*

seen through a green—*Carb. s.*

looking through a lace—*Xanth.*

thick, before eyes—*Ant. t.*

thin, before eyes—*Eupi.*

11

Vision—*Continued*

    objects were covered with a thin—*Nat. m.*

    white, over objects—*Staph.*

—vessel of molten iron even when eyes are closed, looking into
    a—*Phos.*

—violet—*Cann. i., Elaps, Sant.*

—water, drops of—*Tab.*

    running—*Merc.*

    sheets of—*Raph.*

    which produced prismatic colors, one were looking through
      clear—*Oxyt.*

    objects were seen through—*Merc.*

    objects were seen through turbid—*Agar., Stram.*

—waves before eyes—*Phys.*

—web of spider were over objects—*Carb. s.*

—wheels turning and becoming larger, yellow—*Kali c.*

—whirling before eyes—*Psor.*

    before right eye as if it would become dark—*Eug.*

—white—*Alum., Am. c., Ars., Bell., Cann. s., Caust., Chel.,
    Chlol., Coca, Coloc., Con., Dig., Grat., Ign., Kali c., Phos.
    ac., Stry., Sulph.*

    drops falling—*Kali c.*

    gauze—*Ars.*

    blue-white—*Elaps, Nitro. o.*

    flames—*Chlf., Sep.*

    spots—*Acon., Ars., Coca, Gins., Mez., Phys., Rat., Sol. n.,
      Sulph., Ust.*

    stars—*Alum., Am. c., Bell., Kali c., Nat. c.*

    stripes—*Sol. n.*

    stripes when eyes are closed—*Bry.*

    vapor about objects—*Atro.*

    veil—*Staph.*

—wide enough, doorway were not—*Samars.*

—wipe away threads before eyes, she could not—*Sulph.*

    eyes to clear vision, he should—*Nat. m.*

—worm on carpet, he saw a—*Atro.*

—wrapped in fog, eyes were—*Petr.*

—written in red ink, letters were—*Phos.*

—yellow—*Agar., Aloe, Alum., Aml. n., Am. m., Ars., Bell.,
    Cann. i., Canth., Carb. an., Carb. s., Cedr., Chin., Cina, Cot.,
    Cyc., Crot. h., Dig., Digit., Hyos., Kali c., Lachn., Mang.,*

Vision—*Continued*

    Nat. s., Osm., Peti., Phos., Plb., Sant., Sep., Sil., Stront., Sulph., Tab., Zinc.

    during day, objects were—*Cedr.*

    haze of light, objects were in—*Sant.*

    mist enveloped objects—*Kali bi.*

Waking from sleep, lids were—*Mang.*

Warts, surface of eyeball studded with—*Euphr.*

Water in eyes—*Spig.*

  –were before eyes, drop of—*Tab.*

  –were constantly coming into eyes, only in warm room—*Croc.*

  –which produced prismatic colors, one were looking through clear—*Oxyt.*

  –twitched about in eyes—*Stram.*

  –warm, flowing over right to left and from eyes—*Nit. ac.*

  –eyes were swimming in—*Chin., Sil., Squill.*

  –objects were seen through—*Merc.*

  –objects were seen through turbid—*Agar., Stram.*

  –between lids, drops of cold—*Berb.*

  –eyes were full of—*Staph.*

  –would be pressed out of eyes—*Laur.*

  –hot, right eye were bathed in—*Am. br.*

  –left eye were full of—*Sil.*

  –hot, in eye—*Nux v.*

  –running—*Merc.*

  –sheets of—*Raph.*

Waves before eyes—*Phys.*

Weak and dull looking, eyes were—*Rheum*

Web of spider were over objects—*Carb. s.*

Weeping violently, she had been (in conjunctiva)—*Croc.*

  –in left eye, going to right, had been—*Croc.*

  –she had been—*Cedr., Guare., Kali p.*

  –she had been (felt in lids)—*Magnol.*

  –but had not, had been—*Sa:. lac.*

Weight pressed down into eyes—*Phos.*

  –above eyes—*Cist.*

  –heavy, over eyes—*Sil.*

  –heavy, were within eyes—*Aml. n.*

  –behind right orbit—*Rhus t.*

  –at night, eyelids were held down by a—*Croc.*

  –great, on eyelids—*Anan.*

Weight—*Continued*

  —eyeballs and lids were pressed by a heavy—*Corn.*
  —upper lids were pressed down by a heavy—*Con.*
  —heavy, rested on eyes—*Carb. v.*
  —round, were resting on right eye—*Lepi.*
  —were attached to back of eyes—*Sep.*

Wept much, she had—*Croc., Zinc.*

Wheels turning and becoming larger, yellow—*Kali c.*

Whirling before eyes—*Psor.*

  —in eyes—*Bov., Cist.*
  —before right eye as if it would become dark—*Eug.*

White—*Alum., Am. c., Ars., Bell., Cann. s., Caust., Chel., Chlol., Coca, Coloc., Con., Dig., Grat., Ign., Kali c., Phos. ac., Stry., Sulph.*

  —drops falling—*Kali c.*
  —gauze—*Ars.*
  —blue-white—*Elaps, Nitro. o.*
  —flames—*Chlf., Sep.*
  —spots—*Acon., Ars., Coca, Gins., Mez., Phys., Rat., Sol. n., Sulph., Ust.*
  —stars—*Alum., Am. c., Bell., Kali c., Nat. c.*
  —stripes—*Sol. n.*
  —stripes when eyes are closed—*Bry.*
  —vapor about objects—*Atro.*
  —veil—*Staph.*

Wide enough, doorway were not—*Samars.*

Wind, had been out in—*Samars.*

  —biting in eye as from being in—*Merc.*
  —blew out of sockets, eyes were gone and—*Sep., Sulph.*
  —were blowing in them, eyes were opened by force and fresh—*Fl. ac.*
  —cold, blowing in eyes—*Med., Paraf., Syph.*
  —cold, blowing under eyelids—*Fl. ac.*
  —cool, blowing across eyes—*Berb., Croc.*
  —cold, blowing into sore eyes from ears—*Alum.*
  —cold, in eyes—*Berb.*

Wink constantly, he must—*Fl. ac.*

Wipe away threads before eyes, she could not—*Sulph.*

  —eyes to clear vision, he should—*Nat. m.*

Wiped from eyes, something would be—*Croc.*

  —dry, conjunctiva—*Leon.*

Wrapped in a fog, eyes were—*Petr.*
Written in red ink, letters were—*Phos.*
Worm on carpet, he saw a—*Atro.*
Yellow—*Agar., Aloe, Alum., Aml. n., Am. m., Ars., Bell., Cann. i., Canth., Carb. an., Carb. s., Cedr., Chin., Cina, Cot., Cyc., Crot. h., Dig., Digit., Hyos., Kali c., Lachn., Mang., Nat. s., Osm., Peti., Phos., Plb., Sant., Sep., Sil., Stront., Sulph., Tab., Zinc.*
  –during day, objects were—*Cedr.*
  –haze of light, objects were in—*Sant.*
  –mist enveloped objects—*Kali bi.*

EARS AND HEARING

Abscess would form in ear—*Ment.*
  —would open in ears—*Caps.*
Air in ears—*Mez.*
  —cold, in ears—*Dulc., Plat.*
  —cold, were blowing into ears—*Act. sp., Alum., Sanic.*
  —cold, were blowing on ears—*Mag. p. Aust.*
  —were coming out of ears, alternate currents of cold and warm —*Verat. a.*
  —bubble in left ear—*Nat. m.*
  —bubble were pushed through Eustachian tube in middle of ear and burst with tingling—*Sil.*
  —catches itself in left Eustachian tube—*Tell.*
  —tympanum were exposed to cold—*Mez.*
  —distending right external meatus then left—*Mez.*
  —ear were filled with compressed—*Cur.*
  —were forced out of ears—*Puls.*
  —were forced into ears on blowing nose—*Sulph.*
  —were forced through Eustachian tube on eructation—*Graph.*
  —cold, were passing out of ears—*Mill.*
  —could penetrate ears, opening and closing mouth would open a way—*Thuj.*
  —penetrated Eustachian tube—*Graph.*
  —penetrates ear on blowing nose—*Puls.*
  —were pouring into ear or tympanum were exposed—*Mez., Staph.*
  —to ear were prevented, free access of—*Thuj.*
  —were rushing into meatus auditorius—*Amph.*
  —cold, were rushing into ear—*Caust., Lachn.*
  —were streaming into right ear—*Sarr.*
  —whistled through left Eustachian tube—*Tell.*
Alive in ear, something were—*Rhus t., Sil.*
Animals were burrowing in ear—*Am. m., Ant. c.*
  —were crying in ears—*Cur.*
Artery, large, were throbbing behind ear—*Ang.*
Asleep, right ear were—*Calad.*
  —outer ear were—*Sulph.*
Balls, little, circulated in ears—*Galvan.*

Band were about ear—*Mag. p. Arct.*
 −were over ear—*Am. br., Sul. ac.*
 −or cord were drawn tightly from ear to ear—*Anac.*
 −were pressing about ears—*Ther.*
 −were pulling lower part of ear downward—*Thuj.*
Bat in ears, sound of—*Mill., Phos. ac.*
Battery of guns discharged in ear—*Spong.*
Beating in ear, sound of distant—*Mez.*
 −against a door causing a din, sound in ears—*Ant. c.*
 −a drum, something were—*Sil.*
 −on an iron bar, tremulous tingling in ears—*Puls.*
Bee were fluttering in ear—*Sal. ac., Samars.*
Bees buzzing in ears, a swarm of—*Sal. ac.*
 −humming in ears—*Abrot., Nux v.*
Bell struck, forcing him to get up at night—*Sil.*
Bells were ringing in ears—*Am. c., Arund., Chin. s., Coca, Gas., Hyos., Led., Nat. s., Mez., Phos. ac., Sil., Sul. ac., Valer.*
 −were ringing in the distance—*Agar., Coff. t., Der., Nat. s.*
 −were tolling—*Sars.*
Binding up in ears—*Nat. n.*
Bird were fluttering in ear—*Ant. t., Cham., Mag. c., Phos. ac., Plat., Spig., Tab.*
 −large, were fluttering before left ear—*Ant. t.*
 −wings fluttering momentarily in ears—*Nat. m.*
 −wings, rushing in ears of—*Mosch.*
Birds were warbling in ears—*Bell., Bry.*
Biting of electric sparks on ear—*Phel.*
Bladder full of water were cracking in ear—*Sulph.*
Blood would burst through ear—*Meli.*
 −would burst out of ear lobes—*Pyrog.*
 −rushed to right ear—*Lyss.*
 −hot, rushed into ears—*Lyc.*
Blow in inner ears, dull pressure from—*Cham.*
 −below mastoid bone—*Ruta*
Blowing in ears, sound of—*Hydrc., Ox. ac.*
 −into ears, someone were—*Ail., Sep., Rhus t.*
 −horn in ears, sound of—*Kalm.*
Board were before left ear—*Arg. m.*
Body, foreign, in ear—*Astac., Phos.*
 −foreign, before drum—*Calc. ar.*
 −foreign, in Eustachian tube—*Nux m.*

Body—*Continued*

 –foreign, obstructed right ear—*Astac.*

 –hard and large as an egg behind ear—*Graph.*

 –rough, in Eustachian tube—*Nux m.*

 –thick, were being forcibly driven into ear—*Puls.*

Boiling water in ears, sound of—*Cann. i., Lyc., Thuj.*

 –water were hissing before ears—*Dig.*

 –water were roaring in ears—*Chlf.*

Boring in anterior wall of canal, worms were—*Med.*

Breath came from ears instead of respiratory organs—*Psor.*

Breathing, warm, on outer ear—*Mag. p. Aust.*

Break, ear would gather and—*Spong.*

Bruised, ear were—*Arn., Stry., Vib.*

 –cartilage of ear were—*Arn.*

 –beneath ear—*Zinc.*

Bubble of air were pushed through Eustachian tube and burst in middle of ear with tingling—*Sil.*

 –bursting of soap bubble in—*Nat. c., Puls., Sulph.*

Bubbles of air in ears—*Hur., Lyc.*

Bubbling in right ear, liquid were—*Thuj.*

Burning on coming from cold to warm room, ears were—*Kali n.*

 –from a coal in ear—*Tep.*

Burrowing in ears, animals were—*Ant. c.*

 –in ear and would come out, something were—*Am. m.*

Burst in ear, something would—*Card. b., Hell., Psor.*

 –on going to sleep, drums of ears—*Rhus t.*

 –on sneezing, ear would—*Puls.*

Bursting in ears, air bubbles were—*Card. b., Graph., Nat. m.*

 –in ears—*Aml. n., Calc. caust., Caust., Lyc., Nit. ac., Psor.*

 –in ear, leaflet were—*Gamb.*

 –in ears, soap-bubble were—*Nat. c., Puls., Sulph.*

Buzzing—see SOUND

Cannonading in ears, sound of—*Chel., Mosch.*

 –thundering in ears of distant—*Plat.*

Cascade—see also RUSHING and WATER

Cascade, sound of—*Rhus t.*

Cat spitting in ears, sound of—*Nit. ac.*

Chirping in ear, crickets were—*Carb. v., Euph., Ferr., Sil.*

 –in ear, grasshopper were—*Stann., Tarax.*

 –in ear, locust were—*Nux v.*

Cleft behind ear—*Am. c.*

Clinking in ears—*Aml. n.*
Closed—see also the GENERAL REPERTORIES
Closed, ears were—*Brom., Glon., Manc., Mar., Lachn., Merc. i. f., Nat. c., Nit. s. d., Puls. n., Spig., Tab.*
  –ears, something—*Lachn., Tell.*
  –ears suddenly—*Tanac., Tell., Verb.*
  –from within, ear were—*Ars., Lach.*
  –with a finger, ear were—*Spig.*
  –and deaf, ear were—*Cocc., Merc. i. f., Nit. ac.*
  –on blowing nose, ear were—*Calc. c., Con., Mar.*
  –external auditory passages were—*Coc. c.*
  –and opened—*Bor.*
  –or plugged with some foreign substance—*Asar.*
Clucking in ear—*Agar., Cadm. s., Sep.*
Coal, red-hot, in right ear—*Tep.*
Coals glowing in small spots on ear—*Caust.*
Coldness in ears with numbness extending to cheeks and lips—*Tell.*
Come out of right ear, something would—*Am. m.*
Compressed air, ear were filled with—*Cur.*
Connected, ear and throat were—*Am. m.*
Constricted, ear were—*Verat. a.*
Contracted, left ear were—*Caust.*
Cord or band were drawn tightly from ear to ear—*Anac.*
Cotton were in ears—*Cyc., Psor.*
  –or plug were in ear—*Anac.*
Coughed into an empty tube, sounds as if he had—*Osm.*
Cracking, drum had burst with—*Rhus t.*
  –from bladder full of water in ear—*Sulph.*
  –of whip in ear, sound of—*Sulph.*
Crackling in ear—*Alum., Aur., Azad., Bar. c., Calc. c., Carb. v., Coc. c., Dulc., Eup. pur., Glon., Graph., Hep., Hipp., Kali c., Mar., Mosch., Rheum, Saba., Sep., Spig.*
  –of electric sparks in ears—*Ambr., Hep., Spig.*
  –paper in ears, sound of—*Sep.*
  –of straw on motion of jaws, sound of—*Carb. v.*
Crash of breaking glass in ears—*Zinc.*
Crawling in ear—*Psor., Spong.*
  –in right ear—*Med.*
  –in left ear—*Rhod.*
  –over ear—*Pic. ac.*

Crawling—*Continued*
  —out of ear, something were—*Puls.*
  —in ear, worm were—*Med., Pic. ac., Rhod.*
Creaking in ear—*Agar., Graph., Stann., Thuj.*
  —like turning of wooden screw in ear—*Thuj.*
Creeping in ear—*Stry.*
  —into ear, water were—*Rhod.*
  —of worm in left ear—*Rhod.*
Cricket twittering in ear—*Puls.*
Crickets chirping in ear—*Carb. v., Euph., Ferr., Sil.*
  —were singing in ear—*Caust., Cedr.*
Croaking in ear, frogs were—*Mag. s., Mang.*
Crying in ear, animals were—*Cur.*
Cymbals and drums sounded in ear—*Lob.*
Deaf—*Bar. c., Coc. c., Nit. ac.*
  —but could hear everything—*Coca, Merc. i. f.*
Detonating in ears—*Itu*
Digging in ear with blunt piece of wood—*Ruta*
Distended, ear were—*Bell., Kali i., Laur., Nit. ac., Puls., Til.*
Diving, sound in ears as when—*Raph.*
Drawing together and ear would burst—*Hell.*
    —together internally, > boring finger in ear—*Bor., Coloc., Lachn., Mez.*
Drawn inward, left ear would be—*Verb.*
  —out of head, ear were—*Cann. s.*
  —over ear, skin were—*Bell.*
  —over ear on which she was lying, parchment were—*Med.*
  —over ear and tickling, a veil were—*Phos.*
Dropping in ear when lying down, water were—*Nat. p.*
  —from a height into a long round vessel, water were—*Nat. p.*
Drumming in ear, sound of—*Bell., Bor., Canth., Cupr., Dros., Dulc., Manc.*
  —in left ear as over a subterranean vault—*Bor.*
Dry, ears were very—*Sulph.*
Dull, hearing were very; but sensitive to the most minute sounds —*Phyt.*
Echoes in ear—*Ant. c., Caust., Lyc.*
Electric sparks biting on ear—*Phel.*
  —sparks crackling in ear—*Hep., Spig.*
  —sparks snapping in ear—*Ambr.*
Enveloped, ear were—*Bor.*

Explosion and clashing in left ear from breaking glass—*Aloe*
Fallen before ear, something had—*Verb.*
 --in front of drum, something had—*Spig.*
 --to floor and burst ears, something heavy had—*Saba.*
Fanning before ears—*Calc. c.*
Feather were tickling in ear, < opening mouth—*Azad.*
Filled with compressed air, ears were—*Cur.*
 --with water, ears were—*Lac butyr.*
 --with water, left ear were—*Graph.*
 --with water, external meatus were—*Thuj.*
Flapping of wings in ears—*Jac.*
Flea were in ear—*Mosch., Zinc.*
 --in meatus—*Hæm.*
Fluid were pushing outward in ear—*Coc. c.*
Flowing from ear, humor were—*Sil.*
 --in a circle around right ear, warm water were—*Calad.*
Fluttering in ear—*Carl., Cupr., Mag. m., Merc., Merc. d., Puls. n., Sel., Sil., Spig., Sulph.*
 --in ear, bee were—*Sal. ac., Samars.*
 --in ear, bird were—*Ant. t., Cham., Mag. c., Phos. ac., Plat., Spig., Tab.*
 --before left ear like a large bird—*Ant. t.*
 --in ears of bird wings, momentarily—*Nat. m.*
 --butterfly were--*Nat. m.*
 --from opening and shutting in ear—*Iris fœ.*
Fly were enclosed in auditory meatus—*Elaps*
Force out of ear, something were trying to—*Casc., Caust.*
Forced into ear, something were—*Lyc.*
 --out with each pulse beat, membrana tympani would be—*Aml. n.*
Forcing its way out of ear, something were—*Merc., Nat. s., Puls.*
 --ear apart, wedge were—*Par.*
 --toward ear, something were—*Lyc.*
 --hot blood into ear—*Lyc.*
 --of brain through skull (felt in ear)—*Nat. m.*
Frostbitten and tingling, cartilage of ears were—*Sac. lac.*
Frozen, ears had been—*Agar.*
Full, ears were—*Eup. pur., Lac c.*
Galvanic rays were passing through ears—*Galvan.*
Gather and break, ears would—*Spong.*
Gathering in left ear, there were—*Sac. lac.*

Gauze before ear—*Phos.*

Gnawing in ear, something were—*Led.*

Grasshopper were chirping in ear—*Stann., Tarax.*

  —rustling in ear—*Stann.*

Groaning in ear—*Thuj.*

Grunting in ear when swallowing—*Calc. c.*

Guns were discharged in ears, a battery of—*Spong.*

  —in ears, reports of—*Cann. i.*

Gurgling in ears—*Castor.*

  —of water in ears—*Sulph.*

Hand over right ear, he were holding—*Chel.*

Hear but she can, she could not—*Sac. lac.*

Heard with ears not his own—*Psor.*

Heat were escaping from ears—*Æth., Calc. c., Clem., Kali c., Ol an., Par.*

  —burning, were rushing out of ears—*Par.*

  —in ears from standing near stove—*Ant. t., Mang.*

  —were streaming out of ears—*Sulph.*

  —were streaming out of right ear—*Æth.*

Heavy lay before ears, something—*Carb. v.*

  —had fallen to floor and burst ears, something—*Saba.*

Hissing in ears—*Acon., Cahin., Calc. c., Chin. s., Graph., Ill., Lyc., Mar., Nat. s., Pic. ac., Sil., Sumb.*

  —of boiling water before ears—*Dig.*

Hollow, ears were—*Nux v.*

  —and open, ears were—*Aur. m.*

Horn were blowing in ears—*Kalm.*

Hot coal in right ear, red—*Tep.*

  —were streaming from ear, something—*Canth.*

  —were streaming out of right ear, something—*Æth.*

Humming—see Sound

Humming in ear, spinning-wheel were—*Agar.*

Humor were flowing from ear—*Sil.*

Ice were drawn over ear and face—*Til.*

Insect were entering left ear, > boring finger in—*Thlaspi*

Insects were humming in ear—*Meny.*

  —were whizzing in ear—*Lach.*

Instrument in ear, sharp pointed—*Berb.*

  —sharp, were thrust into left ear—*Genist.*

  —someone were quickly pressing tympanum with blunt—*Carb. s.*

umping in ear, flea were—*Zinc.*

–in ear, something were—*Spig.*

Kettledrums in ears, din of—*Bell.*

Knife, dull, were pressing in ear interiorly and superiorly—*Lyss.*

–were stabbing in ears—*Vib.*

Landslide, sound in ears of far-off—*Cinch. b.*

Lay before ear, something heavy—*Carb. v.*

–before ear on blowing nose, something—*Alum.*

–in front of membrana tympani, something—*Calc. c.*

Leaf were lying before ear—*Sul. ac.*

–were lying before tympanum—*Ant. c.*

Leaflet were bursting in ear—*Gamb.*

Liquid were bubbling in right ear—*Thuj.*

–were running from ear—*Mill.*

Locomotive rushing in ear, sound of—*Agar.*

Locusts chirping in ear—*Nux v.*

–singing in ear—*Rhus t.*

Lying before ear, something were—*Mag. m.*

Machinery in ear, sound of—*Hydrs.*

Matter were in ear, or flowing from—*Sil.*

Membrane in front of ear—*Asaf., Cann. s., Sel., Verat. a.*

–of ear would be forced out at each heart beat—*Aml. n.*

–were stretched over ear—*Verat. a.*

Mice, young, were twittering in ear—*Rhus t.*

Mill in ears, sound of—*Cit. v., Iod.*

–in head when waking, sound of—*Naja*

–at a distance, sound of—*Bry., Mez.*

Mist before ear—*Par.*

–were thick in front of ear—*Spig.*

Moisture in ear—*Bry.*

Moved in ear on swallowing, something—*Nat. c.*

Muffled by an obstruction from within, right ear were—*Chen. v.*

Murmuring of water in ear—*Petr.*

–of boiling water in ear—*Mag. p. Arct.*

Music in ears—*Puls., Sal. ac., Sarr.*

Nail were driven from meatus through head—*Tarent.*

–were driven into a board at a distance, sound of—*Agar.*

–were stitching in ear—*Berb.*

Narrow, ear were too—*Lyc.*

Narrowed, meatus were—*Asaf.*

Needle, cold, were stitching in internal ear—*Agar.*

Noise—see Sound
Noise in left ear came from heart—*Glon.*
Noises—see Sound
Numb, ears were—*Plat.*
Obstructed, ears were—*Caust., Chen. v., Lyc., Saba.*
  –by cotton, ears were—*Led.*
  –by plug, ears were—*Elec.*
Open and hollow, ears were—*Aur. m.*
  –ears were too—*Mez.*
Opened and closed, ears—*Bor.*
Opening and closing in right ear like a fluttering—*Iris fœ.*
  –in right ear through which air could penetrate on opening or
      closing mouth, there were—*Thuj.*
  –and closing of valve in left ear, < in afternoon—*Psor.*
Parchment were drawn over ear on which she was lying—*Med.*
Passing from left ear to throat, something were—*Sal. ac.*
  –out of ears, water were—*Calc. c., Spi j., Sulph.*
  –out of ears, wind were—*Æth., Calc. c., Chel., Mill., Psor.*
Penetrated ear, hot water—*Euphr.*
  –ears to meet in center, two plugs—*Anac.*
Piercing outward in ear, sharp pointed instrument were—*Berb.*
Pinned to head, ear were—*Vib.*
Piston were working up and down in ear—*Aml. n.*
Plug or cotton in ear—*Anac.*
  –in right ear—*Lob.*
  –ear were obstructed by—*Elec.*
  –were pressing in ear—*Spig.*
  –right ear were suddenly stopped by—*Lob.*
Plugged by some foreign substance, ears were—*Asar.*
  –up in ears—*Ant. c., Aur. m., Chin. s., Parth., Sep.*
Plugs, two, penetrated ears to meet in center—*Anac.*
Pressed out, ears were—*Par.*
  –outward in ears—*Nux v.*
  –together internally, ears were—*Dros.*
  –in or torn out, ears were alternately—*Bell.*
  –against head, ears were—*Mosch.*
Pressing in ear, dull knife were—*Lyss.*
  –in ear, plug were—*Spig.*
  –on tympanum with dull instrument, someone were quickly—
      Carb. s.
  –of spectacles on ear—*Ant. c.*

Pressure, dull, as from blow in inner ear—*Cham.*
  —of fingers in meatus—*Rheum*
Prevented hearing, something before ear—*Calad.*
Puffed out of ear on swallowing, wind were—*Meli.*
Rain in ears, sound of—*Bov.*
  —striking ground, sound of—*Rhus t.*
Rattling of paper in ear, sound of—*Sep.*
Re-echoing in ears—*Caust., Ether., Gas., Merc., Nit. ac., Phos.,*
    Phos. ac., Puls., Rhod.
Relaxed, ear drums were—*Rheum*
  —meatus were—*Mez.*
Reports in ears—*Eup. pur., Nit. ac., Staph.*
  —of guns in ears—*Cann. i.*
  —of distant shots in ears—*Am. c.*
Reverberation in ears—*Bar. c., Cop.*
Ringing—see the GENERAL REPERTORIES
Ringing, beginning deep then becoming higher—*Berb.*
  —bells were—*Am. c., Arun., Chin. s., Coca, Gas., Hyos., Led.,*
    Nat. s., Mez., Phos. ac., Sil., Sul. ac., Valer.
  —in the distance, bells were—*Agar., Coff. t., Der., Nat. s.*
  —distant, in ears—*All. c., Arg. n., Coca, Spig.*
  —of high-sounding glasses—*Merc.*
  —in ears like music—*Ail., Phos.*
River running in ears, sound of—*Cact.*
Roaring—see the GENERAL REPERTORIES
Roaring would occur—*Mez.*
  —in ears if he takes a few steps—*Colch.*
  —of a conch-shell in ears—*Rumx.*
  —of distant noises in ears—*Pimp., Puls.*
  —in ears like draft through a stove—*Thuj.*
  —as from bird fluttering—*Plat.*
  —like a partridge drumming—*Hydrs.*
  —as of blood rushing to head—*Petr.*
  —of storm in a forest—*Coc. c.*
  —like water in ears—*Mag. s.*
  —of boiling water in ears—*Chlf.*
  —of rushing water in ears—*Cham., Mag. c.*
  —of waterfall in ears—*Sul. ac.*
  —of wind in ears—*Asar., Caust., Chel., Con., Croc., Led., Mag.*
    c., Petr., Verat. a.
Rolled back and forth in ears on shaking head, something—*Ruta*

Running in ears, warm water were—*Glon.*
  –from ears, ice-cold water were, recurring—*Merc.*
  –out of right ear, hot water were—*Cham.*
  –in ears, sound of river—*Cact.*
Rushing in ear of a stream of blood—*Stann.*
  –through small hole in ear, steam were—*Dig.*
  –into ears, water were—*Rhod., Sulph.*
  –of fulling-machine heard in ears—*Nux v.*
  –like locomotive in ear—*Agar.*
  –of escaping steam in ear—*Glon.*
  –of storm in ear—*Bor.*
  –of bird wings in ear—*Mosch.*
  –in ears as when listening at tube—*Cocc.*
  –of water in ears, sound of—*Cham., Cocc., Kali n., Mag. c.,*
      Nitro. o., Petr., Puls.
  –in ears of water falling—*Lyss.*
  –as of waterfall—*Ars., Caust.*
  –of wind out of ears—*Abrot., Mosch., Sulph.*
Rustling of grasshopper in left ear—*Stann.*
Scraping ear with a blunt piece of wood, someone were—*Ruta*
Scratching ear, spear of grain were—*Plb.*
Screaming sound in ear on blowing nose—*Phos. ac., Stann.*
Screw behind each ear—*Ox. ac.*
  –in ears, creaking of a wooden—*Agar.*
Screwed in in front of ears—*Sul. ac.*
Seashell in left ear, sound of—*Ter.*
Sharp instrument were thrust into left ear—*Genist.*
  –pointed instrument in ear—*Berb.*
Singing of crickets in ear—*Caust., Cedr.*
  –of locust in ear—*Rhus t.*
  –in ear like steam escaping—*Phys.*
  –like wind in ear—*Carb. s.*
Skin were stretched over right external ear—*Asar.*
  –were stretched before ears—*Graph.*
  –were drawn over ears—*Bell.*
Snapping in ear—*Puls. n.*
Something were before drum—*Spig.*
  –were in ear—*Card. b., Symph.*
  –were before ear—*Acon., Alum., Ang., Bry., Calad., Card. b.,*
      Chin., Cocc., Cyc., Kali n., Merl., Phos., Sulph.

Sound:
 –air whistled through left Eustachian tube—*Tell.*
 –of animals crying—*Cur.*
 –bat in ear—*Mill., Phos. ac.*
 –beating, distant—*Mez.*
 –beating against a door (a din)—*Ant. c.*
 –bees—*Sal. ac., Samars.*
   humming—*Abrot., Nux v.*
 –bells ringing—*Am. c., Arund., Chin. s., Coca, Gas., Hyos., Led., Mez., Nat. s., Phos. ac., Sil., Sul. ac., Valer.*
   ringing in the distance—*Agar., Coff. t., Der., Nat. s.*
   tolling—*Sars.*
 –bird fluttering—*Ant. t., Cham., Mag. c., Phos. ac., Plat., Spig., Tab.*
   wings fluttering momentarily—*Nat. m.*
   wings rushing—*Mosch.*
 –birds warbling—*Bell., Bry.*
 –blowing—*Hydrc., Ox. ac.*
   of horn—*Kalm.*
 –boiling water—*Bry., Cann. i., Chlf., Lyc., Thuj.*
 –bubbling liquid in right ear—*Thuj.*
 –buzzing—*Acon., Alco., Aloe, Arg. n., Bar. c., Bell., Cact., Cahin., Canch., Cann. i., Carl., Chel., Chen. a., Chin. s., Coff., Cop., Dios., Elaps, Glon., Kalm., Lyss., Mag. m., Nicc., Nux m., Phos., Pic. ac., Psor., Rhod., Ricin., Saba., Sul. i., Tarent., Thuj.*
   of flies—*Sal. ac.*
   insect entering left ear—*Thlaspi*
 –cannonading—*Chel., Mosch.*
 –cascade—*Rhus t.*
 –cat spitting—*Nit. ac.*
 –clashing of breaking glass—*Aloe*
 –clock striking—*Mang., Ter.*
 –clucking—*Agar., Cadm. s., Sep.*
 –coughed into an empty tube, one had—*Osm.*
 –cracking from a bursting drum—*Rhus t.*
   of a whip—*Sulph.*
 –crackling—*Alum., Aur., Bar. c., Bor., Calc. c., Carb. v., Coc. c., Dulc., Eup. pur., Glon., Graph., Hep., Hipp., Kali c., Mar., Mosch., Rheum, Saba., Sep., Spig.*
   of electric sparks—*Hep., Spig.*

Sound—*Continued*

> of paper—*Sep.*
> of straw on motion of jaws—*Carb. v.*
> –crash of breaking glass—*Aloe, Zinc.*
> –creaking—*Agar., Graph., Stann., Thuj.*
> –cricket twittering—*Puls.*
> –crickets chirping—*Carb. v., Euph., Ferr., Sil.*
>> singing—*Caust., Cedr.*
> –croaking of frogs—*Mag. s., Mang.*
> –cymbals and drums—*Lob.*
> –drumming—*Bell., Bor., Canth., Cupr., Dros., Dulc., Manc.*
> –drums and cymbals—*Lob.*
> –explosion and clashing in left ear as breaking glass—*Aloe*
> –fallen on floor, something heavy had—*Saba.*
> –far-off landslide—*Cinch. b.*
> –flies buzzing—*Sal. ac.*
> –fluttering—*Carl., Cupr., Mag. m., Merc., Merc. d., Puls. n., Sel., Sil., Spig., Sulph.*
>> of a bird—*Ant. t., Cham., Mag. c., Phos. ac., Plat., Spig., Tab.*
>> of bird wings, momentarily—*Nat. m.*
>> of butterfly—*Nat. m.*
> –frogs croaking—*Mag. s., Mang.*
> –glass crashing—*Aloe, Zinc.*
> –grasshopper chirping—*Stann., Tarax.*
>> rustling—*Stann.*
> –groaning—*Thuj.*
> –grunting when swallowing—*Calc. c.*
> –guns were discharged, a battery of—*Spong.*
>> reports of—*Cann. i.*
> –gurgling—*Castor.*
>> water—*Sulph.*
> –hissing—*Acon., Cahin., Calc. c., Chin. s., Graph., Ill., Lyc., Mar., Nat. s., Pic. ac., Sil., Sumb.*
> –humming—*Acon., All. s., Amyg., Anac., Arn., Ars., Aur., Bell., Bry., Carb. ac., Calc. c., Carb. s., Carb. v., Card. b., Carl., Chel., Cinch., Cob., Con., Cop., Der., Ferr., Fer. g., Gels., Glon., Graph., Jal., Kali c., Lyc., Merc. c., Mez., Nat. m., Nit. ac., Op., Plb., Puls., Rhod., Ricin., Saba., Sang., Seneg., Sep., Stry., Tab., Verat. v., Zing.*
>> of bees—*Abrot., Nux v.*

Sound—*Continued*

  –insect buzzing and entering left ear—*Thlaspi*
  –insects humming—*Meny.*
  –kettledrum, din of—*Bell.*
  –liquid bubbling in right ear—*Thuj.*
  –locust singing in ear—*Rhus t.*
  –locusts chirping—*Nux v.*
  –machinery—*Hydrs.*
  –mice were twittering—*Rhus t.*
  –mill in ears—*Cit. v., Iod.*
    at a distance—*Bry., Mez.*
    going in head when waking—*Naja*
  –murmuring of water—*Petr.*
    of boiling water—*Mag. p. Arct.*
  –music—*Puls., Sal. ac., Sarr.*
    ringing—*Ail., Phos.*
  –nail were being driven into board at a distance—*Agar.*
  –noises—see the GENERAL REPERTORIES
  –paper crackling—*Sep.*
  –rain—*Bov.*
    striking the ground—*Rhus t.*
  –re-echoing—*Caust., Ether., Gas., Merc., Nit. ac., Phos., Phos.*
    ac., Puls., Rhod.
  –reports—*Eup. pur., Nit. ac., Staph.*
    of distant shots—*Am. c.*
    of gun—*Cann. i.*
  –reverberation—*Bar. c., Cop.*
  –ringing—see the GENERAL REPERTORIES
  –ringing beginning deep then becoming higher—*Berb.*
    distant—*All. c., Arg. n., Coca, Spig.*
    of bells—*Am. c., Arund., Chin. s., Coca, Gas., Hyos., Led.,*
      Nat. s., Mez., Phos. ac., Sil., Sul. ac., Valer.
    in the distance, bells were—*Agar., Coff. t., Der., Nat. s.*
    of high-sounding glasses—*Merc.*
    like music—*Ail., Phos.*
  –roaring—see the GENERAL REPERTORIES
  –roaring if he takes a few steps—*Colch.*
    of distant noise—*Pimp., Puls.*
    like draft through a stove—*Thuj.*
    as from a bird fluttering—*Plat.*
    like a partridge drumming—*Hydrs.*

Sound—*Continued*

as of blood rushing to the head—*Petr.*

of a storm in a forest—*Coc. c.*

like water—*Mag. s.*

of boiling water—*Chlf.*

of rushing water—*Cham., Mag. c.*

of waterfall—*Sul. ac.*

of wind—*Asar., Caust., Chel., Con., Croc., Led., Mag. c., Petr., Verat. a.*

–running of river—*Cact.*

–rushing of fulling-machine—*Nux v.*

like a locomotive—*Agar.*

of escaping steam—*Glon.*

of storm—*Bor.*

of bird wings—*Mosch.*

as when listening at a tube—*Cocc.*

of water—*Cham., Cocc., Kali n., Mag. c., Nitro. o., Petr., Puls.*

of falling water—*Lyss.*

of waterfall—*Ars., Caust.*

of wind out of ears— *Abrot., Mosch., Sulph.*

–rustling of grasshopper in left ear—*Stann.*

–screaming in ear on blowing nose—*Phos. ac., Stann.*

–seashell in left ear—*Ter.*

–singing of crickets—*Caust., Cedr.*

of locusts—*Nux v.*

like steam escaping—*Phys.*

of teakettle—*Tarent.*

like wind—*Carb. s.*

–snapping—*Puls. n.*

–sounding-board when breathing—*Bar. c.*

–spinning-wheel humming—*Agar.*

–spitting of cat—*Nit. ac.*

–spurting liquid—*Thuj.*

–steam in left ear—*Dig., Sal. ac.*

escaping—*Phys.*

rush of escaping—*Glon.*

were rushing through a small hole in ear—*Dig.*

–strange in his ears, his voice were—*Tanac.*

–straw were crackling in ears on motion of jaw—*Carb. v.*

–striking, clock were—*Mang., Ter.*

Sound—*Continued*
 –teakettle beginning to boil at a distance—*Agar.*
   singing—*Tarent.*
 –thunder rumbling—*Elaps*
 –thundering—*Am. m., Carb. o., Caust., Gas., Graph., Lach., Sil.*
   like distant cannonading—*Plat.*
 –ticking—*Chin., Nat. m., Petr., Ter.*
 –tick-tack—*Gad.*
 –tinkling—*Atro.*
 –trumpets, din like—*Bell., Gas.*
 –tube, one had coughed into an empty—*Osm.*
   rushing as when listening at a—*Cocc.*
 –twittering—*Calad.*
   of cricket—*Puls.*
   like young mice—*Rhus t.*
 –vibration of string of an instrument—*Cann. s.*
 –voice sounds strange in his ears, his own—*Tanac.*
   sounds like someone else's voice speaking, her own—*Cann. s.*
   were passing through wool—*Agn.*
 –voices, confused, in his ears—*Benz. ac.*
   were far off—*Sabal*
 –walking at night, he hears someone—*Carb. v.*
 –warbling of birds—*Bell., Bry.*
 –watch, sound of winding—*Ambr.*
 –water boiling—*Bry., Cann. i., Chlf., Lyc., Thuj.*
   boiling and hissing—*Bry., Cann. i.*
   cascade—*Rhus t.*
   roaring of rushing—*Cham., Mag. c.*
   of water-fall—*Sul. ac.*
   running constantly—*Lyss.*
   out of hydrant—*Lyss.*
   rushing—*Cocc., Kali n., Nitro. o., Petr., Puls.*
   of a water-fall—*Ars., Caust.*
 –water-fall—*Cann. i., Chel., Con., Nat. p., Petr.*
   roaring of—*Sul. ac.*
   rushing of—*Ars., Caust.*
 –waves—*Aster.*
 –wheel—*Hydrs.*
 –whip cracking—*Sulph.*

Sound—*Continued*

  —whirring—*Lact., Lyc., Merc. c.*

  —whispering—*Rhod.*

  —whistling—*Æth., Alum., Ambr., Aur., Bell., Carb. an., Caust., Chel., Cur., Elaps, Ferr., Hep., Hura, Lyc., Mag. c., Manc., Mur. ac., Puls., Sarr., Sep., Verat. a., Vinc.*

  —whizzing—*Alum., Arg. n., Berb., Calc. ac., Hura, Lach., Mag. c., Mim., Naja, Olnd., Pedi., Phos., Plb., Sang., Sep., Tarent., Thuj., Zinc.*

    of insects—*Lach.*

  —wind—*Carb. v., Led., Mag. c., Plat., Puls., Spig.*

    roaring—*Asar., Caust., Chel., Con., Croc., Led., Mag. c., Petr., Verat. a.*

    rushing out of ears—*Abrot., Mosch., Sulph.*

    singing—*Carb. s.*

  —wind-storm—*Led.*

Sounding-board when breathing, ear were—*Bar. c.*

Sounds came from a distance—*Caps., Lac c.*

  —came from another world—*Carb. an.*

  —came from heart—*Glon.*

  —came through forehead and brain—*Sulph.*

  —were caused by resonance of contiguous parts—*Osm.*

  —were double—*Med.*

  —enter ears through a thick medium—*Coca*

  —in left ear with feeling as if pharynx were enlarged—*Dig.*

Spark, electric, were snapping in ear—*Ambr.*

Sparks, electric, were biting here and there in ears—*Phel.*

Spinning-wheel were humming in ear—*Agar.*

Spitting of cat in ear, sound of—*Nit. ac.*

Splitting, ear were—*Phos.*

Spurting liquid in ear, sound of—*Thuj.*

Squeezing out of ears, something were—*Thuj.*

  —in front of ears extending to angles of jaws—*Dios.*

Stabbed in ears—*Thuj.*

Stabbing with knife in eyes and ears—*Vib.*

Stabs in hollow of ear—*Alum.*

Steam in left ear, sound of—*Sal. ac.*

  —sound of the rushing of escaping—*Glon.*

  —were rushing through a small hole in ear—*Dig.*

  —sound of the singing of escaping—*Phys.*

Sticking in ear, something were—*Anac., Ang.*

Stitches were passing through tympanum—*Spong.*

Stitching in internal ear, cold needle were—*Agar.*

Stopped—see the GENERAL REPERTORIES

Stopped loosely—*Spig.*

  –suddenly—*Dios.*

  –on blowing nose—*Con., Sulph.*

  –when reading aloud—*Verb.*

  –by sweat—*Tep.*

  –by a swelling—*Merc.*

  –while talking—*Meny.*

  –with a finger when the wind blew in—*Spig.*

  –with cotton wool—*Chin. m.*

Storm in forest, roaring in ears as of—*Coc. c.*

  –rushing, noise in ears as of—*Bor.*

Straighten out lobe of ear, he must—*Vib.*

Strange in his ears, his own voice sounds—*Tanac.*

Straw crackling in ears on motion of jaws, sound of—*Carb. v.*

Stream of blood rushing in ear—*Stann.*

  –of water were running from one ear to the other, small—*Der.*

Streaming from ear, something hot were—*Canth.*

  –from right ear, something hot were—*Æth.*

Stretched across ear, something had been—*Meny.*

  –over ear, membrane were—*Verat. a.*

  –before ear, skin were—*Graph.*

  –over right external ear, skin were—*Asar.*

  –wide open, ear were—*Mez.*

Striking in ears, sound of clock—*Mang., Ter.*

String broke in ear—*Sulph.*

  –were pulled from shoulder to ear—*Lepi.*

Struck with hammer at base of bone behind ear—*Lappa a.*

Stuck behind right ear and pressed it forward on stroking hair, something were—*Ars. s. f.*

Stuffed up, ears were—*Æth., Cann. i., Carb. s., Cot., Lach., Nicot., Psor., Spig., Sulph.*

  –in ear, something were—*Carb. s.*

  –with cotton, ears were—*Psor.*

  –right ear were—*Merc.*

  –during a full moon, ears were—*Graph.*

Stupefied, hearing were—*Hyos.*

Suppurated, ear were—*Coc. c.*

Swarming in ears, animals were—*Ant. c.*

Swashing in ears, water were—*Ant. c., Spig., Sulph.*

Sweat stopped ears—*Tep.*
Swelling, ears were—*Acon.*
  —ears were stopped by—*Merc.*
Swollen, all parts around ear were—*Form.*
  —minor meatus were—*Juncus*
  —bone of ear were—*Plan.*
Teakettle beginning to boil at a distance, sound in ear of—*Agar.*
  —singing in ears—*Tarent.*
Thread were drawn through ear—*Rhus t.*
Thrust into left ear, sharp instrument were—*Genist.*
Thunder were rumbling in ears, sound of—*Elaps*
Thundering in ears, sound of—*Am. m., Carb. o., Gas., Graph., Lach., Sil.*
  —in ears like distant cannonading—*Plat.*
Ticking sound in ears—*Chin., Nat. m., Petr., Ter.*
Tick-tack sound in ears—*Gad.*
Tickling in ear of a feather—*Azad.*
  —from veil drawn over ear—*Phos.*
Tingling as if frost-bitten, cartilage of both ears were—*Sac. lac.*
  —as from beating on an iron bar, tremulous—*Puls.*
Tinkling in ears—*Atro.*
Torn out, ear were—*Bell., Ery. a., Par., Saponin.*
  —out, ears were being—*Sep.*
  —from within, ears were—*Lil. t.*
  —from their location, ears were being—*Ery. a.*
  —out, ears were alternately pressed in and—*Bell.*
  —asunder, middle ear would be—*Con.*
  —out of right ear, bone would be—*Canth.*
Trumpets, din in ears like—*Bell., Gas.*
Tube went through head from ear to ear—*Med.*
  —sound as when coughing into an empty—*Osm.*
  —rushing sound in ears as when listening at—*Cocc.*
Turned around, ear were—*Mag. s.*
Twitched out of ear with hook, something were—*Nat. m.*
Twittering in ear—*Calad.*
  —of crickets in ear—*Puls.*
  —of young mice in ear—*Rhus t.*
Ulcerated in ear—*Anac., Ant. t., Ferr., Kali c., Mur. ac., Sars., Sulph.*
Valve in motion in ear, leather-covered metal—*Agar.*
  —opening and shutting in right ear—*Xanth.*

Valve—*Continued*
  –in ear opening and closing at each step—*Graph.*
  –in left ear opening and closing, < afternoon—*Psor.*
Vapor were going into ears—*Euphr.*
  –hot, coming from ears—*Canth.*
Veil were drawn over ear, tickling—*Phos.*
Vibration of string of instrument in ear—*Cann. s.*
Voice sounds strange in his ears, his own—*Tanac.*
  –sounded like someone else's speaking, her own—*Cann. s.*
  –were passing through wool—*Agn.*
Voices were far off—*Sabal*
  –in ears, sound of confused—*Benz. ac.*
Vomit, he would (sensation starting in front of ear)—*Dios.*
Walking at night, he hears someone—*Carb. v.*
Warbling of birds in ear, sound of—*Bell., Bry.*
Watch, sound of winding—*Ambr.*
Water were in right ear, comes and disappears suddenly—*Chr.
    ac.*
  –in ears, coldness from—*Meny.*
  –boiling, were before ear—*Dig.*
  –were creeping into ear—*Rhod.*
  –were dropping in ear when lying down—*Nat. p.*
  –were dropping from height into a long round vessel in ear—
    Nat. p.
  –ears were filled with—*Lac butyr.*
  –left ear were filled with—*Graph.*
  –external meatus were filled with—*Thuj.*
  –warm, were flowing in circle around right ear—*Calad.*
  –warm, flowing from ears—*Calad.*
  –were gurgling in ears—*Sulph.*
  –were murmuring in ears—*Petr.*
  –murmuring in ears, boiling—*Mag. p. Arct.*
  –were passing out of ear—*Calc. c., Spig., Sulph.*
  –hot, penetrated ears—*Euphr.*
  –warm, running in ears—*Glon.*
  –ice-cold, running from ears (recurring)—*Merc.*
  –hot, were running out of right ear—*Cham.*
  –were rushing into ears—*Petr., Puls., Rhod., Sulph.*
  –sound of falling—*Ars., Cann. i., Caust., Chel., Con., Lyss.,
    Nat. p., Petr., Rhus t., Sul. ac.*
  –of boiling—*Bry., Cann. i., Chlf., Lyc., Thuj.*

Water—*Continued*
  –roar of rushing—*Cham., Mag. c.*
  –of waterfall—*Sul. ac.*
  –of rushing—*Cocc., Kali n., Nitro. o., Puls.*
  –rushing of water-fall—*Ars., Caust.*
  –swashing—*Spig., Sulph.*
  –water-fall—*Cann. i., Chel., Con., Nat. p., Petr.*
Waves in ears, sound of—*Aster.*
Wax were flowing from ear—*Agar.*
  –would flow into mouth—*Crot. h.*
  –would flow out on swallowing saliva—*Coc. c.*
  –hot, were trickling out of ear—*Crot. h.*
Wedge were driven in left ear—*Merc.*
  –were driven in meatus—*Par.*
  –were forcing ear apart—*Par.*
Wheel in ear, sound of—*Hydrs.*
Whip in ear, crack of—*Sulph.*
Whirring sound in ear—*Lact., Lyc., Merc. c.*
Whispering in ear—*Rhod.*
Whistling in ears—*Æth., Alum., Ambr., Aur., Bell., Carb. an., Chel., Caust., Cur., Elaps, Ferr., Hep., Hura, Lyc., Mag. c., Manc., Mur. ac., Puls., Sarr., Sep., Verat. a., Vinc.*
Whizzing in ears—*Alum., Arg. n., Berb., Calc. ac., Hura, Lach., Mag. c., Mim., Naja, Olnd., Pedi., Phos., Plb., Sang., Sep., Tarent., Thuj., Zinc.*
  –of insects in ears—*Lach.*
Wide and hollow inside, ears were—*Aur. m.*
Wind in ears—*Bell., Chel., Eupi., Mez., Mosch., Stann., Stram.*
  –blew into ears—*Staph.*
  –cold, blowing into right ear—*Caust., Mang., Meny., Plat., Staph.*
  –cold, blowing through both ears into sore eyes—*Alum.*
  –were blown with force, pressing on ears and surrounding parts—*Eupi.*
  –cold, in ears—*Stann., Vinc.*
  –hot, in external right ear—*Phys.*
  –passing out of ear—*Æth., Calc. c., Chel., Mill., Psor.*
  –puffed out of ears on swallowing—*Meli.*
  –roaring in ears—*Asar., Caust., Chel., Con., Croc., Led., Mag. c., Petr., Sulph., Verat. a.*
  –were rushing out of ears—*Aphis, Chel., Stram.*

Wind—*Continued*
  –rushing out of ears, sound of—*Abrot., Mosch., Sulph.*
  –strong rushing, as from bird-wing—*Mosch.*
  –in ears, sound of—*Carb. s., Led., Mag. c., Plat., Puls., Spig.*
Wind-storm in ear—*Led.*
Wings were flapping in ear—*Jac.*
  –of a bird were rushing in ear—*Mosch.*
Wood, someone were digging in ear with blunt piece of—*Ruta*
Worm in ear—*Guare., Pic. ac., Rhod.*
  –boring in anterior wall of canal—*Med.*
  –creeping into left ear—*Rhod.*
Worms crawling in ear—*Med., Pic. ac., Rhod.*

NOSE

Air, cold, in nostril—*Hydr.*

  —in nostrils were icy cold—*Anan.*

  —in left nasal fossa, current of cold—*Lepi.*

  —were forced through mucus, squeaking—*Teucr.*

  —passed into nose and mouth, too much—*Ther.*

  —were pressing through posterior nares with violence—*Mag. s.*

  —were too sharp in left nostril—*Brach.*

Band were pressing in root of nose—*Ther.*

Beaten, nasal bone had been—*Sil.*

  —tip of nose had been, and blood pressed out—*Viol. o.*

Biting from something acrid—*Plat.*

  —of mustard in nose—*Mez., Saba.*

Bleed, nose would—*Both. a., Phys., Samb., Sep., Thea, Xanth.*

  —left nostril would—*Sabin.*

Blister on mucous membranes—*Sulph.*

Blood would burst from nose—*Lac. ac.*

  —would burst through—*Meli.*

  —congestion of blood to—*Cupr.*

  —in the nose which she could not blow out, there were a deposit of—*Raph.*

  —would issue through nose when blowing—*Lil. t.*

  —pressed out where tip of nose had been beaten—*Viol. o.*

Blowing across the nose, a gentle wind were—*Spig.*

Board were lying against nose—*Calc. c.*

Body, foreign, in posterior nares—*Stann.*

Breath, hot, came out mouth and nose—*Saba.*

Broken, nose were—*Sal. ac.*

Bruised, nasal cartilage were—*Pers.*

  —nasal bones were—*Arg. n.*

  —soft parts of nose were—*Laur.*

Bubble were bursting in nose—*Sulph.*

Bubbles, small, burst in nose—*Sars.*

Burned by breath, nostrils were—*Ptel.*

  —by the sun, nose had been—*Oxyt.*

Burning in the nostrils—*Cina*

  —from horseradish in nose—*Pall.*

  —and raw, end of nose were—*Carb. s.*

Burst, nose would—*Asaf., Kali bi.*

  —nose seems—*Oxyt.*

  —in nose, small bubbles—*Sars.*

  —in right wing of nose—*Asaf., Asar.*

Bursting in nose, a bubble were—*Sulph.*

Catarrh about to start—*Berb., Ferr. ma.*

  —stopped—*Puls.*

Centipede were crawling in left nostril—*Med.*

Clawing in cavity of nose—*Arg. m.*

Close, nose would—*Echin.*

Cobweb on the nose—*Brom., Sang. n.*

Cold air in nostril—*Hydrs.*

  —in left nasal fossa, a current of—*Lepi.*

  —icy, in nostrils—*Anan.*

  —would set in—*Thuj.*

  —she had taken—*Sol*

Compressed, nasal bones were—*Arg. m.*

Conscious of having a nose—*Merl.*

Cord or hair pressing in nose like spectacles—*Ant. t.*

Coryza were about to come on—*Am. m., Ars. s. r., Aur. m., Carb. an., Cham., Colch., Coloc., Dign., Phos., Psor., Sulph., X-ray*

  —violent, would set in—*Ars. m., Pen.*

  —in looking at bright objects—*Lyss.*

  —severe, had a—*Bry.*

Crackling in temples, forehead and nose—*Acon.*

Crawling in nose—*Arg. m., Aur. m.*

  —in right nostril—*All. c., Samars.*

  —in cavity of nose—*Aur. m.*

  —centipede were crawling in left nostril—*Med.*

Crepitation in the nose—*Acon.*

Crosswise in nose, a pin were—*Ment.*

Crowing in the nose—*Iod.*

Crushed, nasal bones were being—*Pip. n.*

Crushing in nose—*Sep.*

Current of cold air in left nasal fossa—*Lepi.*

Curtain were opening and shutting in right nostril—*Hydrs.*

Cutting into wound in nostril, someone were—*Nux v.*

Deadened in nose—*Ars. h.*

Detached from bone, mucous membrane were—*Sulph.*

Dragging in nose—*Mag. c.*

Drawn tightly across bridge of nose, horsehair were—*Ant. t.*

  —up on face and nose, skin were—*Com.*

  —up with a string and fastened to center of forehead, tip of nose were—*Crot. c.*

Dry, nose were—*Verat. a.*

  —mucus entirely filled nose—*Agar.*

Dull instrument were pressing just above root of nose—*Til.*

Dust in nose—*Verat. a.*

Electric sparks, fine, in left wing of nose—*Carb. ac.*

Enlarged, nose were, and face red—*Acon.*

  —posterior nares and upper part of œsophagus were—*Elat.*

Enlarging and obstructing vision, nose were—*Cann. s.*

Epistaxis would occur, profuse—*Eucal.*

Expanded upon walking out, nasal passages were—*Carb. an.*

Feather, nostril were tickled with a stiff—*Phyt.*

Fastened to center of forehead, tip of nose were drawn up with a string and—*Crot. c.*

Filled with dry mucus, nose were entirely—*Agar.*

Fire, ulcers in mouth and nose were on—*Syph.*

Fish were in nose—*Gels.*

Fishbone in nose—*Nit. ac.*

Fleabites in left side of nose—*Pall.*

Flowed from the nose, acrid matter—*Nat. m.*

Fluid, acrid, running through posterior nares and over palate—*Kali bi.*

Forced through mucus, squeaking, air were—*Mar.*

  —asunder, bones of nose would be—*Puls.*

  —transversely through nose, a plug were—*Ruta*

Full of mucus, posterior nares were—*Pæon.*

Fumes—see SMELL

Hair in nostril—*Hydrs.*

  —high up in left nostril—*Kali bi.*

  —or cord were pressing in like spectacles—*Ant. t.*

  —pulled by a hair in—*Plat.*

  —hair had been pulled out of—*Plat.*

  —tickling from a hair in left nostril—*Kali bi.*

  —tickling in right nostril—*Hydrs.*

  —touched lightly by hair, back of nose were—*Spig.*

Hanging down in posterior nares, something were—*Yuc.*

  —from nose, a weight were—*Kali bi.*

Heavy, nose were too—*Kali bi.*

Horsehair drawn tightly across bridge of nose—*Ant. t.*
Horseradish were burning in nostrils—*Pall.*
　—and it were rising to the nostrils, he had taken—*Sang. n.*
Hot breath came out mouth and nose—*Saba.*
　—expired air felt—*Kali bi.*
Hypersensitive at root of nose, mucous membrane were—*Med.*
Icy cold air in nostrils—*Anan.*
Inflamed, nose were—*Lith.*
Inhaled sulphuric acid—*Carb. s.*
Large, nose were—*Sang. n.*
Leaf at root of nose—*Kali i.*
　—fine, lay before posterior nares—*Bar. c.*
Leaflet were at root of nose obstructing smell—*Kali i.*
Leather, nasal mucous membrane were stiff as—*Stict.*
Lodged in the posterior nares, quantity of mucus were—*Lac. ac.*
Loose, base of nose were thickened and—*Sulph.*
Lump in posterior nares—*Wye.*
Lying against the nose, board were—*Calc. c.*
Mucus, posterior nares were full of—*Pæon.*
　—dry, entirely filled nose—*Agar.*
　—lodged in posterior nares, a large quantity were—*Lac. ac.*
Needle pricking point of nose—*Sars.*
Numb, one side of nose were—*Nat. m.*
Obstructing vision, nose were enlarging and—*Cann. s.*
Open, alæ nasi were spread wide—*Iod.*
　—posterior nares were spread wide—*Fl. ac.*
Opening, a curtain opening and shutting in right nostril—*Hydrs.*
Parchment, nostrils were made of—*Kali bi.*
Passed into nose and mouth, too much air—*Ther.*
Pepper, nose were full of—*Cench.*
　—red, were through nostrils and air passages—*Seneg.*
Pimple would form on septum—*Con., Sel.*
　—sore, below right nostril—*Gamb.*
Pin crosswise in nose, sore and dry—*Ment.*
Pinched, bridge of nose feels—*Lachn.*
Pinching nostrils together—*Lachn.*
Plug were forced transversely through nose—*Ruta*
　—in—*Hydrs., Kali bi., Psor., Sep.*
　—solid plug in—*Sec.*
Pressed together, bones of nose were—*Plan.*
　—asunder, nasal bones were—*Cor. r.*

Pressed—*Continued*

　　—into head, root of nose would be—*Zinc.*

　　—out where tip of nose had been beaten, blood were—*Viol. o.*

　　—through posterior nares while drinking, water were—*Bapt.*

Pressing through posterior nares with violence, air were—*Mag. s.*

　　—band in root of nose—*Ther.*

　　—on root of nose like spectacles, a cord or hair were—*Ant. t.*

　　—just above root of nose, dull instrument were—*Til.*

　　—on root of nose, blunt point were—*Cann. s.*

Pressure on the bridge of nose—*Kali bi., Pic. ac.*

Pricking on tip of nose, needle were—*Sars.*

Prickling in nose—*Hydr. ac.*

Pulled out of nostril, hair had been—*Plat.*

Pushed up nose, something were—*Calc. c.*

Raw and burning, end of nose were—*Carb. s.*

Return through nose on swallowing, water would—*Raph.*

Rubbing against each other in right side of nose when blowing it, two bones were—*Kali bi.*

Running through posterior nares and over palate, acrid fluid were—*Kali bi.*

Screen opening and shutting in right nostril—*Hydrs.*

Sharp in nostrils, air were too—*Brach.*

Shifted, nose were—*Stram.*

Shutting in right nostril, a curtain were opening and—*Hydrs.*

Smell, burnt feathers—*Bapt.*

　　—fumes of iodine—*Iodof.*

　　—herring—*Agn.*

　　—inhaled sulphuric acid—*Carb. s.*

　　—horseradish rising to nose—*Sang. n.*

　　—decayed leaves from a swamp—*Iodof.*

　　—manure—*Verat. a.*

　　—moldy scent—*Mag. p. Ambo*

　　—musk—*Agn.*

　　—onions—*Cor. r., Manc.*

　　—smoke—*Cor. r., Verat. a.*

　　—pine smoke—*Bar. c.*

　　—offensive stool were in room—*Crot. t.*

　　—sulphur vapors in nose and throat—*X-ray*

Snake in nose—*Sulph.*

Sneeze, would—*Kali cy., Sulph.*

Sneezing, before—*Kali cy.*
Snuff in nose—*Osm.*
  –after a pinch of—*Æsc.*
  –fine, in—*Puls.*
  –causing sneezing—*Genist.*
Soldered together, head, nose and teeth were—*Lyss.*
Something were in nasal passages—*Wye.*
  –in nasal passages, no > trying to clear them—*Wye.*
Sore, corners of nostrils were—*Camph.*
  –outside, nose were—*Squill.*
Sparks, fine electric, in left wing of—*Carb. ac.*
Spectacles, he had on heavy—*Cinnb.*
  –cord or hair were pressing in like—*Ant. t.*
Splinter in nose when touched—*Nit. ac.*
  –sticking in the—*Nit. ac.*
Spread wide open and dry, alæ nasi were—*Iod.*
  –wide open, posterior nares were—*Fl. ac.*
Squeezed in a vise at root of—*Plat.*
Squirming in nostril, a small worm were—*Nat. m.*
Squirting at root of—*Nat. c.*
Steamed from nose and mouth, heat—*Stront.*
Sticks, little, or splinters in the nose—*Nit. ac.*
  –in ulcers in—*Nit. ac.*
Stiff, nose were—*Kali bi., Lyss.*
  –as leather, nasal mucous membranes were—*Stict.*
Stone in dorsum of nose—*Agn.*
Stopped, nose were—*Nat. a., Sin., Stram., Verb.*
  –up, right nostril were partly—*Mar.*
Stretched, muscles of nose were—*Lyc.*
Stuck together, nose were—*Phos.*
Stuffed up, nose were—*Cimic., Cupr., Eucal., Graph., Kali n., Merc., Naja, Sep., Stram., Uran.*
  –as from catarrh—*Kali n.*
  –sinuses were—*Hydrs., Iris v.*
Substance, hard, in dry nose—*Kali bi.*
  –hard, in moist nose—*Stict.*
Sulphuric acid, he had inhaled—*Carb. s.*
Sunburnt, nose were—*Oxyt.*
Suppurate, tip of nose would—*Rhus t.*
  –left nostril would—*Staph.*
Suppurating in nasal bones—*Sil.*

Swelling, nose were—*Coloc.*

Swollen, nose were—*Coca, Sulph.*

Thickened and loose, base were—*Sulph.*

Thicker, nose were—*Kali bi., Kali c., Mez.*

Tickled with a stiff feather in nostril—*Phyt.*

Tickling of a hair in right nostril—*Hydrs.*

  –of a hair in left nostril—*Kali bi.*

Tingling on nose—*Sang. n.*

Torn from left nostril, flesh had been—*Conv.*

Touched with a cold metallic substance on bridge of nose—*Cinnb.*

  –by a hair, back of nose were lightly—*Spig.*

Turned up toward the forehead, nose were—*Bell.*

Two noses, she had—*Merl.*

Ulcerate, left nostril would—*Staph.*

Ulcerated, nose were—*Verat. a.*

  –margin of nostril were—*Nux v.*

  –inside of nose were—*Laur.*

Ulcers in mouth and nose were on fire—*Syph.*

Vapors—see SMELL

Vise, pain at root of nose as though parts of nose were squeezed in—*Plat.*

Water, scalding, rushed along nasal passages on left side on inspiration; right side stopped up—*Gels.*

  –pressed through posterior nares while drinking—*Bapt.*

  –acrid, flowed from—*Nat. m.*

  –in left nostril, stream of scalding—*Gels.*

  –would return through nose on swallowing—*Raph.*

Wearing someone else's nose—*Lac c.*

Web were in nose going down to the throat—*Pen.*

Weight hanging from the nose—*Kali bi.*

Wind, gentle, blowing across the nose—*Spig.*

Worm, small, squirming in nostril—*Nat. m.*

FACE AND JAW

Acid, corroding, touched upper lip—*Lyss.*
Air below malar bone were bulging out cheeks, a bubble of—*Sin.*
  –cold, were blowing on face—*Mag. p. Aust.*
  –cool, were blown on face—*Coloc., Mez.*
  –warm, streaming on left side of face—*Ars. m.*
Alive under skin of face, something were—*Til.*
Asleep on side of face—*Caust.*
Beaten across, parts of malar bones were—*Plat.*
Bitten by a mosquito in center of cheek—*Carb. ac.*
  –in left side of face near mouth, she had been—*Lyss.*
Bleeding, lower lip were—*Rhus t.*
Bloated, face were swollen and—*Ferr.*
Blood were all in face and head—*Cur.*
  –would burst through face—*Parth.*
  –pressed into face—*Equis.*
  –would be pressed out of upper lip—*Ill.*
  –were rushing to right side of jaw—*Fl. ac.*
  –would start through skin—*Aml. n.*
Blow on facial bones, one had had—*Berb.*
Blowing on face, cold air were—*Mag. p. Aust.*
Blown on face, cool air were—*Coloc., Mez.*
Boil would form on face—*Plan.*
Bored in left lower jaw, a hole were being—*Mez.*
Break, jaws would—*Rhus t.*
  –lower jaw were going to—*Phos. ac.*
  –out on face, sweat would—*Ferr.*
Broad, face were growing—*Coll.*
Broken, jaws were—*Sars.*
Bruised, face were—*Fago., Plan., Sars., Ter.*
  –in facial bones—*Kali bi., Sulph., Tarent., Zinc.*
  –cheekbones were—*Nat. m.*
  –left zygoma were—*Cor. r.*
  –jaws were—*Arn., Berb., Caust., Crot. h., Kali bi., Laur., Nat. c., Plan., Rhus t., Sil.*
  –lower lips were—*Juni.*
Bubble of air just below malar bone were bulging out cheeks—*Sin.*

187

Bubbling in right jawbone—*Juncus*

Bulging out cheeks just below malar bone, bubble of air were—*Sin.*

Burned by the sun, skin on left side of face had been—*Lach.*

Burning from a coal on right side of chin—*Ant. t.*
  —on face, nettles were—*Chel.*

Burnt, face were—*Guare.*
  —by sun on face—*Clem., Lach.*

Burrowing in zygoma, something were—*Clem.*

Burst, cheeks would—*Bov.*

Candle were held near left cheek, lighted—*Kali p.*

Cast asunder, bones of face were being—*Colch.*

Chap, lips would—*Apis*

Cloud over upper part of face—*Nit. s. d.*

Clucking in lower jaw—*Bell.*

Coal were burning on right side of chin—*Ant. t.*
  —glowing in small spots on face—*Caust.*

Cobweb on face—*Alum., Bar. c., Bor. ac., Bor., Brom., Calad.,
    Carl., Graph., Laur., Mez., Morph., Ran. s., Sumb.*
  —on right side of face—*Bor.*
  —on right cheek—*Con.*
  —on left cheek—*Wies.*
  —covered the face—*Ran. s.*
  —over face, temples and scalp—*Bar. c.*
  —were moving on face—*Sumb.*

Cobwebs on fact constantly—*Graph.*
  —or white of egg dried on face, temples and scalp—*Bar. c.*
  —here and there on face, or fly crawling—*Calad.*
  —at right side of mouth—*Bor., Rat.*
  —tickling below nose—*Brom.*

Cold crawling from temple down right cheek—*Helod.*

Coming off bones of face and edges were separated and sticking
    out, flesh were—*Lac d.*

Compressed from both sides by a heavy weight, face were—*Acon.*

Contracted, muscles of face were firmly—*Acon.*
  —jaws were—*Caust.*

Contraction of skin of forehead between eyebrows—*Franz.*

Contusion, lips had received a—*Apis*

Corroding acid touched upper lip—*Lyss.*

Corrugated, brows were—*Dirc.*

Covered by cobweb, face were—*Ran. s.*
   –with fur, face were—*Caust.*
   –whole face, one large pain—*Sac. lac.*
   –with salt, lips were—*Sulph.*
Crack in upper lip, there were a—*Saba.*
   –jaws would—*Sep.*
Cracked in lip—*Staph.*
Cramped, masseter muscles were painfully—*Cham.*
Crawling over face, something were—*Anac., Camph., Gymn., Lachn., Laur., Plat.*
   –cold, from temple down right cheek—*Helod.*
   –on face, flies and spiders were—*Laur.*
   –on face, fly were—*Calad., Gymn.*
   –on left cheek, fly were—*Cench.*
   –over left side of face, flies were—*Gymn.*
   –on lips, insects were—*Bor.*
   –on chin, something were—*Stram.*
   –in lips during menses—*Graph.*
Creeping on face, insects were—*Apis, Crot. t., Myric.*
Crushed with tongs, face were—*Verb.*
   –jaw were—*Ign.*
Cut had been made around eyes—*Crot. h.*
   –nerves of face were being drawn tighter and tighter then suddenly let loose as if string were—*Puls.*
Darting of electricity in ramus of jaw—*Valer.*
   –in lips and face, needles were—*Coll.*
Dashed with cold water, face were—*Sulph.*
Dead, lower jaw were—*Acet. ac.*
Digging in angle of left jaw—*Dios.*
Dislocated, jawbone were—*Ant. t., Rob., Sac. lac., Spong.*
   –maxillary joint were—*Mag. p. Arct.*
   –jaw had been suddenly—*Thuj.*
   –jaw would be—*Laur., Rhus t.*
Distended, zygomatic process were—*Carl.*
Drawn up shorter, face would be—*Stann.*
   –toward root of nose, then toward occiput by a string, **face** were—*Par.*
   –to a point at tip of nose, head and face were—*Bism.*
   –tighter and tighter then suddenly let loose as if a string **were** cut, nerves of face were being—*Puls.*

Drawn—*Continued*

—over face, a piece of ice were—*Til.*

—to one side, facial muscles would be—*Cist.*

—tight over bones of face, facial muscles were—*Helod.*

—together with a string, upper lip were—*Saba.*

—from both sides toward the middle, lips were—*Coc. c.*

—backward, lower jaw were—*Bell.*

—up on face and nose, skin were—*Com.*

—skin of face were tightly—*Cann. i.*

—tightly over bones of face, skin were—*Acon.*

Dried on forehead, glue had—*Alum.*

—on face, temples and scalp, egg white had—*Bar. c.*

—on face, white of egg had—*Alum., Bar. c., Calad., Graph., Mag. c., Ol. an., Phos. ac., Sul. ac.*

Driven into jaws, nails were—*Phos.*

Drop of water were trickling above left zygoma—*Sumb.*

Dropping under left cheekbone—*Lob. s.*

Drops, cold, were spurted on face when going into open air—*Berb.*

Dryness of lips were caused by heat of breath—*Nat. c.*

Egg white had dried on face—*Alum., Bar. c., Calad., Graph., Mag. c., Ol. an., Phos. ac., Sul. ac.*

—white dried on face, temples and scalp—*Bar. c.*

—white had dried on lips—*Ol. an.*

Electric shocks pricking in face—*Nux m.*

—sparks on face—*Acon.*

Electricity were darting in ramus of jaw—*Valer.*

Enlarged, head and face were—*Stry.*

Eruption were appearing on right malar bone—*Coloc.*

—would appear on chin—*Spong.*

Fall off from piercing, jaws would—*Acon.*

Fatigued jaw muscles by chewing, one had—*Ang.*

Feather were tickling on face—*Aur. m.*

Finger were pressed above left corner of lips—*Sul. ac.*

Fire, face were on—*Sarr.*

—mounted to face—*Stram.*

Fissure were on lower lip but there was none—*Sulph.*

Flies were crawling on face—*Calad., Gymn.*

—were crawling over right face—*Gymn.*

—and spiders were crawling on face—*Laur.*

Fluid were accumulating in jaw—*Daph.*

Fly were crawling on left cheek—*Cench.*

　—were crawling on face or cobwebs here and there—*Calad.*

Form on face, boil would—*Plan.*

　—on chin below jaw, pimple would—*Staph.*

Fractured, jawbone were—*Rob.*

Frostbitten, face were—*Agar.*

Fullness, peculiar, as from pressure inside of face out—*Pip. m.*

Fur, face were covered with—*Caust.*

Glowing coals in small spots on face and hands—*Caust.*

　—cheeks were—*Daph. o.*

Glue had dried on forehead—*Alum.*

Glued together, lips were—*Cann. i.*

Gnawing in jaw, something were—*Naja, Nat. m.*

Grinding in angle of jaw—*Dios.*

Grow together, lips would—*Stram.*

Growing larger, face were—*Acon.*

　—larger, chin were—*Glon.*

Hair on right cheek—*Laur.*

Hairs or minute insects on chin and neck—*Chlol.*

　—on face, > wiping—*Carl.*

Hanging loosely, everything about upper part of face were—
　　Form.

　—right side of face were—*Nux v.*

Heavy, whole face were—*Acon.*

Held near left cheek, lighted candle were—*Kali p.*

Hole in bone of face—*Stram.*

　—were being bored in left lower jaw—*Mez.*

Hot iron were thrust through ramifications of fifth pair of nerves
　　—*Ars.*

　—plate of iron were nearly in contact with face—*Nux v.*

　—iron in right zygomatic process, red—*Canth.*

　—iron, lips were seared by—*Colch.*

Ice in cheeks—*Mag. p. Arct.*

　—were drawn over face and ears, piece of—*Til.*

　—face were pricked with points of—*Helod.*

　—he had a mustache of—*Lach.*

Immovable, skin were—*Ars. m.*

Indurated, spot under right nostril would become—*Thuj.*

　—lips were—*Cyc.*

Insects were crawling on face—*Apis, Crot. t., Myric.*

　—were crawling on lips—*Bor.*

Insects—*Continued*
  —minute, or hairs on chin and neck—*Chlol.*
Iron, hot, were thrust through ramifications of fifth pair of
    nerves—*Ars.*
  —were nearly in contact with face, hot plate of—*Nux v.*
  —red hot, in right zygomatic process—*Canth.*
  —lips were seared by a hot—*Colch.*
Jerking and stitching in face, needles were—*Zinc.*
  —down from head to jaw, pain were—*Calc. ac.*
Knocked up, chin had been—*Plat.*
Lame in condyle of jaws—*Psor.*
Larger, face were growing—*Acon.*
  —after dinner, face were—*Alum.*
  —left cheek were—*Arg. m.*
  —chin were growing—*Glon.*
Living under skin of face, something were—*Til.*
Long, chin were too—*Glon.*
Loose as if strings were cut, nerves of face were being drawn
    tighter and tighter and suddenly let—*Puls.*
Lost, movement of jaw were—*Tab.*
Many teeth for jaw, there were too—*Tub.*
Mesmerized, face were—*Kali i.*
Mobility, lower jaw had lost its—*Tab.*
Molasses, face were smeared with—*Lecith.*
Mosquitoes, face were bitten by—*Carb. ac.*
Mounted to face, fire—*Stram.*
Mustache of ice, he had—*Lach.*
Move jaws, he could not—*Phyt.*
Mumps were coming on—*Puls., Trif.*
Nail in left zygoma, pressure of—*Laur.*
Nails were driven into jaws—*Phos.*
Needle in lower face, pierced with a—*Ind.*
  —stitches in cheeks—*Calad.*
  —or splinter sticking in lips—*Bov.*
  —stuck in upper lip from within out—*Peti.*
Needles in face, fiery burning—*Apis*
  —were darting in face and lips—*Coll.*
  —muscles in left side of face, neck and left axilla were pierced
    by red hot—*Spig.*
  —or pins pricking skin on forehead, neck and arms—*All. c.*
  —stitching and jerking in face—*Zinc.*

Needles—*Continued*
  —red hot, pricking in swollen upper lip—*Ars.*
  —were pricking chin—*Agar.*
  —a hundred little, had been run into tongue and lips—*Arum m.*
Nettles were burning on face—*Chel.*
Opened when chewing, jaws could not be—*Sep.*
Off bones of face and edges separated and sticking out, flesh
    were—*Lac d.*
Pain, face would begin to—*Fl. ac.*
  —covering whole face, one large—*Sac. lac.*
Paralyzed, face were—*Nux m.*
  —entire left side of face were—*Form.*
  —in left half of head and face—*Stry.*
  —in left jaw—*Crot. h.*
Pepper, red, on spot size of silver quarter on left malar bone—
    Culx.
Pierced by red hot needles, muscles in left side of face from
    forehead to neck and axilla were—*Spig.*
  —with a needle in lower face—*Ind.*
  —in angle of jaw—*Phos.*
Piercing, jaws would fall off from—*Acon.*
Pimple over right antrum—*Com.*
  —would form on chin below jaw—*Staph.*
Pincers in both malar bones, face were pressed together with—
    Cina
  —in zygomatic region, face were seized by—*Puls.*
Pinched, skin of cheek and chin were—*Sul. ac.*
Pins or needles were pricking skin on forehead, neck and arms
    —*All. c.*
Plate of iron, hot, nearly in contact with face—*Nux v.*
Pressed together with pincers, both malar bones and face were
    —*Cina*
  —out of upper lip, blood would be—*Ill.*
  —above left corner of lips, finger were—*Sul. ac.*
  —against upper jaw, left ramus of jaw were—*Verb.*
Pressing upon left malar bone, one were violently—*Verb.*
Pressure from inside out caused fullness of face—*Pip. m.*
  —of a nail in left zygoma—*Laur.*
Pricked with points of ice, face were—*Helod.*
Pricking from electric shocks in face—*Nux m.*
  —skin on forehead, neck and arms, needles or pins were—*All. c.*

Pricking—*Continued*
    –in swollen upper lip, red hot needles were—*Ars.*
    –into chin, needles were—*Agar.*
    –in face—*Spire.*
Puckered and causing dizziness, skin of face were—*Com.*
Puffed up, face were all—*Caj.*
Puffy, cheeks were—*Sul. ac.*
Pulled up forcibly at malar bone, face were—*Ol. an.*
Pulling in jaw—*All. s.*
Rain fell on face, cold drops of—*Berb.*
Raised from periosteum by throbbing, muscles of face would be
        —*Arg. m.*
Ranging themselves on one another, muscles and bones of face
        were—*Pip. n.*
Rattling in joints, jaws were loose and—*Saba.*
Raw and sore, inside of lower lip were—*Ign.*
Rent asunder, bones of nose and face were being—*Colch.*
Rheumatism in face, he had—*Act. sp.*
Rough, jaw were—*Phos.*
Rub something away from face, he must constantly—*Carl.*
Run into tongue and lips, a hundred little needles were—*Arum
        m.*
    –into right lower jaw, splinter were—*Agar.*
Rushing to right side of jaw, blood were—*Fl. ac.*
Salt on face—*Caps.*
    –lips were covered with—*Sulph.*
Sand on lips—*Rhus v.*
Sawed through, bones of face were—*Stram.*
Scalded, cheek bones were—*Bell.*
    –lips were—*Arum t., Saba.*
Scorched, left side of face had been—*Spig.*
Screwed in, chin were—*Plat.*
Screws; malar bones, mastoid process and chin were between
        —*Plat.*
Seared by a hot iron, lips were—*Colch.*
Seized by pincers in zygomatic region—*Puls.*
Separated and sticking out, flesh were coming off bones and
        edges were—*Lac d.*
Shivering near nose—*Puls.*
Shocks, electric, pricking in face—*Nux m.*
Short, facial muscles were too—*Mosch.*

Shrunken, features were—*Rob.*
Slapped in face—*Puls.*
Sleep, face had gone to—*Benz. ac.*
  –lower lip had gone to—*Ill.*
Smaller, left side of face were—*Cinnm.*
Smeared with molasses, face were—*Lecith.*
Sore and raw inside of lower lip—*Ign.*
Soreness and tension in skin of face on arising, bruised—*Plan.*
Spasm would occur in face—*Fl. ac.*
Spark, hot, on chin—*Ant. c.*
Sparks, electric, on face—*Acon.*
Spiders and flies were crawling on face—*Laur.*
Spiderwebs on face—*Brom., Calad., Ran. s.*
Splinter sticking into face—*Juncus*
  –were sticking in lips, needle or—*Bov.*
  –were run into right lower jaw—*Agar.*
Sprained in left maxilla—*Arum t.*
  –in articulation of left lower jaw—*Cor. r.*
Sprinkled with cold water, face and back of hands were—*Berb.*
Spurted on face when going into open air, cold drops were—*Berb.*
Sticking out, flesh were coming off bones of face and edges were separated and—*Lac d.*
  –in lips, needle or splinter were—*Bov.*
Stiffness of muscles of face—*Agar.*
  –from a boil forming—*Plan.*
  –in muscles of jaw—*Gels.*
  –in maxillary joints—*Bad.*
Stitches from needle in cheek—*Calad.*
  –from needle or splinter in lips—*Bov.*
Stitching and jerking in face, needles were—*Zinc.*
Streaming on left side of face, warm air were—*Ars. m.*
Stretched tightly over bones of face and immovable, skin were—*Ars. m.*
String, face were drawn toward root of nose then toward occiput by a—*Par.*
  –upper lip were drawn together with a—*Saba.*
Struck in the face with a cloth—*Guai.*
Stuck in upper lip from within out, needle were—*Peti.*
Stung by bees in face—*Stry.*
Suppurate on skin of face, something would—*Rhus t.*

Suppurating, left cheek were—*Staph.*
Swarming in face—*Bart.*
Sweat would break out on face—*Ferr.*
Swelling, cheeks were—*Samb.*
  –muscles of face were (in morning)—*Spig.*
  –bones of face were—*Bell.*
Swollen, face were—*Æth., Bar. c., Daph. o., Euph., Grat., Nicc., Puls.*
  –with coryza, head and face were—*Ars. m.*
  –< washing; face, head and hands were—*Æth.*
  –and bloated, face were—*Ferr.*
  –left side of face were—*Stram.*
  –cheeks were—*Aran., Staph.*
  –malar bones were—*Nat. a.*
  –right cheek bone were—*Chel.*
  –lower lip were—*Glon.*
  –jaw were—*Vichy*
  –maxillary joints were—*Lach.*
  –skin of face were—*Ferr.*
  –glands beneath chin were—*Staph.*
Tense, periosteum were—*Thuj.*
Tension and bruised soreness in skin on arising—*Plan.*
Thick, skin about eyes were—*Par.*
Thrust through ramifications of fifth pair of nerves, hot iron were—*Ars.*
Tickling on face, something were—*Acon., Indg., Merc. i. r.*
  –on face, feather were—*Aur. m.*
  –on face, hair were—*Laur.*
  –below nose, cobwebs were—*Brom.*
Tight, skin on face were too—*Acon., Ars. m., Cann. i., Phos., Sumb.*
  –over bones of face, facial muscles and skin were drawn—*Helod.*
Tighter and tighter and suddenly let loose as if string were cut, nerves of face were drawn—*Puls.*
Tightly drawn, skin of face were—*Acon., Cann. i.*
Tingling in lips and tongue—*Sac. lac.*
  –in jaw—*Mur. ac.*
Tired, jaw were—*Tarent.*
Tongs, face were crushed with—*Verb.*
Tooth would come through at angle of jaw—*Plect.*

Torn from right side, left side of face were—*Coloc.*
   –to pieces by jerking pain in right zygoma—*Chel.*
   –out, bones of face would be—*Phos.*
   –out, lower jaw and malar bone would be—*Sulph.*
   –out of joint, right side of lower jaw would be—*Spig.*
Touched by corroding acid, upper lip were—*Lyss.*
Trembling in face—*Stry.*
   –around lower face—*Ran. s.*
Triangle in face, there were; malar bones the base, apex at vertex—*Irid.*
Trickling above left zygoma, drop of water were—*Sumb.*
Twanging in left side of face and neck, wires were—*Kali bi.*
Twisted, jaw were—*Stry.*
Ulcerated, left side of face were—*Plan.*
   –cheek bones were—*Psor.*
   –lips were—*Sul. ac.*
   –jaw were—*Nicc.*
   –left side of chin were—*Spong.*
Vise, chin were in a—*Daph. o.*
Walked in cold wind, one had (felt in face)—*Arum t.*
Water, face were dashed with cold—*Sulph.*
   –face and back of hands were sprinkled with cold—*Berb.*
   –were trickling above left zygoma, a drop of—*Sumb.*
Weight, face were compressed from both sides by a heavy—*Acon.*
   –hung from jaw in evening—*Kali i.*
Wind, one had walked in cold—*Arum t.*
Wire, hot, were thrust through ramifications of fifth pair of nerves—*Ars.*
Wires twanging in left side of face and neck—*Kali bi.*
Wood, upper lip were made of—*Euph.*

MOUTH, TONGUE, TASTE, TEETH, GUMS

Abscess were at root of tooth and would burst when air touches it or on pressure—*Am. c.*

Accumulate in mouth, water would—*Ruta*

Acid were burning in mouth—*Carb. s.*

—resinous fruit, he had been eating—*Peti.*

—had been gargled over tongue, something—*Fl. ac.*

—in teeth, he had taken—*Ail.*

—vomitus set teeth on edge—*Rob.*

Acids, teeth had been injured by—*Chlor.*

Acrid in mouth—*Æsc., Prim.*

—taste in mouth—*Alumn., Brom., Caj., Carb. s., Chin. s., Fl. ac., Glon., Iris, Lac. ac., Pimp., Plan., Plb., Rhus t., Saponin., Seneg., Thuj., Verat. a.*

—wine were—*Iod.*

—on gums had made them raw, something—*Nux v.*

Adhered like glue, upper and lower teeth—*Arg. m.*

Affected, submaxillary glands were—*Brach.*

Agglutinated, teeth were—*Zinc.*

—in fauces—*Kreos.*

Air in mouth, a draft of cold—*Sars.*

—were cold in mouth, inspired—*Raph.*

—were hot in mouth, expired—*Raph.*

—entered mouth—*Nux v.*

—too much, passed into nose and mouth—*Ther.*

—passed out of mouth—*Lyc.*

—penetrated mouth, cold sharp—*Squill.*

—penetrated a wound in mouth—*Thuj.*

—tongue were chilled by cold water or cold—*Acon., Dulc.*

—that filled mouth tasted of rotten eggs—*Acon.*

—to bursting, tooth were filled with—*Lyss.*

—were forced into hollow back teeth—*Cocc. s.*

—front incisors were chilled by cold—*Plan.*

—nerve in hollow tooth were exposed to—*Bry.*

—teeth were sensitive to—*Tub.*

—were shooting into loose teeth on inhaling—*Sulph.*

—cold, touched teeth on inspiration—*Cedr.*

Alike, everything tasted—*Merc. m., Phos.*

Alive in teeth, something were—*Syph.*
Alkaline taste—*Am. c., Cere. b., Kali chl., Mez., Zinc. m.*
Almonds, he had eaten sweet—*Coff., Crot. t., Dig.*
Alum after he had been smoking, taste of—*Nat. h.*
Animal taste in mouth—*Con.*
Apple-wine taste—*Cahin.*
Aromatic taste—*Bell., Cham., Coc. c., Glon., Pip. m.*
Arrow-root, tongue and fauces were smeared with—*Sul. ac.*
Asleep, mouth were—*Nit. ac., Nitro. o.*
 –teeth were—*Dulc.*
 –tongue were—*Bor.*
 –gums were—*Arn.*
Astringent in mouth—*Arg. n., Gels., Gran., Lob. s., Nit. ac.*
 –in mouth as from metal—*Saba.*
 –on tongue—*Arg. n., Nat. m., Sulph.*
 –taste—*Acon., Acon. l., Agar., Alum., Arg. n., Ars., Brom.,
    Calc. i., Gal. ac., Gent. c., Iod., Kali bi., Kali cy., Kali i.,
    Merc. c., Mur. ac., Musa, Ox. ac., Plb., Salix p.*
Bad taste—see TASTE, BAD
Bad taste came from spot on side of tongue—*Tab.*
Ball of sputum rushed to mouth—*Syph.*
Bent on chewing and were soft, teeth became—*Coch.*
Benumbed, mouth were—*Ther.*
Big and filled whole mouth, tongue were (although swelling
    were but a trifle—*Itu*
Bites, violent, on tongue—*Cinch. b.*
Biting in mouth, peppermint were—*Verat. a.*
Bitten in side of mouth—*Lyss.*
 –in tongue—*Caust.*
 –out, teeth were—*Arn.*
Bitter taste—see the GENERAL REPERTORIES
Blanched, tongue were—*Verat. v.*
Blister on tip of tongue—*Sin.*
Blisters, tongue were full of—*Saba.*
 –tip of tongue were covered with—*Kali c.*
 –on side of tongue—*Bar. c.*
 –inside of gums were full of—*Thlaspi*
Blood were in mouth—*Phos.*
 –saliva were mixed with (taste)—*Aspar.*
 –would crowd into teeth—*Caust.*
 –were forced into teeth—*Chin., Hyos.*

Blood—*Continued*
  –were entering tooth—*Hep.*
  –too much, were pressed into nerves of teeth—*Hep.*
  –were pumped through upper incisor teeth—*Croc.*
Bloody—see TASTE, BLOODY
Blunted, tongue were—*Laur.*
  –papillæ on tongue were—*Nat. m.*
Body, foreign, had stuck in fauces—*Agar.*
  –foreign, in left side of throat at root of tongue—*Cedr.*
  –foreign, between loose molar teeth—*Ran. b.*
  –foreign, in tooth—*Caust.*
  –tenacious, were lodged between teeth—*Cor. r.*
Boring in teeth, hot iron were—*Sulph.*
  –in tooth, something were—*Kali c.*
Bound or tied up, tongue were—*Crot. h., Lach.*
Brassy taste—*Chin. s., Ham., Merc., Ptel.*
Breaking, lower molars were—*Nat. m.*
Breast were coming up into her mouth—*Hedo.*
Breath, hot, came out mouth and nose—*Saba.*
  –were offensive—*Laur.*
Broad, tongue were too—*Par., Plb., Puls., Ziz.*
Broken off, teeth would be—*Sulph.*
  –incisor teeth were—*Fl. ac.*
Bruised, tongue were—*Sec.*
  –teeth were—*Crot. h., Fago.*
  –right upper molar were—*Alum.*
Bubbling in right upper molar—*Prun.*
Bullet, leaden, were pressing in inner surface of gums—*Arn.*
Burned, mouth were—*Alum., Ambr., Bell., Berb., Cinch., Dios., Ferr. ma., Glon., Jatr., Lac. ac., Lyc., Mag. m., Med., Menis., Merc. i. r., Pop., Rumx., Sang., Seneg., Thuj., Tub., Verat. a., Zinc. ac.*
  –roof of mouth were—*Lac. ac.*
  –left side of roof of mouth were—*Calc. s.*
  –with acid, mouth were—*Rhus v.*
  –with creosote, mouth were—*Calad.*
  –tongue were—*Ambr., Am. br., Apis, Arg. n., Ars., Bapt., Chlor., Cund., Daph. o., Dios., Ferr., Fer. g., Glon., Ham., Hydrs., Ign., Kreos., Laur., Mag. m., Phos., Phys., Plat., Podo., Pop., Prun., Psor., Puls., Rumx., Sang., Sep., Sol. n., Sul. ac., Syph., Ther.*

Burned—*Continued*

  –tip of tongue were—*Acon., Bell., Calc. p., Cinch. b., Coloc., Kali c., Kali i., Lact., Nat. s., Psor., Rat.*

  –middle of tongue had been—*Puls.*

  –tongue, palate and anterior gums were—*Cic.*

  –palate had been—*Podo.*

  –on forepart of palate—*Bor.*

  –gums were—*Cimx., Ign., Sep.*

  –and wrinkled, gums were—*Par.*

  –on inner gums after rubbing—*Cimx.*

  –and inflamed around molars—*Aloe*

Burning in mouth and throat—*Verat. a.*

  –from acid in mouth—*Carb. s.*

  –from pepper in mouth—*Nat. s.*

  –as from vesicles on tongue—*Kali i., Phel.*

  –on tongue, pimento were—*Elaps*

  –on tongue, tobacco were—*Agar.*

Burnt taste—*Bry., Coca, Cyc., Franc., Laur., Phos., Puls., Ran. b., Squill., Sulph., Tab., Zinc. m.*

Burst, tooth would—*Sabin.*

Bursting, tooth were filled with air to—*Lyss.*

Calomel, taste of—*Nux m.*

Carrot-tops, taste of—*Nux v.*

Caustic in mouth and throat—*Coll.*

Cedar-pitch, taste of—*Canth.*

Cement, teeth were covered with sticky—*Arg. m.*

Chalk, mouth were dry as from—*Calc. ac.*

  –teeth were covered with—*Nux m.*

Chalky taste—*Arg. n., Nux m.*

Cheesy taste—*Æth., Lyc., Par., Phel., Zinc.*

Chewing cotton batting—*Podo.*

Chilled by cold air or cold water, tongue were—*Dulc.*

  –by cold air, front incisors were—*Plan.*

Chip, tongue were like a—*Com.*

Chips, everything tastes like—*Sang. n.*

Chocolate taste—*Crot. t.*

Cinnamon taste—*Glon.*

Clay, everything tastes like—*Acon. l., Agar., Aloe, Ammc., Arg. n., Carl., Euphr., Lyc., Merc.*

Cleave to roof of mouth, tongue would—*Kali p.*

Clenched, jaws were—*Morph.*

14

Close together, teeth were too—*Cor. r.*

Closing up, roof of mouth were swollen and cavity were—*Gels.*

Coal were on tongue—*Galvan.*

  –small, on edge of tongue—*Semp.*

Coated, mouth were—*Carl., Gnaph., Pip. m., Ther.*

  –with fat, mouth were—*Sabal*

  –but it is not, tongue were thickly—*Puls. n.*

Coffee taste—*Cinnb.*

Cold were placed on tongue, something—*Anag.*

  –teeth were—*Cocc. s., Nit. ac., Spig., Spira.*

  –with heat of gums, teeth were—*Anan.*

  –upper incisors were—*Tax.*

  –tips of incisors were—*Gamb.*

  –fingers, incisor teeth were grasped by—*Coc. c.*

  –cool water on teeth were too—*Ther.*

Coldness in mouth and throat—*Verat. a.*

  –of mint drops in mouth and throat—*Coll.*

  –icy, coming from tips of teeth—*Ol. an.*

  –rushed out of molars—*Rat.*

Come through, a new tooth would—*Hep.*

Coming through, tooth were—*Pip. n.*

Compressed or stretched in lower teeth, nerve were—*Coloc.*

Contact with something hot, tongue were in—*Sang.*

Contracted, buccal cavity were—*Card. b.*

  –mouth were—*Alum., Asar., Fl. ac., Gas., Seneg.*

  –teeth were—*Calc. p.*

Contracting and numb in right half of front of tongue—*Ars. h.*

Coolness like ice in mouth and throat—*Sac. lac.*

Copper, tip of tongue had been touched with—*Con.*

Coppery taste—*Æsc., Agn., Arg. n., Ars., Aspar., Aur. m. n., Bell., Brom., Cann. i., Carb. an., Cerv., Cocc., Con., Cupr., Cupr. ac., Cupr. s., Hura, Jug. c., Kali bi., Lach., Lac. ac., Meph., Merc. c., Merc. n., Myris., Naja, Nat. p., Nit. m. ac., Nux v., Ostrya, Plb., Polyp. o., Polyp. p., Psor., Rhus t., Sulph., Ust., Zinc.*

Coryza, taste of old—*Upas*

Cotton in mouth—*Nux m.*

  –batting, he were chewing—*Podo.*

Covered with blisters, tip of tongue were—*Kali c.*

  –with foreign body, tongue were—*Cann. i., Gels.*

  –with chalk, teeth were—*Nux m.*

Covered—*Continued*

   —with fat, palate were—*Card. m.*

   —with fur, mucous membrane of mouth were—*Pip. m.*

   —with fur, tongue were—*Merc., Pip. m.*

   —with a greasy substance, tongue were—*Iris*

   —with Indian meal, tongue were—*Nit. ac.*

   —with leather, tongue were—*Nux m.*

   —with milk, surface of mouth were—*Kali i.*

   —with viscid mucus causing dryness, tongue were—*Agar.*

   —with oil in mouth, parts had been—*Sabal*

   —with pepper, tongue were—*Cann. i., Lach.*

   —with sand when in open air, tongue were—*Gins.*

   —with the skin of a plum, palate were—*Verat. a.*

   —with sticky cement, teeth were—*Arg. m.*

   —with tallow, tongue were—*Til.*

   —with velvet, mouth were—*Dig.*

   —with velvet, tongue were—*Pip. m.*

Crack, mouth would—*Arum t.*

Cracked, tongue were—*Nat. c.*

Crawling at root of tongue, worm were—*Kali i.*

   —in root of teeth, worms were—*Kali i., Syph.*

Cream of tartar taste—*Tarent.*

Creeping in molars, worm were—*Cast.*

Creosote, mouth were burned with—*Calad.*

   —taste—*Phys.*

Crowd into teeth, blood would—*Caust.*

Crushed to fragments, teeth were—*Ign.*

   —lower molar were—*Lyc.*

   —nerves of tooth were shattered and—*Ign.*

Cupping-glass were drawing on tooth—*Sep.*

Cut at root of tongue—*Syph.*

   —off at root, tongue were—*Anan.*

Darting in mouth with mouth open like a catfish, needle were—*Coll.*

Dead, tongue were—*Ham.*

Decayed internally, tooth were—*Asar., Sel.*

Denuded, tip of tongue were—*Iod.*

Deprived of papillæ, mouth and tongue were—*Ter.*

Detached in palate, skin were—*Seneg.*

Dirty, mouth were—*Plan.*

Distended and swollen, alveoli were—*Cham.*

Doughy taste—*Cerv., Phos., Sulph.*

Draft of cold air in mouth—*Sars.*

Dragged downward, upper molars were—*Cham.*

Drawing in teeth—*All. s.*
  —on tooth, cupping-glass were—*Sep.*
  —out of socket, tooth were—*Com.*

Drawn together in fauces, parts were—*Caps.*
  —together in root of tongue—*Hydr. ac.*
  —down into throat, tongue were—*Linum*
  —down into throat when nervous, tongue were—*Plat.*
  —tight together, throat and tongue were laced and—*Thlaspi*
  —into sockets, teeth were—*Rhus t.*
  —out, tooth were being—*Astac.*
  —up, hollow tooth were being—*Sel.*

Dried up, roof of mouth were—*Carl.*
  —in fauces, egg-white had—*Mag. c.*
  —up, hard palate were completely—*Viol. o.*

Drop out, teeth would—*Eupi.*

Drops of ice water fell on tongue—*Pana.*

Dry during salivation, mouth were—*Cocc., Viol. t.*
  —and numb, mouth were—*Mag. s.*
  —as from chalk, mouth were—*Calc. ac.*
  —upper teeth were—*Bry.*
  —and burnt, tip of tongue were—*Psor.*
  —(but is moist), tongue were—*Arg. m.*

Dull and loose, teeth were—*Spong.*

Earthy things, he had eaten—*Puls.*
  —taste—*Aloe, Bry., Cann. s., Caps., Chin., Euphr., Ferr., Franc., Gent. l., Hep., Ign., Linum, Lyc., Merc., Nux m., Phos., Pimp., Puls., Stront., Tell.*

Eaten acid resinous fruit, he had—*Peti.*
  —pepper, he had—*Bapt., Caust., Coca, Cocc.*
  —peppermint lozenges, he had—*Camph., Lyss., Verat. a.*

Edge, teeth were on—*Amph., Bell., Cinch. b., Coloc., Cor. r., Lyss., Parth., Staph., Tarax.*
  —vomitus were so acid it set teeth on—*Rob.*
  —upper teeth were on—*Parth.*
  —every tooth on left side were set on—*Cor. r.*
  —incisors were set on—*Stel.*
  —molar were on—*Spong.*

Egg-white had dried in fauces—*Mag. c.*

Eggs, air that filled the mouth tasted of rotten—*Acon.*

   –taste of rotten—*Acon., Arn., Ferr., Gas., Graph., Hep., Merc., Mur. ac., Sil., Yuc.*

Electric shock went from mouth straight down to feet—*Nux m.*

   –shocks through tongue—*Aran.*

   –shocks continually from one tooth to another—*Tab.*

   –sparks through teeth—*Tarent.*

Electrically sensitive on tip of tongue—*Crot. t.*

Elevated, papillæ on tongue were—*Bry., Lepi.*

Elm-bark taste—*Guai.*

Elongated, teeth were—*All. c., Alumn., Amph., Anac., Arn., Aur., Bell., Bor., Bov., Brom., Bry., Calad., Calc. c., Camph., Caps., Carb. an., Cast., Caul., Chel., Chr. ac., Clem., Cob., Cocc., Coc. c., Colch., Glon., Gran., Hep., Hyos., Iris, Kali i., Kreos., Lach., Laur., Lil. t., Lyc., Mag. c., Mez., Nat. m., Nicc., Nit. ac., Petr., Phos., Phyt., Plan., Ptel., Rheum, Rhus t., Sabin., Sil., Spira., Spong., Stann., Sulph., Wies.*

   –upper teeth were—*Carb. an., Nat. s., Stry.*

   –and dull, upper teeth were—*Caps.*

   –incisors were—*Gamb., Sep.*

   –upper incisors were—*Pall., Rat.*

   –molars were—*All. c., Amph., Bon., Bry., Hell., Iris, Laur., Rat., Sil., Spong., Sulph.*

   –and swollen, molars were—*Sep.*

Embedded in some soft matter, teeth were—*Eupi.*

Enlarged and stretched out over teeth, tongue were—*Colch.*

   –and starting from gums, two middle incisors were—*Raph.*

Enveloped in saliva, tongue were—*Chen. v.*

Eroded, surface of tongue were—*Bor.*

   –inside of gums were—*Puls.*

Eruption on tongue, there were—*Phos.*

Ether taste—*Glon.*

Excoriated, mouth were—*Æsc.*

   –at edge and scalded at anterior, tongue were—*Rumx.*

Exposed to air, nerve in hollow tooth were—*Bry.*

Extracted, teeth were being—*Mag. p. Arct.*

Fall into powder, tongue would—*Nux m.*

   –out, teeth would—*Acon., Nit. ac., Paraf., Stram.*

   –out, tooth were loose and would—*Ars., Hyos., Psor.*

Fall—*Continued*
　—out, all teeth in lower jaw were going to—*Tarent.*
　—out, incisors would—*Eupi., Cocc.*
　—out of their sockets, incisors would—*Merc.*
Fat, mouth were coated with—*Sabal*
　—palate were covered with—*Card. m.*
　—of mutton were adhering to palate—*Ol. an.*
Fatty taste—*Alum., Ambr., Asaf., Bar. c., Bry., Carb. v., Caust.,*
　　Cham., Euph., Fl. ac., Glon., Ign., Ip., Kali bi., Lach., Laur.,
　　Lyc., Mag. m., Mang., Merc. c., Mur. ac., Ol. an., Petr.,
　　Phos., Phos. ac., Puls., Ran. s., Rhod., Rhus t., Saba., Sabin.,
　　Sang., Sil., Thuj., Valer.
Febrile taste—*Chlor., Laur., Merc., Stry.*
Feverish, mouth were—*Atro., Gels., Sang.*
Fibres in mouth—*Merc. i. r.*
Filled with mucus, fauces were—*Calc. c.*
　—the whole mouth, tongue were so large it—*Caj.*
　—the whole mouth (though swelling were but a trifle), tongue
　　were big and—*Itu*
　—with settlings of his pipe, back of tongue were—*Tab.*
　—with water, palate were—*Apis*
　—with air to bursting, tooth were—*Lyss.*
　—with lead, teeth were—*Verat. a.*
Fingers, incisors were grasped by cold—*Coc. c.*
Fire, mouth and fauces were on—*Iris*
　—ulcers in mouth and nose were on—*Syph.*
Fish, taste of—*Acon., Astac., Sars.*
Fit, teeth do not—*Nat. m.*
Fixed in a mass of pap, teeth were—*Merc.*
Flannel, mouth were lined with—*Ars.*
Fluid, acrid, were running through posterior nares over palate
　　—*Kali bi.*
Fly to pieces on biting teeth together, molar and bicuspid teeth
　　would—*Cinnb.*
Food remained above stomach and were being pressed back into
　　mouth—*Nux v.*
　—lodged between teeth—*Ptel.*
　—remained in cavities of teeth—*Staph.*
Forced into hollow back teeth, air were—*Cocc. s.*
　—into teeth, blood were—*Chin., Hyos.*
　—out of head, teeth would be—*Bell., Polyp. o.*

Forced—*Continued*
  –out, teeth were being—*Bol.*
  –out of sockets, teeth were—*Arn., Puls.*
  –out, left upper molars would be—*Lyc.*
Foreign body, tongue were covered with—*Cann. i., Gels.*
  –body between molars—*Lach.*
  –separated right molars—*Ran. b.*
Fragments, teeth were crushed to—*Ign.*
Fruit, he had eaten acid resinous—*Peti.*
  –taste of unripe—*Saba.*
Full of peas, mouth were—*Pyrog.*
  –of pins and needles, mouth were—*Spig.*
  –teeth were too—*Chlor.*
Fur, tongue were covered with—*Merc., Pip. m.*
  –mucous membrane of mouth were covered with—*Pip. m.*
Furred, mouth were—*Ther.*
Fuzzy, mouth were—*Acon. f.*
  –from mucus, mouth were—*Til.*
  –in spots, mouth were—*Acon.*
  –gums were—*Sul. ac.*
  –molars were—*Calc. caust.*
Galvanic shock in mouth—*Cedr.*
Gargled over tongue, something acid had been—*Fl. ac.*
Garlic, taste of—*Asaf., Calc. ar., Merl.*
Gaseous taste—*Arg. cy., Pic. ac.*
Gas-works, taste like smell of—*Kersln.*
Glass between cheek and teeth, a splinter of—*Stann.*
Glue, upper and lower teeth adhered like—*Arg. m.*
Glued with insipid mucus, mouth were—*Mur. ac.*
  –together, teeth were—*Psor.*
  –together, incisors were soft and—*Zinc. ox.*
Glycerine in mouth, taste of—*Spong.*
Got into tooth, something had—*Kali c.*
Grapes, taste of—*Coca*
Grasped by cold fingers, incisors were—*Coc. c.*
Grease, mouth were lined with rancid—*Euph.*
  –roof of mouth were covered with cold—*Iris*
  –roof of mouth were lined with rancid—*Kali p.*
Greasy, tongue and gums were—*Iris*
  –gums were—*Til.*
Grip, teeth were held in—*Nux m.*

Growing from tongue, hair were—*Nat. m.*

Hair on tongue—*Apis, Arg. n., Ars., Carb. s., Cocc., Lyc., Nat. m., Nit. ac., Ran. b.*

 —on tip of tongue—*Apis, Nat. p., Sil.*

 —extended from tip of tongue to trachea—*Sil.*

 —were growing from tongue—*Nat. m.*

 —on back of tongue and velum—*Kali bi.*

 —in fauces—*Kali bi.*

 —on tongue, with drawing in teeth—*All. s.*

 —lying on fore part of tongue—*Sil.*

 —across base of tongue—*Kali bi.*

Hanging down in mouth, a piece of skin were—*Plat.*

 —loose in mouth and throat, skin were—*Iris*

Hard and stiff as shoe leather, tongue were—*Stram.*

 —and rough were lodged in mouth and fauces, something—*Arn.*

Hazelnuts, taste as after eating—*Coff.*

Heat, pungent, in mouth and throat—*Æth.*

Heavy, tongue were too—*Anac., Bell., Carb. v., Colch., Guare., Hyos., Lyc., Macrot., Merl., Morph., Mur. ac., Nat. m., Nux v., Plb., Sec., Stram., Tep., Verat. a.*

 —and would fall out, incisors were—*Cocc.*

Herby taste—*Calad., Carb. s., Nat. m., Nux v., Phos. ac., Ptel., Puls., Sars., Stann., Verat. a.*

Held in a grip, teeth were—*Nux m.*

Herring taste—*Coca*

Herring-brine taste—*Anac.*

Hollow, teeth were—*Cocc. s., Staph.*

 —teeth on left side were—*Asar.*

Honey, beer tastes like—*Mur. ac.*

Hook, teeth would be torn out by—*Cocc. s.*

Horse-chestnuts, taste in mouth of—*Sumb.*

Horse-radish, he had been eating—*Sin. n.*

Hot breath came from mouth and heated neighboring parts—*Saba.*

 —iron in center, tongue were scored by—*Ter.*

 —tongue were in contact with something—*Sang.*

 —iron boring in teeth—*Sulph.*

 —iron, all teeth were suddenly pierced by—*Tep.*

Ice were in mouth and throat—*Sac. lac.*

 —water fell on tongue, drops of—*Pana.*

Inhaled hot steam from root of tongue to bronchi, one had—*Med.*

Injured by acids, teeth had been—*Chlor.*
Ink, taste of—*Aloe, Arg. n., Bart., Calc. c., Ferr. i.*
Insipid—see the GENERAL REPERTORIES
Iron in center, tongue were scored by hot—*Ter.*
  –hot, boring in teeth—*Sulph.*
  –all teeth were suddenly pierced by a hot—*Tep.*
  –taste of—*Aloe, Calc. c., Cedr., Cimx.*
Jammed between teeth, something had become—*Spong.*
  –together, there were too many teeth and they were—*Tub.*
Jerking, teeth were torn out with—*Euph.*
Laced and drawn tight together, throat and tongue were—*Thlaspi*
Lame, speech were thick as if tongue were—*Æsc. g.*
Large, tongue were too—*Acon., Ars., Colch., Crot. t., Cupr. n.,
      Dign., Get., Glon., Hydrs., Kali bi., Kali i., Lac. ac., Merc.
      c., Nat. ar., Ox. ac., Par., Phos., Plb., Sep.*
  –for mouth, tongue were too—*Kali ar.*
  –it fills the whole mouth, tongue were so—*Caj.*
  –and numb, tongue were too—*Crot. t.*
  –teeth were—*Nux m.*
  –and too long, teeth were too—*Sil.*
  –right molars were soft and too—*Cinnb.*
Lay deeper in mouth than usual, tongue—*Bell.*
Lead, teeth were filled with—*Verat. a.*
  –taste of—*Calc. c.*
Leather, tongue were covered with—*Nux m.*
Leathery, mouth were—*Stann.*
  –mouth were dry and—*Tan.*
Lifeless, tongue were—*Bell.*
Lifted, teeth were being—*Mez., Spong.*
Light, tongue were—*Dirc., Kali cy.*
Lime water, taste of—*Verat. a.*
Lined with mucus, fauces were—*Crot. h., Rhod., Verat. a.*
  –with flannel, mouth were—*Ars.*
  –with rancid grease, mouth were—*Euph.*
  –with rancid grease, roof of mouth were—*Kali p.*
Linen, taste of old—*Colch.*
Liver, taste of fried—*Podo.*
Lobelia, taste of—*Lac. ac.*
Lodged in fauces, something had—*Ham., Saba.*
  –in fauces causing constant inclination to swallow, something
      had—*Æsc.*

Lodged—*Continued*

–in fauces, something rough—*Arn.*

–at root of tongue, something had—*Phyt.*

–between teeth, a tenacious body were—*Cor. r.*

–between teeth, food were—*Ptel.*

–between teeth, tenacious substance—*Rhus t.*

Long, palate were too—*Hyos.*

–tongue were too—*Æth.*

–teeth were too—*Agar., Alum., Aur., Berb., Bor., Cham., Cob., Coc. c., Colch., Hep., Hyos., Iodof., Lachn., Mag. c., Merc., Mez., Nat. m., Nicc., Nux v., Parth., Phyt., Plan., Rhus t., Sanic., Spig., Spira., Sulph., Wild., Zinc.*

–and too large for her, teeth were—*Sil.*

–and loose, teeth were—*Zinc.*

–front teeth were too—*Lyc.*

–incisors were too—*Agar., Lyc., Rat., Stann., Tep.*

–upper incisors were too—*Mag. m.*

–right eye tooth were too—*Mez.*

–back teeth were too—*All. c., Helod.*

–molar teeth were too—*Merc. i. f., Rat.*

–lower molars were too—*Sil.*

–hollow tooth were too—*Clem., Hep., Lach.*

–painful teeth were too—*Chr. ac.*

Loose, teeth were—*Ars., Ars. s. f., Con., Eupi., Glon., Lith., Merc., Nicc., Nux v., Psor., Rhus t., Scroph., Sol. t. æ., Sulph., Tub., Zinc.*

–during mastication, teeth were—*Ars. s. f., Con., Hyos.*

–incisor teeth were—*Lachn.*

–incisor teeth were when chewing—*Coff.*

–teeth were dull and—*Spong.*

–and would fall out, teeth were—*Ars., Hyos., Psor.*

–teeth were long and—*Zinc.*

–and numb, teeth were—*Lith.*

–right molar teeth were—*Com.*

–nerve of tooth were put on stretch and then let—*Puls.*

Loosened during menses, mucous membrane in mouth were— *Mag. c.*

Lump in tooth—*Bell.*

Lumps in mouth, there were—*Lyss.*

Lye, taste of—*Caj., Nit. s. d.*

Lying on fore part of tongue, hair were—*Sil.*

Manure, taste of—*Calc. c., Carb. an., Hell. f., Merc., Plb., Sep., Verat. a.*

Many teeth and they were jammed together, there were too —*Tub.*

Meal, tongue were covered with Indian—*Nit. ac.*

Mealy taste—*Bry., Grat., Lach., Nicc.*

Meat between teeth, shreds of—*Caust.*

  –taste of bad—*Bry., Puls., Rhus t.*

Metal, astringent sensation in mouth came from—*Saba.*

Metallic in right half of tongue—*Cann. i.*

  –taste—see TASTE, METALLIC

Mercury, he had taken—*Lach.*

Milk, surface of mouth were covered with—*Kali i.*

Milky taste—*Aur.*

Morsel were still sticking in mouth after swallowing—*Merl.*

Moldy taste—*Lyc., Mar., Pimp., Tab.*

Move tongue to speak, it were difficult to—*Nux m.*

Mucus in mouth—*Glon., Lyc., Mag. c., Mag. m., Squill.*

  –roof of mouth were covered with tenacious—*Puls.*

  –mouth were fuzzy from—*Til.*

  –fauces were filled with—*Calc. c.*

  –fauces were lined with—*Crot. h., Rhod., Verat. a.*

  –tongue were covered with viscid—*Agar.*

Mud, tongue were smeared with—*Myric.*

Musty taste—*Bor., Kali bi., Led., Lyc., Phos. ac., Rhus t.*

Narrow, mouth were—*Am. c.*

Nauseous taste—see the GENERAL REPERTORIES

Near each other, teeth were too—*Cor. r.*

Needle were darting in mouth, with mouth open like a catfish— *Coll.*

  –membrane in right side of mouth were raised with—*Canth.*

  –hot, were thrust into tip of tongue—*Lach.*

Needles and pins, mouth were full of—*Spig.*

  –tongue were pierced by—*Nux v.*

  –had been run into tongue and lips, a hundred little—*Arum m.*

Nerve, bare, were touched in teeth—*Dios.*

Nitre, taste of—*Spira.*

Nuts, he had been eating—*Phyt., Spong.*

Numb, mouth were—*Bov., Mag. s.*

  –tongue were—*Eup. pur.*

  –and too large, tongue were—*Crot. t.*

Numb—*Continued*

  –tip of tongue were—*Adren., Ign.*

  –and contracting in right front of tongue—*Ars. h.*

  –gums were—*Apis*

  –teeth were loose and—*Lith.*

Object were between teeth, some—*Cor. r.*

Oil, parts in mouth had been covered with—*Sabal*

  –teeth were covered with—*Æsc.*

  –taste of—*Glon., Mang., Psor., Sec., Sil., Tab.*

  –taste of rancid—*Euphr., Tab.*

Oily, tongue were—*Phys.*

Onions, he had taken—*Æth., All. c., Carb. s., Crot. c., Meph., Merl., Mosch., Par., Sin. n.*

Open, passage from mouth to nose were wide—*Fl. ac.*

Oysters, taste of raw—*Zinc. m.*

Painted in morning on waking, mouth were—*Carb. v.*

Pap, teeth were fixed in a mass of—*Merc.*

Papier mache, teeth were made of—*Raph.*

Papillæ, mouth and tongue were deprived of—*Ter.*

Paralyzed, tongue were—*Ars., Cedr., Cocc., Cupr. s., Phys., Sec., Syph.*

Parched in mouth and fauces—*Aml. n.*

Partaken of raw or yellow sugar, he had—*Nat. p.*

Passed into nose and mouth, too much air—*Ther.*

Passing over tongue, cold air were—*Acon.*

Peach brandy taste—*Laur.*

  –pits, taste of—*Ang.*

Peas, mouth were full of—*Pyrog.*

  –taste of raw—*Zinc.*

Pebbles were in mouth—*Merc. i. f.*

Peel, tongue were going to—*Lach.*

Peeled off, mucous membranes of roof of mouth were—*Lach.*

Peeling off gums, epithelium were—*Lach.*

Penetrated mouth, cold sharp air—*Squill.*

  –a wound in mouth, air—*Thuj.*

  –teeth, every sound—*Ther.*

  –teeth, cold water—*Staph.*

Pepper, he had eaten—*Bapt., Caust., Coca, Cocc.*

  –were in mouth—*Mez.*

  –mouth were full of—*Manc.*

  –from mouth to stomach, full of—*Euph.*

Pepper—*Continued*

  —were burning in mouth—*Nat. s.*

  —on palate—*Mez.*

  —on tongue—*Agar.*

  —tongue were covered with—*Cann. i., Lach.*

  —on front of tongue—*Chin., Coc. c., Mez.*

  —on sides on tongue—*Mar.*

  —on back of tongue—*Sep.*

  —or spice on tip of tongue—*Malar.*

Peppers in mouth and throat—*Sang. n., Xanth.*

Peppermint were biting in mouth—*Verat. a.*

  —lozenges, he had eaten—*Camph., Ferr. i., Lyss., Verat. a.*

Peppery taste—*Acon., Cahin., Hydrs., Iris, Mez., Polyg., Raph., Tarax., Xanth.*

Pieces on biting teeth together, molar and bicuspid teeth would fly to—*Cinnb.*

Pierced, tongue were—*Galvan.*

  —by needles, tongue were—*Nux v.*

  —by a hot iron, all teeth were suddenly—*Tep.*

Pimento were burning on tongue—*Elaps*

  —taste of—*Crot. t.*

Pine roots or wood, taste of—*Glon.*

Pinned together, teeth were—*Tub.*

Pins and needles; mouth were full of—*Spig.*

  —a thousand, were pricking tongue—*Carb. ac.*

  —were sticking in tongue—*Samars.*

Pitch taste in mouth—*Cadm. s., Calc. s., Canth.*

Pithy, front of tongue were—*Am. c.*

Place, teeth were all out of—*Syph.*

Plug of mucus in mouth—*Scroph.*

Plum, palate were covered with skin of—*Verat. a.*

Polished away, mucous membrane of tongue were—*Phos.*

Potatoes, taste of raw—*Sol. t. æ.*

Powder, tongue would fall into—*Nux m.*

Pressed back into mouth, food remained above stomach and were being—*Nux v.*

  —into nerves of teeth, too much blood—*Hep.*

  —deeper into gum when biting, teeth were—*Staph.*

  —out of sockets, teeth were—*Coc. c.*

  —together, teeth were—*Merc. i. f., Stram.*

  —together with pincers, molar teeth were—*Cina*

Pressing it up, something under root of tongue were—*Ust.*

   –inner surface of gums, leaden bullet were—*Arn.*

Pressure, teeth were very sensitive to—*Hecla*

Pricked with needles, tongue were—*Nux v.*

Pricking in mouth, pins were—*Spig.*

   –tongue, a thousand pins were—*Carb. ac.*

   –gums would aggravate toothache—*Sanic.*

Prickling, tongue were—*Ptel.*

Protruded, teeth—*Carb. v.*

Puckered, fauces were—*Brom.*

   –tongue were—*Calc. s.*

Pulled by the roots, tongue were—*Rhus v.*

   –out, teeth had been—*Laur.*

   –out, teeth would be—*Zinc.*

   –upper and lower teeth were being gently—*Chim. umb.*

   –out, carious teeth were being—*Mag. p. Arct.*

   –out, a tooth were screwed in and then—*Bry.*

   –out, lower teeth were being—*Der.*

   –then left in sockets, teeth were—*Sanic.*

   –out of teeth, nerves were suddenly—*Stry.*

Pulling center of tongue toward hyoid bone, string were—*Cast.*

Pumped through upper incisor teeth, blood were—*Croc.*

Pungent heat in mouth—*Æth.*

Pushed from sockets on biting, stumps of teeth were—*Alum.*

   –up, lower incisors were—*Con.*

Radish were stinging on back of tongue—*Agar.*

Raised with a needle, mucous membrane in right side of mouth were—*Canth.*

   –tooth would be—*Prun.*

Rancid grease, mouth were lined with—*Euph.*

   –grease, roof of mouth were lined with—*Kali p.*

   –taste—*Agar., Alum., Asaf., Bry., Ferr. m., Form., Hell., Kali bi., Kali i., Nat. c., Petr., Scroph., Sulph., Zing.*

Raw, inner mouth were—*Stram.*

   –whole mucous membrane of mouth would become—*Ign.*

   –palate were—*Puls.*

   –tongue were—*Alco., Ammc., Am. caust., Apis, Ars., Bar. c., Canth., Carb. v., Cinnb., Cist., Coloc., Coniin., Cupr., Glon., Graph., Grat., Hydrs., Kali c., Lac. ac., Laur., Lob. s., Lyc., Mag. s., Menis., Merc., Naja, Nit. m. ac., Petr., Phos., Phys., Sin. n., Sul. ac., Tarax., Thuj., Vip., Zinc. ac.*

Raw—*Continued*
–and sore, tongue were—*Kali c.*
–middle of tongue were—*Acon.*
–tip of tongue were—*Phos.*
–taste in mouth—*Naja*
Resinous taste—*Agar., Cocc., Kali bi., Thuj.*
Rested upon tongue, uvula—*Saba.*
Resting upon a vibrating board, teeth were—*Phys.*
Rinsed his mouth in the morning, he had not—*Cyc.*
Rough and hard were lodged in mouth and fauces, something —*Arn.*
Rubbed against teeth, papillæ of tongue—*Graph.*
Rum, he had taken—*Brom.*
Run into mouth, ear-wax would—*Crot. h.*
–into tongue and lips, a hundred little needles had been—*Arum m.*
Running through posterior nares over palate, acrid fluid were —*Kali bi.*
–from vulva up to mouth, boiling water were—*Sec.*
Rushed out of molars, coldness—*Rat.*
Saliva were cold—*Chen. v.*
–tongue were enveloped in—*Chen. v.*
Salivated, mouth were sore and—*Sec.*
Salt water collected in mouth—*Verb.*
–on tongue, after—*Nux m.*
–on tip of tongue—*Croc., Nat. c.*
–food lacked—*Cocc., Sac. lac.*
–food were saturated with—*Puls.*
–taste—*Agar., Ail., Alco., Alum., Alumn., Ambr., Am. c., Anac., Ant. c., Ant. t., Arn., Ars., Atro., Bar. c., Bell., Benz. ac., Bov., Brom., Bry., Caj., Calc. c., Cann. s., Carb. s., Carb. v., Carl., Caust., Chin., Coca, Coff., Cop., Croc., Cupr., Cyc., Dig., Dros., Elaps, Euph., Fl. ac., Graph., Hyos., Iod., Kali bi., Kali br., Kali chl., Lach., Lith. m., Lyc., Mag. c., Mag. m., Merc., Merc. c., Merc. cy., Mez., Nat. c., Nat. m., Nit. ac., Nux m., Nux v., Op., Phos., Puls., Rhod., Rhus t., Rhus v., Sep., Spig., Stann., Stram., Sulph., Sul. ac., Tarent., Verat. a., Verb., Zinc.*
Salted too little, food were—*Thuj.*
–food were not—*Ars., Calc. c., Canth., Card. m., Cocc., Lyss., Merc. i. r., Sulph., Thuj.*

Sand in mouth—*Ars., Bov., Rhus v.*

–were sticking in palate, hard grain of—*Coloc.*

–on tongue—*Coloc.*

–(in open air) tongue were covered with—*Gins.*

–between teeth—*Rhod.*

Sandy taste—*Stram.*

Sawdust, taste of—*Atro., Cor. r., Nux m.*

Scalded, mouth were—*All. c., Apis, Bad., Bell., Eupi., Eriod., Hura, Hydrs., Iris, Jatr., Mag. m., Merc. c., Peti., Rhus v., Saba., Sin. n., Stict., Thea, Wye.*

–mouth and fauces were—*Am. br., Rhus v.*

–mouth and throat had been—*Rhus v., Stict.*

–by fat, mouth were—*Eupi.*

–from strong cigars, mouth were—*Mag. p.*

–from warm drinks or food, roof of mouth were—*Sanic.*

–on palate—*Cimx.*

–gums were—*Ars. m., Merc. c.*

–mouth and tongue were—*Sep., Tub.*

–tongue were—*Æsc., All. c., Ambr., Am. br., Apis, Ars., Azad., Bad., Bapt., Caj., Caust., Cimx., Coca, Coloc., Conv., Cupr., s., Eriod., Graph., Hydrs., Iris, Lac f., Lach., Lyc., Mag. m., Merc. d., Merc. i. r., Pen., Phys., Phyt., Plat., Podo., Prun., Ptel., Puls., Rhus v., Rumx., Saba., Samb., Sang., Sep., Sin. n., Sol. n., Still., Sumb., Thea, Tub., Verat. a., Verat. v.*

–fauces and tongue were—*Am. br.*

–tip of tongue were—*Ham., Merc., Rumx., Saba., Sang., Sep.*

–tongue were excoriated and—*Rumx.*

–edge of tongue had been—*Puls.*

–sides and surface of tongue were—*Azad.*

–round spots on tongue, there were—*Arum t.*

Scale off, tongue would—*Spig.*

Scored by a hot iron in center of tongue—*Ter.*

Scraped, tongue were—*Sumb.*

–in morning, front of tongue were—*Caps.*

Scraping in mouth—*Æsc., Alum., Am. c., Arn., Bell., Caust., Cedr., Colch., Croc., Crot. t., Kali i., Nit. ac., Phos., Sal. ac.*

Screwed together, teeth were—*Euph., Stront.*

–in and then pulled out, tooth were—*Bry.*

Seltzer-water, he had taken—*Iod.*

Senna leaves, taste of—*Aloe*

Sensitive to air, teeth were—*Tub.*
  —to pressure, teeth were very—*Hecla*
Separated from teeth, gums were—*Raph.*
  —teeth were forcibly—*Anan.*
  —molars, foreign body—*Lach., Ran. b.*
Shattered and crushed, nerves of tooth were—*Ign.*
Shavings, taste in mouth of—*Alumn.*
Shock, electric, went from mouth down to feet—*Nux m.*
Shocks, galvanic, in mouth—*Cedr.*
  —electric, through tongue—*Aran.*
  —electric, continually from one tooth to another—*Tab.*
Shooting into loose teeth on inhaling, air were—*Sulph.*
Short and throat too tight, tongue were too—*Zinc. ac.*
Shreds of meat between teeth—*Caust.*
Skinned, tongue had been—*Rhus t.*
Sleep, tongue had gone to—*Nux m.*
Slime, teeth were full of—*Thea*
Sloe, taste of—*Cahin.*
Small, tongue were—*Vip. l. f.*
Smeared with arrow-root, tongue and fauces were—*Sul. ac.*
  —with mud, tongue were—*Myric.*
Smoked tobacco too long, he had—*Sec.*
Smoky taste—*Benz. ac., Hura, Mez., Nux v., Phos. ac.*
Soapy taste—*Arg. n., Benz. ac., Cact., Calc. s., Chlor., Dulc., Iod., Merc., Merl., Sil.*
Soft on motion, tongue were too—*Mez.*
  —on edge, teeth were—*Lepi.*
  —and bent when chewing, teeth were—*Coch.*
  —and glued together, incisors were—*Zinc. ox.*
  —and too large, right molars were—*Cinnb.*
  —on separating, molars were—*Zinc.*
  —and spongy, teeth were—*Nit. ac.*
Soldered together, head, nose and teeth were—*Lyss.*
Sooty taste—*Ars.*
Sore and thick, mouth were—*Lachn.*
  —tongue were quite—*Mez.*
  —and raw, tongue were—*Kali c.*
  —and swollen, gums were—*Gamb.*
  —and swollen, upper gums were—*Ruta*
  —gums and molars were—*Clem.*
Sounds penetrated teeth—*Ther.*

Sour taste—see the GENERAL REPERTORIES

Sparks, electric, through teeth—*Tarent.*

Speaking with a full mouth—*Nux v.*

Spice on tongue—*Sil.*
  —or pepper on tip of tongue—*Lepi., Malar.*

Spirituous taste—*Chel.*

Splinter in mouth—*Nit. ac., Upas*
  —of glass between cheek and teeth—*Stann.*
  —in tooth or gums—*Hep.*

Split asunder, left lower molars were—*Thuj.*

Spongy tissue, tongue were mostly—*Merc.*
  —teeth were soft and—*Nit. ac.*

Sprained, teeth were—*Arn.*

Stale taste—*Chin. s., Stann.*

Start from jaw, tooth would—*Puls.*

Starting from gums, two middle incisors were enlarged and—*Raph.*

Steam extending from root of tongue to bronchi, he had inhaled hot—*Med.*

Steamed from nose and mouth, heat—*Stront.*

Sticking in mouth after swallowing, morsel were still—*Merl.*
  —to roof of mouth, tongue were—*Con.*
  —in tongue, pins were—*Samars.*
  —in tongue, something were—*Laur.*

Stiff, tongue were—*Phys.*
  —as shoe leather, tongue were hard and—*Stram.*
  —gums were—*Plan.*
  —and sore, nerves of teeth were—*Stry.*

Still, she cannot keep her tongue—*Stict.*

Stinging on back part of tongue, radish were—*Agar.*

Straw, everything tasted like—*Alumn., Arg. n., Chin., Cor. r., Kali i., Kreos., Mag. c., Mez., Rhod., Rhus t., Stram., Sulph.*

Stretch and then let loose, nerve of tooth were put on—*Puls.*

Stretched out over teeth, tongue were enlarged and—*Colch.*
  —torn or compressed in teeth, nerves were—*Coloc.*

String were pulling center of tongue toward hyoid bone—*Cast.*

Stuck together, mouth were—*Spig.*
  —to roof of mouth, tongue were—*Nux v.*
  —in fauces, foreign body were—*Agar.*

Styptic in mouth—*Arum d., Merc. c., Plb.*

Sugar, he had partaken of raw or yellow—*Nat. p.*

Sulphate of iron, taste of—*Ferr. i.*

Sulphur taste—*Plb., Stram.*

Supper, felt in mouth in morning he had no—*Eupi.*

Suppurate, gums were beginning to—*Sep.*

Swallowed, something at root of tongue ought to be—*Pip. m.*

Sweet taste—see the GENERAL REPERTORIES

Swelled interfering with speech, tongue were—*Mag. p. Aust.*

Swelling, left side of tongue were—*Arum m.*

  –teeth were—*Vip.*

  –about teeth, gums were—*Cham.*

Swollen, mouth were—*Am. c., Aml. n.*

  –with burning and numbness, lips and mouth were—*Aml. n.*

  –and cavity closing up, roof of mouth were—*Gels.*

  –tongue were—*Anac., Caj., Cimx., Crot. h., Glon., Lepi., Lyss., Phys., Rat., Spig.*

  –palate were—*Gels., Puls.*

  –gums were—*Aran., Eupi., Gamb., Lach., Spong., Stront.*

  –gums and cheeks were—*Aran.*

  –gums were sore and—*Gamb.*

  –upper gums were sore and—*Ruta*

  –alveoli were distended and—*Cham.*

Taken from mouth, mucous membrane would be—*Juni.*

  –out, teeth would be—*Prun.*

  –out, roots of teeth were being—*Ant. t.*

Tallow, tongue were covered with—*Til.*

  –taste of—*Nat. m., Valer.*

  –taste of fetid—*Sulph.*

Tar, taste of—*Con.*

Taste came from teeth—*Linar.*

  –bad, came from spot on side of tongue—*Tab.*

  –acrid—*Alumn., Brom., Caj., Carb. s., Chin. s., Fl. ac., Glon., Iris, Lac. ac., Pimp., Plan., Plb., Rhus t., Saponin., Seneg., Thuj., Verat. a.*

  –acrid, wine were—*Iod.*

  –alike, everything—*Merc. m., Phos.*

  –alkaline—*Am. c., Cere. b., Kali chl., Mez., Zinc. m.*

  –almonds, sweet—*Coff., Crot. t., Dig.*

  –alum after he had been smoking—*Nat. h.*

  –animal—*Con.*

  –apple-wine—*Cahin.*

  –aromatic—*Bell., Cham., Coc. c., Glon., Pip. m.*

Taste—*Continued*

–astringent—*Acon., Acon. l., Agar., Alum., Arg. n., Ars., Brom., Calc. i., Gal. ac., Gent. c., Iod., Kali bi., Kali cy., Kali i., Merc. c., Mur. ac., Musa, Ox. ac., Plb., Salix p.*

–bad—*Acon., Agar., Anac., Ant. t., Arn., Ars., Asar., Aur., Bar. c., Bell., Bov., Bry., Calc. c., Canth., Caps., Carb. an., Carb. v., Carb. s., Caust., Cham., Chin., Cocc., Coff., Coloc., Con., Cupr., Cyc., Dros., Euph., Ferr., Graph., Hep., Hyos., Ign., Kali br., Kali c., Kreos., Lob., Lyc., Mag. c., Mag. m., Mar., Merc., Mosch., Mur. ac., Nat. m., Nux m., Nux v., Olnd., Petr., Phos., Phos. ac., Psor., Puls., Rheum, Rhus t., Ruta, Sep., Spig., Stann., Staph., Sulph., Sul. ac., Thuj., Valer., Verat. a., Zinc., Zing.*

–bitter—see the GENERAL REPERTORIES

–bitter-sour—*Aloe, Carb. an., Kali c., Kali chl., Petr., Ran. b., Rhus t., Saba., Sep., Sulph.*

–bitter-sweet—*Arg. n., Aspar., Chim. umb., Crot. t., Kali i., Mag. c., Mag. s., Meny.*

–bloody—*Acon., Alum., Am. c., Anan., Asc. t., Ars., Bell., Berb., Benz. ac., Bism., Bov., Bufo, Canth., Carb. v., Chel., Dol., Elaps, Ferr., Ham., Hyper., Ip., Jatr., Kali c., Kalm., Lil. t., Manc., Nat. c., Osm., Phos., Puls., Rhus t., Sabin., Sil., Sulph., Thuj., Zinc.*

–brassy—*Chin. s., Ham., Merc., Ptel.*

–burnt—*Bry., Coca, Cyc., Franc., Laur., Phos., Puls., Ran. b., Squill., Sulph., Tab., Zinc. m.*

–carrot-tops—*Nux v.*

–calomel—*Nux m.*

–cedar-pitch—*Canth.*

–chalky—*Arg. n., Nux m.*

–cheesy—*Æth., Lyc., Par., Phel., Zinc.*

–chips—*Sang. n.*

–chocolate—*Crot. t.*

–cinnamon—*Glon.*

–clay—*Acon. l., Agar., Aloe, Ammc., Arg. n., Carl., Euphr., Lyc., Merc.*

–coffee—*Cinnb.*

–coppery—*Æsc., Agn., Arg. n., Ars., Aspar., Aur. m. n., Bell., Brom., Cann. i., Carb. an., Cerv., Cocc., Con., Cupr., Cupr. ac., Cupr. s., Hura, Jug. c., Kali bi., Lach., Lac. ac., Meph., Merc. c., Merc. n., Myris., Naja, Nat. p., Nit. m. ac., Nux*

Taste—*Continued*

v., *Ostrya, Plb., Polyp. o., Polyp. p., Psor., Rhus t., Sulph., Ust., Zinc.*

–coryza, old—*Upas*

–cream of tartar—*Tarent.*

–creosote—*Phys.*

–doughy—*Cerv., Phos., Sulph.*

–earthy—*Aloe, Bry., Cann. s., Caps., Chin., Euphr., Ferr., Franc., Gent. l., Hep., Ign., Linum, Lyc., Merc., Nux m., Phos., Pimp., Puls., Stront., Tell.*

–eggs, rotten—*Acon., Arn., Ferr., Gas., Graph., Hep., Merc., Mur. ac., Sil., Yuc.*

–elm-bark—*Guai.*

–ether—*Glon.*

–fatty—*Alum., Ambr., Asaf., Bar. c., Bry., Carb. v., Caust., Cham., Euph., Fl. ac., Glon., Ign., Ip., Kali bi., Lach., Laur., Lyc., Mag. m., Mang., Merc. c., Mur. ac., Ol. an., Petr., Phos., Phos. ac., Puls., Ran. s., Rhod., Rhus t., Saba., Sabin., Sang., Sil., Thuj., Valer.*

–febrile—*Chlor., Laur., Merc., Stry.*

–fish—*Acon., Astac., Sars.*

–fruit, unripe—*Saba.*

–garlic—*Asaf., Calc. ar., Merl.*

–gaseous—*Arg. cy., Pic. ac.*

–gas-works, like smell of—*Kersln.*

–glycerine—*Spong.*

–grapes—*Coca*

–hazel-nuts—*Coff.*

–herby—*Calad., Carb. s., Nat. m., Nux v., Phos. ac., Ptel., Puls., Sars., Stann., Verat. a.*

–herring—*Coca*

–herring-brine—*Anac.*

–honey, beer tastes like—*Mur. ac.*

–horse-chestnuts—*Sumb.*

–horse-radish—*Sin. n.*

–ink—*Aloe, Arg. n., Bart., Calc. c., Ferr. i.*

–insipid—see the GENERAL REPERTORIES

–iron—*Aloe, Calc. c., Cedr., Cimx.*

–lead—*Calc. c.*

–lime-water—*Verat. a.*

–linen, old—*Colch.*

Taste—*Continued*

–liver, fried—*Podo.*

–lobelia—*Lac. ac.*

–lye—*Caj., Nit. s. d.*

–manure—*Calc. c., Carb. an., Hell. f., Merc., Plb., Sep., Verat. a.*

–mealy—*Bry., Grat., Lach., Nicc.*

–meat, bad—*Bry., Puls., Rhus t.*

–metallic—*Æsc., Æth., Agar., Agn., Aloe, Alum., Am. c., Ant. t., Arg. n., Ars., Arum d., Aur. m. n., Bell., Bism., Calc. c., Calc. i., Cann. i., Carb. s., Carl., Cedr., Chel., Chr. ox., Chin., Cinnb., Cocc., Coc. c., Coloc., Colocn., Cupr., Cupr. ar., Cupr. s., Hep., Hyos., Indg., Iod., Ip., Jatr., Kali bi., Kali i., Kersln., Lac. ac., Linum, Lyc., Manc., Merc., Merc. c., Merc. i. r., Naja, Nat. ar., Nat. c., Nux v., Phos., Phys., Phyt., Plat., Plb., Polyp. o., Rhus t., Sars., Seneg., Sil., Stram., Sulph., Zinc., Zinc. m.*

–mercury, he had taken—*Lach.*

–milky—*Aur.*

–moldy—*Lyc., Mar., Pimp., Tab.*

–musty—*Bor., Kali bi., Led., Lyc., Phos. ac., Rhus t.*

–nauseous—see the GENERAL REPERTORIES

–nitre—*Spira.*

–nuts—*Phyt., Spong.*

–oil—*Glon., Mang., Psor., Sec., Sil., Tab.*

–oil, rancid—*Euphr., Tab.*

–onions—*Æth., All. c., Carb. s., Crot. c., Meph., Merl., Mosch., Par., Sin. n.*

–oysters, raw—*Zinc. m.*

–peach brandy—*Laur.*

–pits—*Ang.*

–peas, raw—*Zinc.*

–pepper—*Bapt., Caust., Coca, Cocc., Mez., Malar., Sang. n. Xanth.*

–peppermint—*Camph., Ferr. i., Lyss., Verat. a.*

–peppery—*Acon., Cahin., Hydrs., Iris, Mez., Polyg., Raph., Tarax., Xanth.*

–pimento—*Crot. t.*

–pine roots or wood—*Glon.*

–pitch—*Cadm. s., Calc. c., Canth.*

–potatoes, raw—*Sol. t. æ.*

Taste—*Continued*

  —rancid—*Agar., Alum., Asaf., Bry., Ferr. m., Form., Hell., Kali bi., Kali i., Nat. c., Petr., Scroph., Sulph., Zing.*

  —raw—*Naja*

  —resinous—*Agar., Cocc., Kali bi., Thuj.*

  —rum—*Brom.*

  —salt—*Agar., Ail., Alco., Alum., Alumn., Ambr., Am. c., Anac., Ant. c., Ant. t., Arn., Ars., Atro., Bar. c., Bell., Benz. ac., Bov., Brom., Bry., Caj., Calc. c., Cann. s., Carb. s., Carb. v., Carl., Caust., Chin., Coca, Coff., Cop., Croc., Cupr., Cyc., Dig., Dros., Elaps, Euph., Fl. ac., Graph., Hyos., Iod., Kali bi., Kali br., Kali chl., Lach., Lith. m., Lyc., Mag. c., Mag. m., Merc., Merc. c., Merc. cy., Mez., Nat. c., Nat. m., Nit. ac., Nux m., Nux v., Op., Phos., Puls., Rhod., Rhus t., Rhus v., Sep., Spig., Stann., Stram., Sulph., Sul. ac., Tarent., Verat. a., Verb., Zinc.*

  —food lacked—*Cocc., Sac. lac., Thuj.*

  —food were saturated with—*Puls.*

  —food were unsalted—*Ars., Calc. c., Canth., Card. m., Cocc., Lyss., Merc. i. r., Sulph., Thuj.*

  —sandy—*Stram.*

  —sawdust—*Atro., Cor. r., Nux m.*

  —seltzer-water—*Iod.*

  —senna leaves—*Aloe*

  —shavings—*Alumn.*

  —sloe—*Cahin.*

  —smoky—*Benz. ac., Hura, Mez., Nux v., Phos. ac.*

  —soapy—*Arg. n., Benz. ac., Cact., Calc. s., Chlor., Dulc., Iod., Merc., Merl., Sil.*

  —sooty—*Ars.*

  —sour—see the GENERAL REPERTORIES

  —spice—*Lepi., Malar., Sil.*

  —spirituous—*Chel.*

  —stale—*Chin. s., Stann.*

  —straw—*Alumn., Arg. n., Chin., Cor. r., Kali i., Kreos., Mag. c., Mez., Rhod., Rhus t., Stram., Sulph.*

  —styptic—*Arum d., Merc. c., Plb.*

  —sugar, raw or yellow—*Nat. p.*

  —sulphate of iron—*Ferr. i.*

  —sulphur—*Plb., Stram.*

  —sweet—see the GENERAL REPERTORIES

Taste—*Continued*
  –tallow—*Nat. m., Valer.*
  –fetid—*Sulph.*
  –tar—*Con.*
  –tea—*Verat. v.*
  –tobacco—*Agar., Cinnb., Kali i., Nat. c.*
  –unable to—*Merl.*
  –urine—*Psor., Seneg.*
  –vegetables, green—*Cere. b.*
  –verdigris—*Arg. n.*
  –vinegar—*Chel., Dig., Lyc., Jac., Sulph.*
  –wine were—*Cina*
  –violet-root—*Inul.*
  –weedy—*Caps.*
  –wine—*Seneg., Tab.*
  –wood—*Ars., Ruta, Sulph.*
    pine—*Glon.*
Tastes like chips, everything—*Sang. n.*
Tea on tongue, ĩe had taken—*Verat. v.*
Thick, mouth were sore and—*Lachn.*
  –tongue were—*Berb., Lach.*
  –middle of tongue were—*Chim. umb.*
  –teeth were—*Morph., Paull., Stram.*
Thin, teeth were very—*Sanic.*
Thread of mucus on tongue—*Cere. b.*
  –were rolling into a ball in fauces—*Ars.*
Throb, left upper molar would—*Plan.*
Thrust into tip of tongue, hot needle were—*Lach.*
Thrusts from a fist in teeth—*Calc. c.*
Tied up, tongue and throat were—*Crot. h.*
  –up, tongue were—*Lach.*
Tingling in lips and tongue—*Sac. lac.*
Tobacco were burning on tongue—*Agar.*
  –taste of—*Cinnb., Kali i., Nat. c.*
Toothache would develop—*Rhus t.*
Torn out, tongue would be—*Puls.*
  –out by the roots, tongue were being—*Rhus v.*
  –out, tooth would be—*Cyc., Euph.*
  –out, teeth were being—*Rhus t.*
  –out by a hook, tooth would be—*Cocc. s.*
  –out, roots of teeth would be—*Bov., Calc. c.*

Torn—*Continued*
 —out, left molars would be—*Cyc.*
 —out, left lower molars would be—*Prun.*
 —out with jerking, teeth would be—*Euph.*
 —nerves in teeth were—*Ant. c.*
 —and stretched, nerves in teeth were—*Coloc.*
Touched with copper, tip of tongue had been—*Con.*
 —by salt or spicy things, tongue were—*Bor.*
 —teeth on inspiration, cold air—*Cedr.*
 —in teeth, bare nerve were—*Dios.*
Trembling, tip of tongue were—*Nat. m.*
Twisted, teeth were—*Lach.*
Ulcer would form in molar, < cold water—*Lipp.*
Ulcerate, molar would—*Cob.*
Ulcerated, gums were—*Bell., Cob., Graph., Phel., Sulph.*
 —at root of teeth—*Am. c., Sanic.*
Ulcerating, tip of tongue were—*Æsc.*
 —molars were—*Sil.*
Ulcers, little, were about to form on palate—*Kali bi.*
 —beneath teeth—*Eupi.*
Urine, taste of—*Psor., Seneg.*
Vacillating, right lower molars were—*Arg. n.*
Varnished or glazed, tongue were—*Apis, Ter.*
Vegetables, taste of green—*Cere. b.*
Velvet, mouth were covered with—*Coc. c., Dig., Nux m.*
 —tongue were covered with—*Pip. m.*
Verdigris, taste of—*Arg. n.*
Vesicle were on tip of tongue—*Bell.*
Vesicles on tongue, burning came from—*Kali i., Phel.*
Vibrating board, teeth were resting on—*Phys.*
Vinegar in mouth—*Dig.*
 —he had taken sharp—*Iod.*
 —on tongue—*Chel.*
 —when drinking wine it were—*Cina*
 —taste—*Chel., Dig., Lyc., Jac., Sulph.*
Violet-root, he had eaten—*Inul.*
Water would accumulate in mouth—*Ruta*
 —salt, collected in mouth—*Verb.*
 —in mouth, a draft of cold—*Sars.*
 —cool, on teeth were too cold—*Ther.*
 —fell on tongue, drops of ice—*Pana.*

Water—*Continued*
   –palate were filled with—*Apis*
   –cold, penetrated teeth—*Staph.*
   –boiling, were running from vulva up to mouth—*Sec.*
Wax would run into mouth—*Crot. h.*
Wedge were between teeth—*Cor. r.*
Wedged, teeth were—*Lach.*
Weedy taste—*Caps.*
Wind, cold, in mouth—*Rhus t.*
   –strong, in mouth—*Sil.*
   –sockets of teeth were distended by—*Cham.*
   –cold, on teeth—*Coc. c.*
Wine freely, he had been drinking—*Carb. v.*
   –taste of—*Seneg., Tab.*
Wobbling, teeth were—*Arn.*
Wood, hard palate were made of—*Mez.*
   –tongue were made of—*Apis*
   –taste of—*Ars., Ruta, Sulph.*
Worm were crawling at root of tongue—*Kali i.*
   –were crawling in root of tooth—*Kali i., Syph.*
   –were creeping in right molars—*Cast.*
Wrenched out, tooth were—*Nux v.*
Wrinkled and burnt, gums were—*Par.*

THROAT

Abscess would break in throat—*Caps.*

Abraded, membrane in œsophagus had been—*Seneg.*

Acid fruit, had been eating—*Peti.*

Acids were rising in throat—*Hep.*

Acrid in region of epiglottis—*Hydrs., Iris*

  –in œsophagus—*Crot. t., Sars.*

  –fluid were running through posterior nares over palate, causing cough—*Kali bi.*

  –in throat, something—*Saba.*

  –and corroding causing suffocative cough, something—*Carb. v.*

Across throat, finger were—*Lac c.*

Adherent mucus in throat—*Kali bi.*

Adhering to uvula, muscles of throat were—*Ferr. ma.*

Air ascended spirally in throat—*Sumb.*

  –ascending from stomach through œsophagus—*Com.*

  –slowly ascending expanding throat—*Com.*

  –were raised into throat by contraction of œsophagus, ball filled with—*Cham.*

  –dryness and pain as from; constant inclination to swallow—*Merc.*

  –forced in and out in region of thyroid—*Spong.*

  –could not pass through throat, on rising—*Mag. c.*

  –passed into glands of neck on breathing—*Spong.*

  –were passing through posterior nares—*Mag. s.*

  –hot, passing up right side of throat although stomach feels cold—*Am. br.*

  –cold, penetrating to throat though warm—*Ol. an.*

  –something in throat prevented free passage of—*Fel tauri*

Alcohol, throat had been burned with—*Zinc.*

Alive when air reaches it, throat were—*Raph.*

  –goiter were—*Spong.*

  –in tonsils, uvula, behind nasal fossa and along œsophagus—*Raph.*

  –were running from stomach to throat, something—*Verat. a.*

Apoplexy were extending to throat—*Fl. ac.*

Apple core in throat, had a large—*Nit. ac., Phyt., Verat. a.*

  –core were sticking in throat—*Merc.*

Ascended spirally in throat, air—*Sumb.*

Ascending slowly, expanding œsophagus, air were—*Com.*

–from stomach through œsophagus, air were—*Com.*

–from stomach impeding speech, constriction were—*Manc.*

–in throat, a half fluid body were—*Spig.*

–to throat, heart were—*Podo.*

–in throat, lump or body were—*Asaf.*

–in œsophagus, preceded by something cold, something hot were—*All. s.*

Ascends on swallowing, and returns at once, a lump in throat—*Rumx.*

Astringent, he had eaten something—*Peti.*

–drink, he had swallowed—*Saba.*

Attached to epiglottis, something were—*Arum m.*

Awn, throat were scraped by an—*Mag. c.*

Bacon in throat, a piece of—*Nux m.*

Ball—see also LUMP

Ball or lump in throat—*All. c., Cham., Lac c., Lach., Nat. s., Nit. ac., Nux v., Par., Still., Sulph.*

–in œsophagus—*Der.*

–œsophagus were distended by a large—*Anac.*

–filled with air rose into throat by contraction of œsophagus—*Cham.*

–lodged in throat—*Linar., Par.*

–of mucus lodged in throat—*Ars.*

–of red hot iron had lodged in fauces and whole length of œsophagus—*Phyt.*

–were pressed through left wall of œsophagus on swallowing—*Crot. t.*

–were rising into the throat with spasmodic constriction of œsophagus—*Ars., Cham.*

–were rising in throat—*Ars., Asaf., Ign., Kali p., Kalm., Lyc., Nit. ac., Phys., Senec., Still., Stram., Sulph.*

–were rising from throat to brain—*Plb.*

–hard, were rising in throat—*Sulph.*

–were rising into œsophagus—*Verat. v.*

–were rising from stomach to throat, > by eructations—*Mag. m.*

–large, rising from lower end of sternum to upper end of œsophagus—*Lac d.*

–rose from stomach into throat—*Asaf., Lyc., Lyss., Senec.*

Ball—*Continued*

   –were sticking in throat—*Coc. c.*

   –were sticking in pharynx—*Stram.*

   –in throat stopped swallowing—*Senec.*

   –in throat which she could take hold of with fingers—*Lac c.*

Band were tight around throat—*Dios., Op.*

Bar across back part of throat—*Lac c.*

Barley sticking in throat, grain of—*Mag. c.*

   –in right throat, a split of—*Sars.*

Beaten, throat were—*Lyss.*

Biting in œsophagus—*Iod.*

Blend, opposing parts would not—*Sep.*

Blood would come from œsophagus while hawking—*Fl. ac.*

   –were rushing to throat—*Chel., Kali bi.*

Blotting paper, throat had been dried with—*Carb. v.*

Board, throat were stiff as a—*Lac c.*

Body—see also BALL and LUMP

Body or lump were ascending in throat—*Asaf.*

   –were ascending in throat, a half fluid—*Spig.*

   –round, were ascending from stomach—*Con.*

   –foreign, in throat—*Ail., Ambr., Am. c., Ant. c., Apis, Aqua m., Bry., Carb. v., Chin. s., Cic., Cob., Con., Graph., Hæm., Ham., Kreos., Led., Lob., Mag. c., Merc., Merc. s., Myric., Nat. c., Olnd., Phos., Plant., Plb., Rhus r., Saba., Sol. t. æ., Spira., Sulph., Tab., Thea, Zinc.*

   –foreign, in left side of throat at root of tongue—*Cedr.*

   –foreign, in pharynx—*Cop.*

   –foreign, in œsophagus—*Bell., Saba.*

   –foreign, in lower part of œsophagus—*Pic. ac., Vinc.*

   –hard, in œsophagus—*Lyc.*

   –large, in throat—*Con.*

   –soft, in œsophagus—*Scroph.*

   –throat were covered with a dry soft—*Cann. i.*

   –hard, forcing through œsophagus while eating—*Spire.*

   –hard, forcing through œsophagus after eating—*Caj.*

   –round, suddenly impelled upward to throat where it feels like a morsel too large to swallow—*Raph.*

   –irritated in throat from a foreign—*Kali bi.*

   –lodged in throat—*Apis*

   –lodged in œsophagus—*Alco., Gels.*

   –lodged in upper part of œsophagus—*Erig.*

Body—*Continued*

—foreign, were lodged in throat—*Ant. c., Apis, Nux m.*

—hard, lodged in back part of throat—*Lyc.*

—were lodged in pharynx, long narrow foreign—*X-ray*

—hard, were lying near manubrium—*Sin. a.*

—hard, were opposing pressure from pharynx into abdomen—
     Zinc.

—in throat, food had to pass over a foreign—*Merc.*

—foreign, rising to throat—*Chel.*

—living, in stomach rising into throat—*Tarent.*

—foreign, stopped the voice—*Arg. m.*

—he had to swallow over a foreign—*Sabin.*

—in throat that he tries to swallow but he cannot—*Sabin.*

—soft, in throat, which he must swallow—*Saba.*

—foreign, had been swallowed—*Merc., Sabin.*

—foreign, in œsophagus, preventing swallowing—*Upas*

Bone were in throat—*Calc. c., Carb. s., Hep., Ign., Lach., Nit.
     ac., Phys.*

—swallowing over a bone with a rolling around—*Ign.*

—had lodged in upper œsophagus with severe stinging, contract-
     ing pain, piece of—*Carb. s.*

Bone—see also FISHBONE

Bound in throat—*Caust.*

—tightly, whole throat were—*Ars. h.*

—muscles of throat and neck were; stiffness—*Caust.*

—together, throat and chest were—*Ars.*

Bread were too dry to swallow—*Ign.*

—crumb in throat causing choking—*Sanic.*

—had swallowed too large a morsel of—*Puls.*

Break when coughing, uvula would—*Ham.*

—in throat, abscess would—*Caps.*

—when coughing, throat would—*Ham.*

Breathing through a sponge in throat—*Brom.*

Broad substance covered with prickles impeded swallowing—
     Kali bi.

Bruised in throat—*Arg. m., Rhus t.*

—external throat were—*Cic.*

—muscles of throat were—*Hep.*

Brush were brought in contact with epiglottis—*Anag.*

—sharp, had been drawn through œsophagus to stomach—
     Nicot.

Bunch in throat—*Rumx., Xanth.*
 –in left side of throat, shifts to right side on swallowing—*Xanth.*
Burned in left upper throat—*Calc. s.*
 –palate had been—*Podo.*
Burning in throat—*Verat. a.*
 –cavern, throat were—*Iris*
 –in throat, pepper were—*Sal. ac.*
Burnt in throat—*Cupr. s., Pic. ac., Podo., Sol. n.*
 –anteriorly, palate were—*Bor., Sep.*
 –with alcohol, throat had been—*Zinc.*
 –with caustic, throat were—*Lac c.*
 –with hot drinks, throat were—*Chin. s.*
 –in pharynx—*Sang.*
 –a spot in pharynx were—*Merc.*
 –lard in throat caused scraping—*Hep.*
Burst, throat would—*Upas*
 –by force of gas, throat would—*Coca*
Button stuck fast in throat, he had a—*Lach.*
Cat were purring in throat—*Spig.*
Catarrh in back part of throat—*Coff.*
Caustic, throat were burned with—*Lac c.*
Cavern, throat and pharynx were a—*Phyt.*
 –burning, in throat—*Iris*
Choke, she would—*Chel., Nux v.*
 –if he did not swallow, he would—*Bell.*
 –throat were closing and she would—*Lac c.*
 –her, something were coming up to—*Con.*
 –pear in pharynx, had eaten—*Phyt.*
Choked, she would be—*Puls.*
 –were being—*Glon., Œna.*
 –with something that would not go down—*Sep.*
 –throat were so full it—*Phyt.*
Choking, he were—*Caj., Crot. h., Graph., Sac. lac.*
 –in throat—*Cot., Phys.*
 –in throat, with fullness and heat—*Iber.*
 –in right side of throat, only when not swallowing—*Zinc.*
 –lump in throat pit, suddenly—*Dol.*
 –rising in throat when speaking—*Manc.*
 –were rising in throat—*Hedo.*
 –rising up from stomach—*Manc.*

Close up and leave no space for swallowing, œsophagus would —*Caj.*

Closed, throat were—*Calad., Merc. i. f., Nat. p., Tarax., Vacc., Vario., Vip.*

–larynx and throat were—*Tarax.*

–pharynx were—*Sulph.*

–œsophagus would be—*Saba.*

–epiglottis were—*Med.*

–epiglottis were nearly—*Calc. ar.*

–the throat, preventing speech, something—*Nat. p.*

–it like a valve, something rolled into throat and—*Ferr.*

–by a swelling, throat would be—*Nat. m.*

–with a plug, throat would be—*Nat. m.*

–by a spasm, pharynx would be—*Kali i.*

Closing and she would choke, throat were—*Lac c.*

Closure of œsophagus—*Caj.*

Clumsy, posterior organs of speech were covered and—*Plat.*

Clutched and twisted, œsophagus were being—*Lyc.*

Coal, hot, in throat—*Euph.*

Coated with thick sticky mucus—*Samars.*

Cold in throat, had taken—*Plan.*

–in œsophagus—*Spire.*

–then hot and stinging ascended the œsophagus, something —*All. s.*

–air penetrating to throat, though warm—*Ol. an.*

–as from a piece of ice in throat—*Sanic.*

–were rising in throat, something—*Caust.*

Coldness in throat and mouth—*Verat. a.*

–extends up sternum and œsophagus—*Pyrus*

–in throat from peppermint—*Form., Verat. a.*

–in œsophagus from cress or radishes—*Agar.*

Compressed between thumb and finger, thyroid were—*Nat. a.*

Compression of œsophagus during deglutition—*Alum.*

Connected, ear and throat were—*Am. m.*

Constricted in throat and fauces—*Kali per.*

–throat were—*Ars., Bapt., Carb. v., Chel., Chin. b., Cocc., Crot. h., Cupr., Glon., Par., Plat., Puls., Sang. n., Thuj., Tub.*

–entrance to pharynx were—*Lyc.*

–pharynx were—*Nit. ac., Nux v., Thuj.*

–by a string, throat were—*Saba.*

Constricted—*Continued*
    –from above down to stomach, œsophagus were—*Bapt.*
    –continually, everything were knotted up or a hard lump of
        food remained there—*Kali bi., Lac. ac.*

Constriction, loose, in throat—*Cocc.*
    –of throat, food would not pass for—*Alum.*
    –in throat ascending from stomach and impeding speech—
        Manc.
    –of œsophagus from below upward—*Lob.*
    –from string or thread in throat—*Saba.*

Contracted in throat—*Arg. n., Uran.*
    –on swallowing, throat were—*Arg. n., Calc. c., Cupr., Grat.*
    –œsophagus were—*Cimx., Dros., Grat., Thuj.*
    –a part of the œsophagus were—*Alum.*
    –from below upward, œsophagus were—*Lob.*
    –or swollen in pharynx—*Carb. v.*

Cooling substance were rising in throat—*Camph.*

Coolness like ice in mouth and throat—*Sac. lac., Sanic.*

Cord were tied around throat—*Lach., Saba.*

Core of an apple were sticking in throat—*Merc.*
    –of a large apple were in throat—*Nit. ac., Phyt., Verat. a.*

Corkscrew while swallowing, food turned like a—*Elaps*

Corn husk in upper part of throat—*Mag. p.*

Coryza were approaching, in throat—*Graph.*

Cotton in throat—*Phos.*

Covered with dry soft body, throat were—*Cann. i.*
    –with fat, mucous membranes of throat were—*Card. m.*
    –and clumsy, posterior organs of speech were—*Plat.*
    –with mucus, pharynx were—*Cot.*
    –with tenacious mucus, palate were—*Puls.*

Crack, membrane of throat were so dry it would—*Sang.*
    –pharynx would—*Myric., Sang.*

Cramped, œsophagus were being—*Pyrog.*

Crawling in œsophagus, insects were—*Plb.*

Creeping up to throat from burning in stomach—*Carb. v.*
    –up into throat, worm were—*Puls., Zinc.*
    –up into throat causing coughing, worm were—*Zinc.*

Cress or radishes, coldness in œsophagus from—*Agar.*

Crumb or hair lodged in throat—*Ars., Coc. c., Pall.*
    –small, lodged in throat—*Lach.*

Crumb—*Continued*
    —above larynx—*Coc. c.*
    —of bread in throat causing choking—*Sanic.*
    —of bread in pharynx—*Dros., Sanic.*
Crumbs of bread remained in throat—*Dros.*
Crust in upper throat—*Calc. ar.*
Curling or rolling up on itself from tip to base, soft palate were
    —*Nux m.*
Cut to pieces on coughing, throat were—*Sulph.*
Cutting from knife in throat—*Merc. c., Stann.*
    —in lower part of œsophagus when swallowing, continuing
        after—*Vinc.*
Denuded, throat were—*Am. caust., Juni., Merc. c., Pen., Stann.,
    Sul. ac.*
Deprived of epithelium, throat were—*Still.*
Descends on swallowing but returns, lump in throat—*Lac c.,
    Lach., Rumx.*
Desquamation were about to take place in velum palati—*Lach.*
Digging in throat from before back, something were—*Ars.*
Discharge pus, tonsils were about to—*Calc. s.*
Dissolved in throat, a particle of sugar were—*Bad.*
Distended, pharynx were—*Verat. a.*
    —by a large ball, œsophagus were—*Anac.*
Down in throat, causing cough—*Phos. ac.*
Drawn down, soft palate were—*Stram.*
    —up, soft palate were—*Glon.*
    —tight together, throat and tongue were laced and—*Thlaspi*
    —together spasmodically, parts in throat were sore and—*Caps.*
    —from œsophagus to stomach, a sharp brush had been—*Nicot.*
    —across throat, web were—*Zinc.*
    —up from stomach toward throat, œsophagus were being—
        Asaf.
    —snuff through throat, one had—*Staph.*
Dried up in throat—*Paraf.*
    —with blotting paper, throat had been—*Carb. v.*
    —in fauces, causing tension, egg white had—*Mag. p.*
Drink were poured down throat like an empty barrel—*Hydr. ac.*
Drinking, water ran down outside of throat when—*Verat. a.*
Dry, throat were—*Ars., Rhus t., Tell.*
    —leather, soft palate were—*Stict.*
    —that it would crack, membrane of throat were so—*Sang.*

Dry—*Continued*
 --had collected in throat, something—*Cob.*
 --soft body, throat were covered with—*Cann. i.*
 --spot in throat—*Crot. h., Lach.*
 --to swallow, bread were too—*Ign.*
 --everything he swallowed were too—*Raph.*
 --in pharynx, intensely—*Lat. m.*
Dull point were pressing on right wall of œsophagus—*Olnd.*
Dust in throat—*Calc. c., Chel., Crot. c., Iber., Ign., Pic. ac., Rad. br., Saponin., Verat. a.*
 --in throat causing cough—*Am. c., Cist.*
 --in trachea, throat and behind sternum—*Chel.*
 --in throat, larynx and lungs—*Calc. c.*
 --throat were filled with—*Iber.*
Ear-wax were running down throat—*Crot. h.*
Eaten something astringent, he had—*Peti.*
 --choke pear in pharynx, he had—*Phyt.*
 --nuts, in throat, he had—*Calc. ar.*
 --rancid substances, she had—*Camph.*
Eating acid fruit, after—*Peti.*
 --too much, causing fullness in chest and throat—*Phos.*
Egg white had dried in fauces, causing tension—*Mag. c.*
Eggs in throat, lump like two—*Lac c.*
Elasticity of vocal cords, want of—*Sul. ac.*
Electric shock in throat—*Samars.*
 --thrusts in upper throat—*Manc.*
Elevation on left side, had to swallow over—*Graph.*
Elongated, uvula were—*Acon., Coc. c., Cocc. s., Croc., Crot. h., Crot. t., Dulc., Plat., Wye.*
Emphysematous extending to nipples, throat were—*Vip.*
Emptiness in throat—*Calc. p., Lyc., Nat. a.*
 --in œsophagus—*Chin., Mur. ac., Ptel.*
Enlarged, tonsils were—*Iber., Xanth.*
 --and a burning cavern, throat were—*Iris*
 --and swollen, throat were—*Xanth.*
 --and wide open and swollen, pharynx were—*Dig.*
 --something in throat had—*Lac c.*
 --or relaxed, something in throat were—*Lac c.*
 --upper part of œsophagus and posterior nares were—*Elat.*
Erosion in throat—*Apis, Ars., Plan., Sumb.*
Everything were up in throat—*Sil.*

Excoriated, throat were—*Hydrs., Mang., Sulph.*
Expanded, throat and abdomen were—*Hyper.*
Expanding throat, air were slowly ascending and—*Com.*
Expectorate a hair, trying to—*Colch.*
Exposed to heat of brisk fire, throat were internally—*Lact.*
Fat, mucous membranes were covered with—*Card. m.*
Feather in throat—*Cina, Iod.*
  —or down in throat—*Am. c., Cina, Iod.*
  —were tickling in throat—*Calc. c., Cinnb., Dros., Ign.*
  —were tickling in back of throat—*Æsc.*
Fermentation in œsophagus—*Kalm.*
File scratching in throat—*Nit. ac.*
Filled with water, palate were—*Apis*
  —up, throat were—*Lac. ac., Sil.*
  —with lump, throat were—*Lach.*
  —with gurgling mucus, throat were—*Graph.*
  —with mucus, posterior part of throat were—*Mez.*
  —with phlegm, throat were—*Lac c., Sep.*
  —with food, stomach and œsophagus were—*Arg. n.*
Film around upper part of œsophagus—*Sumb.*
Finger were across throat—*Lac c.*
Fire, throat were on—*Canth., Iris, Tart. ac.*
  —throat were exposed to heat of brisk—*Lact.*
Fishbone in throat—*Apis, Chel., Hep., Kali c., Lach., Nit. ac.,*
      Phys., Sac. lac.
  —large, in throat when swallowing—*Apis, Sac. lac.*
  —loose in throat—*Apis*
  —in pharynx, if he gets cold—*Kali c.*
Fist were in throat and chest, something size of—*Cic.*
Flame were running out of throat and stomach—*Euph.*
Flatus rising would rend œsophagus—*Coca*
Flesh would be raised when coughing, a piece of—*Phos.*
Fluid had gone into wrong passage—*Lach.*
  —were running through posterior nares over palate, causing
      cough, an acrid—*Kali bi.*
  —poured down throat—*Glon.*
  —throat were scalded by hot—*Lac c., Psor.*
  —œsophagus were full of rancid—*Crot. h.*
Fold of tissue, mucous membrane of throat were a loose—*Med.*
Food about epiglottis, particles of—*Hepat.*
  —stomach and œsophagus were filled with—*Arg. n.*

Food—*Continued*

    –had to force over a sore spot in throat—*Bar. c.*

    –would not go down—*Arn., Graph., Nit. ac., Sulph.*

    –goes down the wrong way—*Nat. m.*

    –pharynx could not grasp—*Nit. ac.*

    –had lodged in throat or œsophagus—*Arg. n., Bar. c., Benz. ac., Calc. c., Caust., Merc., Zinc.*

    –were lodged in upper end of œsophagus—*Ars.*

    –had lodged in œsophagus, morsel of—*Abies c., Bar. c., Chin., Puls.*

    –were lying in œsophagus—*Abies c., Chin., Puls.*

    –passed over lump in throat—*Graph., Merc., Nat. m., Puls., Sabin.*

    –solid, passes over lump in throat—*Lac c.*

    –passes over sore spot in throat—*Bar. c., Nat. m.*

    –were pushed up as if it had not been swallowed—*Ferr. i.*

    –rancid, caused rawness in throat—*Phos.*

    –remained in throat, hard lump of—*Kali bi., Lac ac., Zinc.*

    –remained in upper part of œsophagus—*Dig.*

    –remained sticking in pharynx—*Calc. c., Zinc.*

    –were sticking in throat—*Aqua pet., Bry., Caust., Croc., Crot. t., Ferr., Ign., Iris, Lach., Plect., Til.*

    –stuck in throat after swallowing, morsel of—*Pip. n.*

    –were stuck in throat, a large morsel of—*Ign.*

    –were stuck in throat and would not go down—*Ambr.*

    –were stuck at base of throat—*Samars.*

    –he had swallowed too large a morsel of—*Cimx., Ferr. ma., Puls., Sin. a.*

    –swallowing suddenly a large piece of—*Phys.*

    –turned like a corkscrew on swallowing—*Elaps*

Force itself over a sore spot, food had to—*Bar. c.*

    –of gas would burst throat—*Coca*

    –out of goiter, everything would; with working, distension and pressure—*Spong.*

    –through pharynx, water would—*Staph.*

Forced asunder, larynx and throat were—*Kali a.*

    –in and out in region of thyroid, air were—*Spong.*

    –into throat, stopper were—*Croc.*

Forcing through œsophagus while eating, a hard body were—*Spire.*

    –through œsophagus after eating, hard body were—*Caj.*

Foreign body—see BODY
Fruit in throat, after eating acid—*Peti.*
Full of peas, throat and mouth were—*Pyrog.*
  –of rancid grease, œsophagus were—*Crot. h.*
  –of sticks, throat were—*Lac c.*
Fullness behind palate—*All. c.*
  –in œsophagus—*Am. m., Zinc.*
  –in chest and throat as if eating too much—*Phos.*
Fumes of sulphur in throat—*Ign., Puls.*
Funnel, pharynx were open like—*Lob. s.*
Glass were in throat, a piece of—*Nit. ac.*
Glued to throat, rough body were—*Arg. m.*
Glutinous in œsophagus—*Kali n.*
Go down, food would not—*Arn., Graph., Nit. ac., Sulph.*
Goes down wrong way, food—*Nat. m.*
Goiter which she could not see over, she had a large—*Zinc.*
Grain husk in throat—*Kali p.*
  –of barley in throat—*Mag. c.*
  –of sand were sticking in palate—*Coloc.*
Grasp food, pharynx could not—*Nit. ac.*
Grasped him by the throat, someone had—*Atro., Lach.*
Grease, œsophagus were full of rancid—*Crot. h.*
Gripped by a hand, throat were—*Tab.*
Grown up, throat were—*Aml. n., Cic., Merc. c.*
  -together internally, throat had—*Cic.*
Growth in throat, in which particles stick on swallowing—*Graph.*
  –in throat, there were a fleshy—*Sol. t. æ.*
Hair on back part of tongue and velum—*Kali bi.*
  –he were trying to expectorate a—*Colch.*
  –were lodged in throat—*Ars., Calc. s., Carb. s., Coc. c., Kali bi., Sulph., Valer.*
  –or crumb lodged in throat—*Coc. c., Pall.*
Hairs in back of throat—*Rhus v.*
  –in throat, interferes with swallowing, a tangle of—*Cent.*
Hand had gripped the throat—*Tab.*
Hanging in throat, something were—*Samars.*
  –in throat, mucus were—*Laur.*
  –in throat, a sponge were—*Lac c., Lach.*
  –in throat near hyoid bone, on swallowing, something were—*Pall.*

Hanging—*Continued*
  –down in throat, string or thread were—*Coc. c., Valer.*
  –in throat, skin, leaf or valve were—*Ant. c., Bar. c., Ferr.,*
    Mang., Phos., Saba., Spong.
  –in throat, loose skin were—*Alum.*
  –in throat, a piece of skin were—*Plat.*
  –loosely in throat, skin were, and must swallow over it—*Saba.*
Hard, he were swallowing something—*Kali c.*
  –all down œsophagus, something were—*Kali bi.*
  –body forcing through œsophagus while eating—*Spire.*
  –body forcing through œsophagus after eating—*Caj.*
  –body in œsophagus—*Lyc.*
  –body were lodged in back part of throat—*Lyc.*
  –body were lying near manubrium—*Sin. a.*
  –body were opposing pressure from pharynx into abdomen—
    Zinc.
  –lump in throat—*Spig.*
  –small lump in throat—*Zinc.*
Hardened, thyroid gland were—*Spong.*
Hardness and heaviness of tonsils—*Cham.*
Heart were ascending to throat—*Podo.*
  –came into throat—*Stry.*
Heartburn caused rawness in throat—*Kali i.*
Heat, pungent, in mouth and throat—*Æth.*
  –down œsophagus to stomach, < eating—*Wye.*
  –of brisk fire, throat were exposed to—*Lact.*
Heaviness and hardness of tonsils—*Cham.*
Held tightly around throat, something were—*Stry.*
Hoarse and lose her voice, she would become—*Prun.*
  –from scraping in throat, she would become—*Psor.*
Hollow, pharynx were—*X-ray*
Hoop around throat, one chest and one around the diaphragm—
    Cact.
Hot air passing up right side of throat though stomach feels cold
    —*Am. br.*
  –coal in throat—*Euph.*
  –drinks, throat were burned with—*Chin. s.*
  –fluid in throat, scalded by—*Lac c., Psor.*
  –iron ball lodged in œsophagus on swallowing—*Phyt.*
  –marble in throat near palate—*Kali p.*

Hot—*Continued*
  –were in throat, something—*Arum t.*
  –steam were rising in throat—*Merc. i. r.*
  –and stinging ascended the œsophagus, following something cold—*All. s.*
  –stone in pharynx—*Stram.*
Hull of wheat in throat—*Plb.*
Husk in throat—*Ast. r., Berb., Croc., Maland.*
  –in left tonsil—*Berb.*
  –of barley in right throat—*Sars.*
  –of corn lodged in upper part of throat, with constant desire to swallow—*Mag. p.*
  –of grain in throat—*Kali p.*
Ice had been held in mouth and throat, a piece of—*Sac. lac., Sanic.*
  –had slipped down throat, a piece of—*Coc. c.*
Imbedded in right side of throat near angle of jaw, a large splinter were—*Dol.*
Impeded swallowing, broad substance covered with prickles—*Kali bi.*
Impelled upward to throat, a round body were; where it feels like a morsel too large to swallow—*Raph.*
Inactive or paralyzed, pharynx were—*Rhus t.*
Inflame, right side of throat were about to—*Thuj.*
Inflamed, œsophagus were—*Cocc.*
Inflammation would follow aching in throat—*Grat.*
Insects were crawling in œsophagus—*Plb.*
Interrupting passage, something in throat were—*Lyss.*
Iron ring around throat, < swallowing—*Nit. m. ac.*
  –ring, rima glottidis were composed of an—*Chlor.*
  –tube, throat were an—*Pip. n.*
Irritated, œsophagus were—*Arg. n.*
  –from a foreign body in throat—*Kali bi.*
Kernel in left tonsil—*Samars.*
Knife were cutting in throat—*Merc. c., Stann.*
  –body in left side of throat could be removed with a—*Lac c.*
Knives, throat were rubbed over with hot—*Lach.*
Knotted up in throat, everything were—*Kali bi., Lac. ac., Zinc.*
Laced and drawn tight together, throat and tongue were—*Thlaspi*
Lard, burnt, in throat causing scraping—*Hep.*

Large, throat were too—*Sanic.*

  –when swallowing, throat were very—*Pulx.*

  –body were in throat—*Con.*

Leaf, valve or skin were lodged in throat—*Ant. c., Bar. c., Ferr., Mang., Phos., Saba., Spong.*

Leather, throat were lined with wash—*Kali bi.*

  –soft palate were dry—*Stict.*

Leave no space for swallowing, œsophagus would close up and —*Caj.*

Lined with mucus, fauces were—*Rhod.*

  –with wash leather, throat were—*Kali bi.*

Live things in œsophagus—*Anan.*

Living body were in stomach rising into throat—*Tarent.*

Lodged in throat, an apple core had—*Merc., Nit. ac., Phyt., Verat. a.*

  –in throat, a ball had—*Linar., Par.*

  –in throat on swallowing, a ball of red hot iron had—*Phyt.*

  –in throat, a ball of mucus were—*Ars.*

  –in œsophagus, everything he swallowed were—*Ars.*

  –in œsophagus, a body were—*Alco., Gels.*

  –in throat, a foreign body were—*Ant. c., Apis, Nux m.*

  –in pharynx, a long narrow foreign body were—*X-ray*

  –in back part of throat, a hard body were—*Lyc.*

  –in upper part of œsophagus, body were—*Erig.*

  –in upper part of œsophagus, a piece of bone were—*Carb. s.*

  –in throat, a small crumb were—*Lach.*

  –in throat, a hair or crumb were—*Coc. c., Pall.*

  –in œsophagus after eating, a sponge were—*Elaps*

  –in throat, food were—*Arg. n., Benz. ac., Calc. c., Caust., Merc.*

  –in œsophagus, food had—*Arg. n., Bar. c., Calc. c., Zinc.*

  –in œsophagus, morsel of food were—*Abies c., Bar. c., Chin., Puls.*

  –in upper end of œsophagus, food were—*Ars.*

  –in throat, a hair were—*Ars., Calc. s., Carb. s., Coc. c., Kali p., Pall., Sulph., Valer.*

  –in throat, a lump were—*Berb.*

  –in throat, a morsel had—*Saba.*

  –in throat, mucus had—*Ars., Hyos.*

  –in throat, something were—*Am. c., Chin. s., Cob., Con., Corn. a., Gels., Kali i., Nat. a., Sep.*

Lodged—*Continued*

    –in throat, something were; wakens in fright from sleep but sensation remains after waking—*Sep.*

    –in throat, something size of a fist had—*Cic.*

    –in right side of throat, something were—*Lach.*

    –in upper part of œsophagus, something were—*Erig.*

    –in throat, a splinter were—*Arg. n.*

    –in throat, valve, leaf or skin were—*Ant. c., Bar. c., Ferr., Mang., Phos., Saba., Spong.*

Long, palate were too—*Hyos.*

    –uvula were too—*Coc. c., Dulc., Lyss.*

Loose in throat, fishbone were—*Apis*

    –fold of tissue, mucous membrane of throat were—*Med.*

    –goiter were—*Spong.*

    –skin were hanging in throat—*Alum.*

Loosen but it does not, lump in throat might—*Lach.*

Lose her voice, she would become hoarse and—*Prun.*

Lump were in throat—*All. c., Alum., Ambr., Am. c., Bell., Berb., Calc. c., Caust., Crot. c., Gels., Ign., Kali bi., Kali c., Lac c., Lach., Lac. ac., Laur., Led., Lyss., Merc. i. f., Merc. i. r., Nat. a., Nat. p., Nat. s., Nux v., Phyt., Psor., Puls. n., Rad. br., Rumx., Ruta, Saba., Sabin., Scut., Stry., Sulph., Sul. ac., Tub., Ust., Zinc.*

    –were in upper part of throat—*Dulc., Lob. s.*

    –were in right side of throat—*Sil., Vacc., Vario.*

    –were in left side of throat—*Ovi g. p., Sil.*

    –in left side of throat below tonsil—*Ferr.*

    –in right tonsil—*Lycpr.*

    –in back of thyroid cartilage—*Pic. ac.*

    –in pharynx—*Itu, Kali c.*

    –in pit of throat—*Benz. ac., Lob. s.*

    –in œsophagus—*Fago., Lob. s., Naja, Raph.*

    –in upper œsophagus—*Lob. s.*

    –or body were ascending in throat—*Asaf.*

    –he had to swallow over—*Nat. m., Puls.*

    –in throat ascending on swallowing and returns at once—*Rumx.*

    –like a button in throat pit—*Lach.*

    –in throat pit, suddenly a choking—*Dol.*

    –hard, of food remained in throat, or throat were constricted or knotted up—*Kali bi., Lac. ac., Zinc.*

Lump—*Continued*

–in throat, descends on swallowing but returns—*Lac. c., Lach., Rumx.*

–like two eggs in throat—*Lac c.*

–filled with lump, throat were—*Lach.*

–or food were lodged in throat—*Caust.*

–in throat, food passes over—*Graph., Merc., Nat. m., Puls., Sabin.*

–in throat, solid food passes over a—*Lac c.*

–hard, in throat—*Spig.*

–hard small, in throat—*Zinc.*

–lodged on side of throat—*Berb.*

–might loosen but it does not—*Lach.*

–moving up and down during eructations—*Bar. c.*

–or globule of mucus in throat which she must swallow—*Hyos.*

–of mucus in throat tasting of blood—*Ars.*

–painful, about left tonsil, < swallowing—*X-ray*

–painful, in œsophagus—*Gels.*

–on right side; feels that she could take hold of it and take it out—*Lac c.*

–in throat cannot be removed—*Bell., Carb. v.*

–in left side of throat could be removed by a knife—*Lac c.*

–in throat returns like a puffball—*Lac. ac., Lac c.*

–rolling over and over when coughing, rising to throat through back—*Kali c.*

–rose to meet food—*Lob. s.*

–were sticking in throat—*Rumx.*

–size of walnut sticking behind larynx—*Calc. c.*

–he had to swallow over a—*Graph., Merc., Nat. m., Puls., Sabin.*

–that could not be swallowed—*Nat. m., Scut.*

–in throat when not swallowing—*Ign.*

–disappears on swallowing but returns—*Lac c.*

–in throat not > by swallowing—*Ign., Lac. ac., Rumx.*

–in throat, he would vomit up—*Lach.*

Lumps, two, as large as the fists came together in throat, > eating—*Lach.*

Lumpy in middle of throat—*Lac c.*

Lungs came into throat—*Kali c., Lach.*

Lying in œsophagus, food were—*Abies c., Chin., Puls.*

  –near manubrium, hard body were—*Sin. a.*

Marble, hot, in throat near palate—*Kali p.*

Meat during empty deglutition, swallowing pieces of—*Sulph.*
Membrane in œsophagus had been abraded—*Seneg.*
　–tough, were moved about by cough—*Kali c.*
　–mucous, of throat were a loose fold of tissue—*Med.*
Moldy taste in throat when hawking up mucus—*Mar.*
Morsel had lodged in throat—*Saba.*
　–of food had lodged in œsophagus—*Abies c., Bar. c., Chin., Puls.*
　–remained in throat—*Lach.*
　–large, of food stuck in throat—*Ign.*
　–in throat too large to swallow—*Raph.*
　–in throat, unable to swallow—*Crot. h., Crot. t.*
　–stuck in throat after swallowing—*Pip. n.*
　–of bread, she swallowed too large a—*Puls.*
　–she had swallowed too large a—*Cimx., Ferr. ma., Sin. a.*
　–she were swallowing too large a—*Rhus t., Sulph.*
Moved up and down in throat causing cough, a plug—*Calc. c.*
　–about by cough, tough membrane were—*Kali c.*
Moving about goiter, everything were—*Spong.*
　–up and down during eructations, a lump were—*Bar. c.*
　–in throat, a worm were—*Hyper.*
Mucus were in back of pharynx—*Coca*
　–throat were coated with thick sticky—*Samars.*
　–collected in throat, large mass of—*Lac c., Lach., Tub.*
　–palate were covered with tenacious—*Puls.*
　–pharynx were covered with—*Cot.*
　–throat were filled with gurgling—*Graph.*
　–posterior part of throat were filled with—*Mez.*
　–were hanging in throat—*Laur.*
　–had lodged in throat—*Ars., Hyos.*
　–tasting of blood in throat, a lump of—*Ars.*
　–in throat which he must swallow, a lump or globule of—*Hyos.*
　–in throat, a plug of—*Hep.*
　–he could not swallow on account of—*Thuj.*
Narrow, throat were too—*Arum t., Bell., Caust., Nux v.*
　–when swallowing, throat were too—*Bell.*
Narrowing, throat were—*Mez., Psor.*
Nausea in soft palate—*Phos. ac.*
Needle pricking in throat—*Merc. c.*
Needles in throat—*Merc. c.*
　–in tonsils—*Naja*

Needles—*Continued*
  –in throat, sticking with fine—*Cinch. s.*
  –or thorn in throat—*Lach.*
  –sticking in throat, a thousand—*Lach.*
Numb, throat were—*Mag. s.*
Nuts, he had eaten—*Calc. ar.*
Obstacle in throat to swallow over, there were—*Zing.*
Obstructed, voice were—*Rumx.*
Obstruction must be pulled out of throat—*Mur. ac.*
Open like a funnel, pharynx were—*Lob. s.*
  –wide and swollen or enlarged, pharynx were—*Dig.*
Outside when swallowing, water ran down—*Verat. a.*
Overloaded stomach caused pressure in œsophagus—*Bry.*
Paper, he had swallowed a piece of—*Carb. an.*
Paralyzed or inactive, pharynx were—*Rhus t.*
  –epiglottis were—*Lyss., Rhus t.*
Parched, throat were—*Alum.*
Particle of tobacco were stuck in throat—*Raph.*
Particles stick in throat on swallowing—*Graph.*
Pass over a foreign body in throat, food had to—*Merc.*
  –for constriction of throat, food could not—*Alum.*
  –in throat, nothing would—*Bell.*
Passed into glands of neck on breathing, air—*Spong.*
  –over a lump in throat, food—*Graph., Merc., Nat. m., Puls., Sabin.*
Passes over sore spot in throat, food—*Bar. c., Nat. m.*
  –over lump in throat, solid food—*Lac c.*
Passing through posterior nares, air were—*Mag. s.*
  –up right side of throat, hot air were; although stomach feels cold—*Am. br.*
  –through posterior nares while drinking, water were—*Bapt.*
Peas, mouth and throat were full of—*Pyrog.*
Peeled off, skin of throat had—*Dios.*
Peeling off œsophagus, mucous membrane were—*Caj.*
Penetrating to throat, cold air were (though warm)—*Ol. an.*
Pepper in throat—*Calc. ar., Samars., Xanth.*
  –on palate—*Mez.*
  –burning in throat—*Sal. ac.*
Peppers, swallowing red hot—*Lyss.*
Peppermint in throat, coldness from—*Form., Verat. a.*
  –he had swallowed—*Sanic.*

Peristaltic motion in œsophagus were reversed—*Asaf.*

Phlegm, throat were filled with—*Lac c., Sep.*

–were constantly in throat—*Eucal.*

Pierced, tonsils were being—*Pip. n.*

Pin in throat—*Nat. p., Sil.*

–were crosswise in throat—*Ment.*

–pricked throat—*Sil.*

–pricking in right tonsil—*Nat. p.*

–sticking in throat—*Nat. a., Nat. p.*

Plug in throat—*Alum., Ant. s. aur., Aur., Bar. c., Cham., Coff., Croc., Crot. h., Graph., Hipp., Ign., Kali bi., Lac. ac., Lac v., Nat. m., Nux v., Phyt., Pic. ac., Plb., Psor., Saba., Sep., Tab., Thuj.*

–in right side of throat—*Berb.*

–in lower part of throat—*Puls.*

–in œsophagus, periodically—*Tab.*

–in pharynx—*Hep.*

–throat would be closed with—*Nat. m.*

–moved up and down in throat causing cough—*Calc. c.*

–of mucus in throat—*Hep.*

–stuck in throat—*Ant. s. aur.*

–in throat that had to be swallowed—*Crot. h.*

–in throat when swallowing—*Hep., Nat. s., Nux v.*

–in throat, not > by swallowing (with relaxed uvula)—*Kali bi., Lach.*

–in throat, < when not swallowing—*Ign.*

Plugged, throat were—*Anan.*

Point, dull, were pressing on right wall of œsophagus—*Olnd.*

Poured down throat like an empty barrel, drink were—*Hydr. ac.*

–down throat, fluid were—*Glon.*

–out of a bottle from throat to abdomen, water were—*Cinc*

Pressed outward in throat, something were being—*Spong.*

–on something hard, uvula—*Caps.*

–through left wall of œsophagus on swallowing, a ball were—*Crot. t.*

–against trachea, pit of throat were—*Brom.*

–in, thyroid cartilage were—*Bar. c.*

Pressing on right wall of œsophagus, dull point were—*Olnd.*

–on throat, eyes would spring out of head when—*Lach.*

–out left side of throat, a ball were—*Crot. t.*

–on something hard in uvula—*Caps.*

Pressure in œsophagus came from overloaded stomach—*Bry.*
Prevented free passage of air, something in throat—*Fel tauri*
Preventing speech, something closed the throat—*Nat. p.*
 –swallowing, a foreign body in œsophagus were—*Upas*
 –swallowing, a sponge in œsophagus were—*Elaps*
Pricked with a pin, throat were—*Sil.* .
Pricking on both sides of throat—*Alumn.*
 –of needle in throat—*Merc. c.*
 –of needle in tonsil—*Naja*
 –of pin in right tonsil—*Nat. p.*
Prickles impeded swallowing, broad substance covered with—
  Kali bi.
Projected into throat on swallowing, submaxillary glands were
  —*Puls.*
Puffball, small, in throat, not > by swallowing—*Lac. ac.*
 –lump in throat returns like—*Lac c.*
Pulled out of throat, some obstruction must be—*Mur. ac.*
Pungent heat in mouth and throat—*Æth.*
 –heat in throat—*Tril.*
Purring of a cat in throat—*Spig.*
Pus, uvula contained—*Lach.*
 –tonsils were about to discharge—*Calc. s.*
Pushed up to throat as if it had not been swallowed, food were
  —*Ferr. i.*
 –against pharynx below, round waves—*Tell.*
Quivering in œsophagus and stomach, nerve were—*Ferr.*
Radishes or cress, coldness in œsophagus from—*Agar.*
Raised into throat by contraction of œsophagus, ball filled with
  air were—*Cham.*
 –when coughing, a piece of flesh would be—*Phos.*
Ran down outside of throat when drinking, water—*Verat. a.*
Rancid fat caused scraping in throat—*Hall*
 –fluid, œsophagus were full of—*Crot. h.*
 –food caused rawness in throat—*Phos.*
 –grease in morning on swallowing first mouthful—*Ars.*
 –substances, she had eaten—*Camph.*
Rattling in throat—*Tub.*
Raw in throat—*Apis, Hep., Lach., Lyss., Sep.*
 –on the left side—*Fl. ac.*
 –posterior throat were—*Puls.*
 –palate were—*Puls.*

Raw—*Continued*

  –pharynx were—*Chlor.*

  –epiglottis were—*Bell.*

Rawness in throat, heartburn caused—*Kali i.*

  –in throat caused by rancid food—*Phos.*

  –in throat caused by snuff—*Thuj.*

  –in œsophagus—*Calc. c., Carb. an., Guare.*

Relax and rub together, walls of throat—*Aral.*

Relaxation in œsophagus and stomach as from drinking much lukewarm water—*Spong.*

Relaxed or enlarged, something in throat were—*Lac c.*

Remained in throat, crumbs or bread had—*Dros.*

  –in throat, a hard lump of food—*Kali bi., Lac. ac., Zinc.*

  –in upper part of œsophagus, food—*Dig.*

  –sticking in pharynx, food—*Calc. c., Zinc.*

  –in throat, a morsel—*Lach.*

  –in chest, something rose in œsophagus and—*Crot. h.*

Remove something from throat, trying to—*Puls.*

Removed with a knife, body in left side of throat could be— *Lac c.*

  –lump in throat cannot be—*Bell., Carb. v.*

Rend œsophagus, rising flatus would—*Coca*

Resistance to overcome in speech, there were some (in throat) —*Sec.*

Rested upon tongue, uvula—*Saba.*

Restlessness in throat—*Ant. c., Ars., Arum d., Hydr. ac., Merc. c., Nit. m. ac., Ox. ac., Pin. s., Plan., Stram.*

Returns like a puffball, lump in throat—*Lac c.*

Reversed in œsophagus, peristaltic motion had been—*Asaf.*

Ring, rima glottidis were composed of an iron—*Chlor.*

  –iron, around the throat causing constant sense of constriction, < from empty swallowing—*Nit. m. ac.*

Rising in throat, acids were—*Hep.*

  –to throat, ball were—*Kalm., Phys., Still., Stram., Sulph.*

  –in throat, a ball were—*Ars., Asaf., Ign., Kali p., Kalm., Lyc., Nit. ac., Phys., Senec.*

  –from stomach to throat, ball were, > by eructations—*Mag. m.*

  –in throat into œsophagus, a ball were—*Verat. v.*

  –in throat, a hard ball were—*Sulph.*

  –in throat when speaking, a choking—*Manc.*

  –in throat, something cold were—*Caust.*

Rising—*Continued*

    –in throat, a cooling substance were—*Camph.*

    –up into throat and choking, foreign substance were—*Hedo.,*
       Zinc.

    –in throat, something warm were—*Zinc.*

    –from stomach, something warm were—*Valer.*

    –in throat, boiling water were—*Stram.*

    –in œsophagus, water were—*Hep.*

    –into throat, worm were—*Spig.*

Rolled into throat and closed it like a valve, something—*Ferr.*

Rolling over and over when coughing, lump were; and rising to
       throat through back—*Kali c.*

    –or curling upon itself from tip to base, soft palate were—
       Nux m.

Rose into throat, something—*Cit. v.*

    –to pit of throat, something—*Ruta*

    –in œsophagus and remained in chest, something—*Crot. h.*

    –from stomach into throat, ball—*Asaf., Lyc., Lyss., Senec.*

    –to meet food, lump in throat—*Lob. s.*

    –in throat, hot steam—*Merc. i. r.*

    –in throat after sour things, water—*Hep.*

Rough body were glued to throat—*Arg. m.*

    –were sticking into soft palate, something—*Arg. m.*

Rub together, walls of throat relax and—*Aral.*

Rubbed over with hot knives, throat were—*Lach.*

Running through posterior nares over palate causing cough,
       acrid fluid were—*Kali bi.*

    –down throat, ear-wax were—*Crot. h.*

    –out of throat and stomach, flame were—*Euph.*

    –from stomach to throat, something alive were—*Verat. a.*

Rushing to throat, blood were—*Chel., Kali bi.*

Sand in throat—*Berb., Cist.*

    –were sticking in palate, hard grain of—*Coloc.*

Scab in upper part of throat—*Calc. ar.*

Scalded, throat were—*Absin., Æsc., Apis, Cinch. s., Elat., Eup.*
      pur., Hura, Kali ox., Lac c., Ovi g. p., Merc. i. r., Merc. s.,
      Mez., Sec., Stict., Ther., Trif. p.

    –mouth and throat were—*Stict.*

    –mouth and throat had been—*Rhus v.*

    –on palate—*Cimx.*

    –pharynx were—*Sang.*

Scalded—*Continued*

  –by a hot fluid in throat—*Lac c., Psor.*

  –after vomiting—*Ther.*

Scalding water flowing from throat to nose, a stream of—*Gels.*

Scraped with an awn, throat were—*Mag. c.*

Scraping in throat—*Med., Psor.*

  –from burnt lard in throat—*Hep.*

  –in throat were caused by rancid fat—*Hall*

  –from swallowing a rose-hip—*Mag. c.*

Scratched off with a sharp instrument, lining of throat were— *Nux v.*

Scratching in throat on attempting to sing—*Agar.*

  –in throat, a file were—*Nit. ac.*

Seed were sticking in throat—*Berb.*

  –in throat, a watermelon—*Tub. lar.*

Seized, throat were—*Atro.*

Sewed together, throat were—*Graph.*

Sharp were in throat, something—*Calad., Saba.*

  –instrument, lining of throat were scratched off with—*Nux v.*

  –brush had been drawn through œsophagus to stomach—*Nicot.*

  –were sticking in throat, something—*Acon., Alum., Iod., Sang.*

  –were sticking in throat on coughing, something—*Nux v.*

Shock in throat, electric—*Samars.*

Short, tongue were; and throat too tight—*Zinc. ac.*

Skin covered posterior part of throat, a piece of chamois—*Merc. i. f.*

  –leaf or valve hanging in throat—*Ant. c., Bar. c., Ferr., Mang., Phos., Saba., Spong.*

  –loose, hanging in throat—*Alum.*

  –hanging down in throat, with rawness, piece of—*Plat.*

  –hanging loosely in throat, must swallow over it—*Saba.*

Skinned, throat were—*Nux v., Sep.*

Slipped down throat, a piece of ice had—*Coc. c.*

Slipping toward stomach, something in œsophagus were—*Ther.*

Small for food, throat were too—*Tab.*

  –œsophagus were too—*Spire.*

Smoking, he had been—*Nux v.*

Snake in throat—*Lach.*

Snuff through throat, one had drawn—*Staph.*

  –caused rawness in throat—*Thuj.*

Soft body in throat which he must swallow—*Saba.*

–body in œsophagus—*Scroph.*

Something in throat interrupting passage—*Lyss.*

–in the way in throat—*Pimp.*

–in lower œsophagus—*Pic. ac.*

Sore, throat would become—*Lith. c.*

–from sour eructations in throat—*Sulph.*

–and spasmodically drawn together, parts of throat were—
Caps.

–spot, food had to force its way over—*Bar. c.*

–spot, food passes over—*Nat. m.*

–spot in throat, swallowed over—*Sil.*

–and torn, throat were—*Camph.*

Spasm would close pharynx—*Kali i.*

Splinter in throat—*Alum., Alum. s., Arg. n., Hep., Nat. m., Nit. ac., Zinc. i.*

–in throat merging into heat and burning—*Ars.*

–in left side of throat—*Upas*

–in left side of throat on swallowing—*Dub.*

–in right tonsil—*Sol. n.*

–in left tonsil—*Samars.*

–in œsophagus—*Ars.*

–were lodged in throat—*Arg. n.*

–were sticking near carotid artery—*Dol.*

–three-fourths of an inch long imbedded vertically in right side
of throat near angle of jaw—*Dol.*

Split open, throat would—*Pic. ac.*

–open on swallowing, throat were—*Mag. c.*

–of barley in right throat—*Sars.*

Sponge were hanging in throat—*Lac c., Lach.*

–in throat, breathing through—*Brom.*

–lodged in œsophagus after eating—*Elaps*

–in œsophagus preventing swallowing—*Elaps*

Spot in pharynx, there were a burnt—*Merc.*

–dry, in throat—*Crot. h.*

–small dry, in throat, pain extending to ear, > swallowing—
Lach.

–food had to force its way over a sore—*Bar. c.*

–food passes over a sore—*Nat. m.*

–in throat, swallowed over a sore—*Sil.*

Sprinkled with sulphur, throat were—*Sulph.*

Squeezed in throat—*Ferr., Kali c., Lach.*

–throat between thumb and finger, someone—*Kalm.*

Squirming in throat causing cough, worms were—*Cist.*

Steam in throat—*Nux v.*

–hot, rising in throat—*Merc. i. r.*

–hot, wavelike, moving through abdomen, chest and throat—*Lyss.*

Stick in throat when swallowing—*Arg. n.*

–in throat reaching to stomach, a burning—*Anan.*

–with a ball on each end extended from throat to left side of abdomen—*Kali c.*

Sticks in throat—*Alum., Arg. n., Cham., Hep., Lac c., Nat. m.*

–throat were full of—*Lac c.*

–little, in throat and vocal cords—*Nit. ac.*

Sticking in uvula—*Nicc.*

–in throat, an apple core were—*Merc.*

–in throat, a ball were—*Coc. c.*

–in pharynx, a ball were—*Stram.*

–in throat, a fishbone were—*Apis, Hep., Kali c., Lach., Nit. ac., Phys., Sac. lac.*

–in throat, food were—*Aqua pet., Bry., Caust., Croc., Crot. t., Ferr., Ign., Iris, Lach., Plect., Til.*

–in pharynx, food remained—*Zinc.*

–in pharynx and could not get to stomach, food remains—*Calc. c.*

–in palate, hard grain of sand were—*Coloc.*

–in throat, a grain of barley were—*Mag. c.*

–in throat, a husk were—*Berb.*

–in throat, a lump were—*Rumx.*

–behind pharynx, lump size of walnut were—*Calc. c.*

–in throat with fine needles—*Cinch. s.*

–in throat, a thousand needles were—*Lach.*

–in tonsils, needles were—*Naja*

–in throat, a pin were—*Nat. a., Nat. p.*

–in throat, a seed were—*Berb.*

–in throat, something were—*Cham., Sol. t. æ., Tab.*

–in pharynx, something were—*Cinch. s.*

–in upper end of œsophagus, something were—*Lac. ac.*

–low down in œsophagus, something were—*Abies n., Vinc.*

–into soft palate, something rough were—*Arg. m.*

Sticking—*Continued*
 –in throat, something sharp were—*Acon., Alum., Iod., Sang.*
 –in throat on coughing, something sharp were—*Nux v.*
 –near carotid artery, a splinter were—*Dol.*
Sticky mucus, throat were coated with thick—*Samars.*
Stiff as a board, throat were—*Lac c.*
 –uvula were—*Crot. h.*
 –rima glottidis were—*Chlor.*
Stiffened, throat were—*Nux m.*
Stinging and hot ascended œsophagus, preceded by something
     cold, something—*All. s.*
Stitches in throat—*Acon., Arum m., Apis, Asar., Bar. c., Bon.,
     Brom., Bry., Calad., Carb. v., Carl., Caust., Chel., Cist.,
     Cupr. a., Dig., Ether., Gamb., Grat., Gymn., Hell., Hep.,
     Ign., Kali i., Kali n., Led., Lyc., Mag. s., Merc. i. r., Nat.
     c., Nicc., Nit. ac., Nux m., Phel., Plect., Ptel., Rat., Sars.,
     Sulph., Tarax., Thuj., Zinc., Zinc. ac.*
 –in throat when coughing—*Bry., Hep., Lyc., Sil.*
 –in throat on exertion—*Manc.*
 –in throat on inspiration—*Hep.*
 –in throat on hawking—*Plat.*
 –in throat when sneezing—*Mag. c.*
 –in throat when swallowing—*Alumn., Bar. c., Bov., Bry., Calc.
     c., Chin., Cinch., Elæis guin., Gamb., Graph., Hep., Kali c.,
     Lach., Led., Lob., Lyc., Nit. ac., Petr., Phos. ac., Plect.,
     Rhus t., Sil., Stram., Sulph.*
 –in throat when not swallowing—*Æth.*
 –in throat when talking—*Nit. ac.*
 –in throat when touched externally—*Agar.*
 –in throat when yawning—*Am. m., Rhus t.*
 –in throat in evening—*Carb. an.*
 –in throat from noise—*Tarent.*
 –in throat > eating—*Caust., Phel.*
 –in throat causing cough—*Cist., Sol. t. æ.*
Stone in throat—*Bufo*
 –hot, were in pharynx—*Stram.*
Stony hard foreign substance in throat—*Zinc.*
Stoppage in pharynx—*Sol. t. æ.*
Stopped swallowing, a ball in throat—*Senec.*
 –the voice, a foreign body in throat—*Arg. m.*

Stopper in throat—*Arg. m.*
  —were forced into throat—*Croc.*
Strangled—*Stry.*
  —she were being—*Zinc.*
Strangling—*Hyos.*
Stream of scalding water from throat into nose—*Gels.*
Stretched, pharynx were—*Sulph.*
String or thread in throat, constriction from—*Saba.*
  —pharynx were constricted by—*Nit. ac., Nux v., Thuj.*
  —or thread hanging down in throat—*Coc. c., Valer.*
  —were tied around throat—*Crot. c.*
  —or cord, throat were tied with—*Lach., Saba.*
Stuck fast in throat pit, a button were—*Lach.*
  —at base of throat, food were—*Samars.*
  —and would not go down, food were—*Ambr.*
  —in throat after swallowing, morsel of food were—*Pip. n.*
  —in throat, large morsel of food were—*Ign.*
  —in pharynx, food remained—*Calc. c.*
  —in throat, plug were—*Ant. s. aur.*
  —in throat, particle of tobacco were—*Raph.*
  —in throat, something were—*Acon., Hep.*
  —in throat pit, something were—*Æsc.*
  —in pharynx, something were—*Sulph.*
  —in upper end of œsophagus, something were—*Lac. ac.*
Substance, cooling, were rising in throat—*Camph.*
  —foreign, in throat—*Trif. p.*
  —foreign, rising up into throat—*Hedo., Zinc.*
  —foreign, stony hard, in throat—*Zinc.*
  —thick, in throat—*Lach.*
Substances in throat, she had eaten rancid—*Camph.*
Suffocate, she would—*Cham., Ferr. i.*
Suffocating, with throat complaints—*Daph. o.*
  —as from a quantity of water poured into windpipe—*Spig.*
Sugar were dissolved in throat, a particle of—*Bad.*
Sulphur fumes in throat—*Croc., Ign., Puls.*
  —throat were sprinkled with—*Sulph.*
  —vapors in throat—*Lyc., X-ray*
Suppurate, tonsils were about to—*Merc. cy.*
  —submaxillary glands would—*Clem.*
Swallow, something were constantly in throat to—*Lach.*
  —he would choke if he did not—*Bell.*

Swallow—*Continued*
 –he could not—*Sil.*
 –a body in throat which he tries to (but cannot)—*Sabin.*
 –round body were suddenly impelled upward to throat where it
   feels like a morsel too large to—*Raph.*
 –a soft body in throat which he must—*Saba.*
 –bread were too dry to—*Ign.*
 –over an elevation on left side of throat, he had to—*Graph.*
 –over a foreign body, he had to—*Sabin.*
 –a morsel, he were unable to—*Crot. h., Crot. t.*
 –on account of mucus, he could not—*Thuj.*
 –over a lump, he had to—*Nat. m., Puls.*
 –over an obstacle in throat, he must—*Zing.*
 –over something, he had to—*Hep.*
 –over a swelling, she had to—*Hep.*
Swallowed an astringent, she had—*Peti., Saba.*
 –a foreign body, he had—*Merc., Sabin.*
 –were too dry, everything he—*Raph.*
 –lodged in œsophagus, everything—*Ars.*
 –food had not been; seems pushed up—*Ferr. i.*
 –too large morsel of bread, one had—*Puls.*
 –a large morsel of food had been—*Sin. a.*
 –too large a morsel of food, she had—*Cimx., Ferr. ma.*
 –lump that could not be—*Nat. m., Scut.*
 –peppermint, he had—*Sanic.*
 –a piece of paper, he had—*Carb. an.*
 –plug in throat that had to be—*Crot. h.*
 –something ought to be—*Pip. m.*
 –something, wakens in fright from first sleep—*Sep.*
 –over a sore spot—*Sil.*
 –tobacco, he had—*Eup. pur.*
Swallowing stopped by a ball in throat—*Senec.*
 –over a bone—*Ign.*
 –impeded by broad substance covered with prickles—*Kali bi.*
 –food turned like corkscrew on—*Elaps*
 –morsel of food stuck in throat after—*Pip. n.*
 –suddenly a large piece of food—*Phys.*
 –a lump in throat when not—*Ign.*
 –a lump in throat ascending on swallowing and returns at once
   —*Rumx.*
 –a lump in throat disappears on swallowing but returns—*Lac c.*

Swallowing—*Continued*

 –lump in throat not > by—*Ign., Lac. ac., Rumx.*

 –too large a morsel—*Rhus t., Sulph.*

 –throat were very large when—*Pulx.*

 –a piece of meat, during empty deglutition—*Sulph.*

 –red hot peppers—*Lyss.*

 –plug in throat when—*Hep., Nat. s., Nux v.*

 –rose-hip, scraping were from—*Mag. c.*

 –something hard—*Kali c.*

 –something remaining in pharynx after—*Kali bi.*

 –œsophagus would close up and leave no space—*Caj.*

 –a sponge in œsophagus were preventing—*Elaps*

 –splinter in left side of throat when—*Dub.*

 –tangle of hairs in throat interferes with—*Cent.*

 –water ran down outside when—*Verat. a.*

Swelled, throat were—*Lyss., Sul. i.*

Swelling in throat—*Casc., Glon., Saba.*

 –throat were—*Bar. c., Glon.*

 –œsophagus were—*Caj., Chel., Ferr. i.*

 –uvula were—*Arum t., Crot. h.*

 –in glands, near larynx and trachea—*Spong.*

 –throat would be closed by—*Nat. m.*

 –she had to swallow over a—*Hep.*

Swollen in throat—*Ambr., Caust., Cocc., Nit. ac., Puls., Sang.*

 –and enlarged, throat were—*Xanth.*

 –right side of throat were—*Tub.*

 –in throat pit—*Lach.*

 –palate were—*Puls., Sulph., Til.*

 –tonsils were—*Juncus, Rhus t., Sulph.*

 –right tonsil were—*Am. c., Merc. i. f., Upas*

 –in throat to suffocation—*Sang.*

 –outside, choking sensation—*Ferr.*

 –pharynx were—*Carb. v., Dig., Iod., Sang.*

 –pharynx were, or wide open and enlarged—*Dig.*

 –walls of pharynx were—*Dig.*

 –or contracted in pharynx—*Carb. v.*

 –cervical glands were greatly—*Daph. o.*

Tangle of hairs in throat interferes with swallowing—*Cent.*

Taste, moldy, in throat when hawking up mucus—*Mar.*

Tearing to pieces on swallowing, throat were—*Syph.*

Thick, throat were—*Ail., Kali n., Sep.*
   —substance in throat—*Lach.*
Things, live, in œsophagus—*Anan.*
Thread or string in throat—*Saba.*
   —hanging down in throat—*Coc. c., Valer.*
   —hanging down in throat, tickling deep in—*Valer.*
   —from œsophagus to abdomen, there were—*Valer.*
Thorn or needles in throat—*Lach.*
Throttled in throat—*Glon.*
Thrusts, electric, in upper part of throat—*Manc.*
Tickling in throat—*Crot. h.*
   —would provoke cough—*Verat. a.*
   —of feather in throat—*Calc. c., Cinnb., Dros., Ign.*
   —of feather in back part of throat—*Æsc.*
   —as of sugar dissolved in throat—*Bad.*
   —from thread in throat—*Valer.*
Tied with cord or string, throat were—*Lach., Saba.*
   —on attempting to eat, throat were—*Lach.*
   —together in throat—*Arum t.*
   —up, throat and tongue were—*Crot. h.*
   —around thyroid, a string were—*Crot. c.*
Tight around throat, a band were—*Dios., Op.*
   —and tongue were too short, throat were too—*Zinc. ac.*
   —posteriorly, throat were too—*Merc.*
Tightly around throat, something were held—*Stry.*
Tired, throat were—*Camph.*
Tobacco stuck in throat, a particle of—*Raph.*
   —he had swallowed—*Eup. pur., Lac. ac.*
Torn in throat (accompanying mental exertion)—*Caust.*
   —and sore, throat were—*Camph.*
Tube, throat were an iron; with stiffness—*Pip. n.*
Tumor in throat—*Tub.*
   —were growing in throat, large—*Bell.*
Turned like a corkscrew on swallowing, food—*Elaps*
Turning about in throat—*Lach.*
Twisted and clutched, œsophagus were—*Lyc.*
Ulcer were cut out in throat—*Merc. cy.*
   —would form in throat—*Fl. ac.*
   —would form on palate, a little—*Kali bi.*
Ulcerated, throat were—*Gels., Graph., Nicc.*

Uneasy in œsophagus—*Æth., Kali i., Kali m.*
Uvula would break when coughing—*Ham.*
--were elongated—*Acon., Coc. c., Croc., Crot. h., Plat.*
--were too long—*Cocc. s.*
--sticking in—*Nicc.*
Valve, leaf or skin lodged in throat—*Ant. c., Bar. c., Ferr., Mang., Phos., Saba., Spong.*
--something rolled into throat and closed it like—*Ferr.*
--rose in throat—*Ferr.*
Vapor ascended to throat, an acrid—*Pæon.*
--rises from throat, hot—*Camph.*
--rising in throat—*Saba.*
--hot, rising from stomach—*Merc., Zinc.*
--hot or smarting, rising in throat—*All. s.*
--rising from throat through head—*Aml. n.*
Vapors of sulphur in throat—*Ign., Lyc., Puls., X-ray*
Varicose veins in throat—*Berb.*
Voice were obstructed—*Rumx.*
--were passing through wool, sounds of—*Agn.*
Vomit up lump in throat, he would—*Lach.*
Warm were rising in throat, something—*Zinc.*
--rising from stomach, something—*Valer.*
Water, palate were filled with—*Apis*
--would force through pharynx—*Staph.*
--were passing through posterior nares while drinking—*Bapt.*
--poured out of a bottle from throat to abdomen—*Cina*
--ran down outside of throat when drinking—*Verat. a.*
--relaxation in œsophagus and stomach as from drinking much lukewarm—*Spong.*
--rising in œsophagus—*Hep.*
--boiling, rising in pharynx and throat—*Stram.*
--rose in throat after sour things—*Hep.*
--from throat up into nose, a stream of scalding—*Gels.*
Watermelon seed in throat—*Tub. lar.*
Wave from uterus to throat—*Gels.*
Waves, round, pushed against pharynx below—*Tell.*
Wax, ear, were running down throat—*Crot. h.*
Weak, organs of speech were—*Nat. m.*
Wearied pharynx, speaking—*Apis*
Web were drawn across throat—*Zinc.*
Weight above cuneiform cartilage—*Nat. p.*

Wheat hull in throat—*Plb.*

Worm in throat—*Bry., Calc. c., Hyper., Merc. s., Puls.*
 –in œsophagus—*Saba.*
 –were creeping up into throat—*Puls., Zinc.*
 –were creeping up into throat causing coughing—*Zinc.*
 –were moving in throat—*Hyper.*
 –were rising in throat—*Spig.*

Worms were creeping in œsophagus—*Puls., Zinc.*
 –squirming in throat causing cough—*Cist.*

STOMACH

Absent, stomach were; had been removed—*Phos.*

Aching in stomach before diarrhœa—*Brom.*

Acrid, pungent exhalations rising from stomach—*Phel.*

Adherent to stomach, diaphragm were—*Mez.*

Air, cold, blew into stomach—*Coc. c.*

  –stomach were filled with—*Cob.*

  –were forcing its way through stomach causing soreness—*Bar. c.*

  –became imprisoned at epigastrium—*Rhus t.*

  –passed through an opening in stomach—*Crot. c.*

  –passed through a hole in epigastrium to back—*Med., Rhus t.*

  –hot, passes up right side of throat although stomach feels cold—*Am. br.*

  –he had swallowed too much—*Plat.*

  –in stomach, every particle of food he ate turned into—*Iod.*

Alive in stomach, something were—*Croc., Manc., Saba., Sabin., Sang., Thuj.*

  –jerking in stomach, something were—*Sang.*

  –jumping about in region of stomach, something were—*Sang.*

  –and jumping about in stomach, something were—*Croc.*

  –in stomach moving toward throat—*Tarent.*

  –and rising from stomach to throat, something were—*Verat. a.*

Animal were moving about in stomach—*Sep.*

  –were wriggling in epigastrium—*Chel.*

Appetite had vanished forever—*Rhus t.*

Apple cores, rice water were—*Stram.*

Ascended toward stomach, something—*Coc. c.*

Ascending from region of stomach to throat, a ball were—*Plb.*

  –from stomach, a round body were—*Con.*

Asleep, stomach would go to—*Castor.*

Astringent earth, stomach were coated with—*Mill.*

  –were contracting stomach—*Acon.*

Bag, stomach hangs like an empty—*Thea*

  –of water which turns as she turns over in bed, stomach were—*Ornith.*

Ball in stomach—*Coc. c., Ter.*

  –ascending from region of stomach to throat—*Plb.*

Ball—*Continued*

    –burning, in stomach—*Bell.*

    –food collected into a—*Merc.*

    –gases collected into—*Hydrc.*

    –hard, like a potato in epigastrium—*Ovi g. p.*

    –hot, in stomach—*Lob.*

    –something in stomach were drawn up into a—*Lach.*

    –or stone lying in stomach—*Coc. c.*

    –rises from stomach to throat and seems to threaten suffocation —*Lyss.*

    –in stomach causing suffocation—*Pana.*

    –in stomach rising up in throat—*Asaf., Kali ar., Mag. m., Senec.*

    –rising from stomach and spreading cool air over vertex and occiput—*Acon.*

    –were rising from pit of stomach to larynx—*Kali ar.*

    –stomach were rolled up into a—*Bry.*

    –were rolling about in stomach during menses—*Tong.*

    –something in stomach were rolling up into—*Arn.*

    –rose in pit of stomach—*Con.*

    –he had swallowed a—*Ter.*

    –of lead or cold iron, he had swallowed—*Samars.*

    –twisted in epigastrium—*Inul.*

Balls extending from stomach to throat, a chain of hard—*Abies n.*

Band tightly drawn around body at stomach—*Mag. p.*

    –laced tight around lower part of stomach region—*Ign.*

    –stomach were squeezed by—*Tarent.*

Balanced up and down, stomach were being—*Phos. ac.*

Bar were laid over stomach, with anguish—*Ricin.*

Bathed in hot water, region of stomach were—*Coc. c.*

Beaten in epigastrium—*Stann.*

Beating in stomach—*Paraf.*

    –in stomach, two hammers were—*Graph.*

Belching were caused by wind on stomach—*Lyc.*

Bent, he had been sitting—*Lact.*

Bile, stomach were full of—*Kali i.*

Bird were fluttering in stomach—*Calad.*

Biting in stomach—*Arn., Cast., Hell., Sulph.*

    –in stomach when fasting—*Hell.*

    –in stomach as from worms—*Hell.*

Bitter were in stomach, something—*Cupr., Stann., Sul. ac.*

Blew into stomach, cold air—*Coc. c.*

Blood could not circulate in back opposite pit of stomach—*Thuj.*

—in stomach, there were too much—*Æsc.*

—ran cold in stomach—*Stry.*

—would rush to stomach—*Stann.*

—streaming from stomach to head, warm—*Calc. c.*

Blow deep in epigastrium—*Cic.*

—in stomach—*Merc. i. f.*

—across stomach—*Paraf.*

—on stomach—*Magnol.*

Blows in pit of stomach—*Nat. c., Nux v., Plat.*

—in epigastrium, he were struck by—*Lac c.*

Board across stomach, with a cord extending into throat which moves up and down in breathing—*Hæm.*

Body, foreign, in stomach—*Agar., Cupr., Fago., Grat., Nat. m., Thuj.*

—foreign, pressed stomach—*Cahin.*

—foreign, sticking in cardiac orifice and behind the sternum—*Nat. m.*

—hard, were pressed into stomach—*Aur. m.*

—hard, lay in stomach—*Sin. a.*

—heavy, hard, in stomach—*Lith.*

—lead, in pit of stomach—*Hep.*

—living, were in the stomach rising into throat—*Tarent.*

—round, were ascending from stomach—*Con.*

—round foreign, difficult of digestion—*Raph.*

—round foreign, rising to stomach—*Pip. n.*

—large round, twisting about in stomach—*Phel.*

Boring in stomach—*Agar., Caps., Carb. an., Nat. s., Plb.*

—in stomach and it would be perforated, something were—*Nat. s.*

—tearing in stomach—*Ars.*

Bottom had fallen out of stomach; temporary > by eating—*Ox. ac.*

Brandy, he had drunk hot—*Laps. c.*

Breaking loose in stomach at every step, something were—*Ictod.*

Breath were retained in stomach—*Eupi.*

—were stopped at pit of stomach—*Rhus t.*

Breeze, cool, blowing on face when heated, were felt in stomach—*Gamb.*

Brick, an iron, were being forced from stomach to chest—*Ornith.*

Bruised in stomach—*Camph., Carb. an., Cupr. ar., Euph., Eupi., Fago., Guare., Indg., Lyc., Mag. m., Merc. i. f., Nux v., Phyt.*

–by coughing, stomach were—*Asc. t.*

–on pressure, stomach were—*Caust.*

–and screwing together, stomach were—*Sulph.*

Bubbling in an angle beneath pit of stomach—*Sabin.*

–from dissolving lime—*Caust.*

Bullet which lodged in pit of stomach, he had swallowed—*Ter.*

Burned up with lime in stomach—*Caust.*

–up with liquor, stomach were—*Chim. umb.*

Burning ball in stomach—*Bell.*

–bitter, in stomach—*Card. b.*

–from corrosive acid—*Carb. ac.*

–cooling—*Agar., Camph., Laur., Nat. m.*

–gnawing in stomach—*Ox. ac.*

–from liquor in stomach—*Chim. umb.*

–from pepper in stomach—*Caust.*

–from vitriol in stomach—*Ir. fœ.*

–from worms in stomach—*Hell.*

–after food followed by pressure as of a foreign body—*Agar.*

–would be > by eating—*Sep.*

Burnt, stomach were—*Pop.*

–in the stomach, lime were being—*Caust.*

–up with whiskey, stomach were—*Pyrus*

Burrowing in stomach—*Grat., Kali c., Nat. m., Staph., Stront.*

–of a worm in stomach—*Lach.*

–in region of stomach—*Chin.*

Burst, stomach would—*Asc. t., Berb., Kali c., Lyc., Sul. ac.*

–with gas, stomach would—*Arg. n.*

–while laughing, stomach would—*Asc. t.*

Bursting from eating and drinking, stomach were—*Tab.*

–after yawning, stomach were—*Arg. m.*

Calomel were operating in stomach, a full dose of—*Verat. v.*

Cat were purring in stomach—*Ferr. s.*

Choked in stomach while eating—*Ornith.*

Cholera, he had—*Ars.*

Clawing in pit of stomach—*Carb. v., Caust., Dros., Lyc., Nit. ac., Nux v., Petr., Puls., Rhod., Sil., Sulph., Tab., Zinc. m.*

–in stomach with cold sweat—*Euph.*

–from a purge—*Nux v.*

Clenched by a hand, region of stomach were—*Morph.*

Clogged, stomach were—*Sumb.*

Closed, stomach were—*Cact.*

 —and being split open with a knife—*Rhus t.*

Clothes were too tight about stomach—*Caust., Crot. h., Gins., Lyc., Spong., Tub.*

Clutched by a hand in abdomen and stomach—*Bell.*

Clutching in stomach, something were—*Cann. i.*

Coals, red hot, in stomach—*Ars., Ars. s. r., Tep.*

 —of fire in stomach—*Ars., Ars. s. r.*

Coated with astringent earth, stomach were—*Mill.*

Cold in pit of stomach—*Cinch. s.*

 —stomach were icy—*Colch.*

 —air blew into stomach—*Coc. c.*

 —in stomach, blood ran—*Stry.*

 —in stomach, he had taken—*Cann. s.*

Coldness in stomach after eating—*Crot. c.*

 —icy, in stomach—*Caps., Colch., Lact.*

Collapsed, stomach were, alternating with distension—*Acon.*

Collected into a ball in stomach, flatus were—*Hydrc.*

Comfort radiating from stomach over whole body as from wine—*Coca*

Compressed, stomach were—*Arg. n., Der., Op., Phos., Sulph., Zinc.*

 —from both sides, stomach were—*Phos.*

 —the heart, pressure came from stomach and—*Nat. m.*

Conscious of stomach after eating—*Nat. ar.*

Constricted in stomach—*Chin. s.*

 —stomach were—*Jab.*

 —from both sides, stomach were—*Zinc.*

Constriction and suffocation in stomach—*Sang.*

 —and rugæ were puckered up—*Jab.*

 —in stomach from a tightly drawn string—*Spig.*

Contracted, stomach were—*Con.*

 —in region of stomach—*Sec.*

 —in pit of stomach—*Daph. o.*

 —gradually, muscular fibres of stomach were—*Verat. v.*

Contracting spasmodically, coats of stomach were—*Arn.*

 —slowly on contents, forcing them into œsophagus, stomach were—*Verat. v.*

 —stomach, something living were moving in—*Chion.*

Contracting—*Continued*
  –from an astringent in stomach—*Acon.*
Convulsion in stomach—*Phos., Sars.*
  –nerves in stomach were in motion causing—*Bell.*
Cooking in stomach, something were—*Phos.*
. **Cooling,** burning in stomach—*Agar., Camph., Laur., Nat. m.*
Cord extending from board across stomach to throat—*Hæm.*
Corrosive burning in stomach—*Saba.*
Cough came from stomach—*Bry., Sep.*
  –were excited by something in pit of stomach—*Bell.*
  –re-echoed in stomach—*Cupr.*
Cramp in orifice of stomach—*Eug.*
Craving in epigastrium—*Thea*
Crawling from stomach to throat—*Sulph.*
  –of a worm in stomach—*Alum.*
Creeping up throat from burning in stomach—*Carb. v.*
Cut to pieces, stomach were—*Kali c , Mag. m., Rat.*
  –through, stomach were—*Lepi.*
Cutting in stomach, glass were—*Calad.*
  –of knife in pit of stomach—*Cupr.*
  –with a sharp knife—*Paraf.*
  –from knives after eating—*Kali bi.*
Dead, stomach were—*Nux v.*
Deathlike sensation in stomach—*Pic. ac.*
Deranged, stomach were—*Thuj.*
Diarrhœa were coming on—*Æth., Plan.*
  –would come on, aching in stomach—*Brom.*
Die with nausea in stomach, she would—*Dig.*
Digest, meat would not—*Pyrus*
  –nothing would—*Pyrus*
Digestion had stopped—*Spong.*
  –were suspended—*Kali bi.*
Digging in stomach—*Chel., Kali c., Nicc.*
Disemboweled, he had been—*Paraf.*
Disordered, stomach were—*Caust., Colch., Iod., Lyc., Mag. c., Phyt., Puls., Stann., Sul. ac., Thuj.*
  –from fatty food, stomach were—*Asaf.*
  –by decayed fruit, stomach were—*Mag. s.*
  –and soured by grapes, stomach were—*Lipp.*
  –by sour wine, stomach were—*Hyper.*
Dissolved after drinking water, stomach would be—*Erech.*

Distended, stomach were—*Ars., Bry., Calc. ar., Calc. c., Calc. p., Card. m., Dig., Dign., Eriod., Euphr., Fl. ac., Gins., Hell., Lob. s., Merl., Petr., Phos., Rhus t., Rumx., Serp.*

–after vomiting, stomach were—*Bry.*

–in pit of stomach—*Camph.*

–walls of stomach would be—*Ign.*

Dragging three hours after eating, stomach were—*Bism.*

Drawn inward, stomach would be—*Eug.*

–inward, everything would be—*Dros.*

–together, stomach were—*Rhus t.*

–upward and backward, stomach were—*Plb.*

–up into a ball, something in stomach were—*Lach.*

–together spasmodically, coats of stomach were—*Arn.*

–through stomach, thread were—*Kreos.*

–against spine, stomach were tightly—*Verat. v.*

Drew together in a lump and suddenly opened—*Manc.*

Drunk a great deal of lukewarm water, she had—*Spong.*

–hot brandy, he had—*Laps. c.*

–too much, he had—*Eucal.*

Dry and wrinkled, stomach were—*Pyrus*

–in stomach, food lay—*Calad.*

Dryness in pit of stomach, great—*Cupr.*

Dull instrument were pressing in stomach—*Nit. s. d.*

Earth, stomach were coated with astringent—*Mill.*

Eat because of faintness, she must not—*Colch.*

–pork, she could not—*Crot. h.*

Eaten herring, she had—*Nux m.*

–too much fat, he had—*Cyc.*

–something indigestible, he had—*Sac. lac., Wye.*

–tough meat, he had—*Chin. a.*

–too much, one had—*Colch., Con., Cyc., Eucal., Ferr. i., Kreos., Op., Paraf., Puls., Rheum, Sabin., Sil., Staph., Sulph.*

–too much, she could not lean forward because she had—*Ferr. i.*

–too much and too rapidly, he had—*Croc.*

–too much and must vomit—*Calad.*

–peppermint lozenges, he had—*Camph.*

–nothing, he had—*Sars.*

–nothing for a long time—*Bruc.*

–nothing for two days, she had—*Sol*

–nuts in solar plexus, he had—*Chin. a.*

–were rising up, everything—*Lyc.*

Eaten—*Continued*
  –spice, he had—*Rumx.*
  –tallow, he had—*Saba.*
  –vegetable acid, he had—*Chlor.*
Eating would relieve burning in stomach—*Sep.*
  –choked while—*Ornith.*
Eats a little, yet hungry; satiety if he—*Rhus t.*
Egg in stomach, hard boiled—*Abies n.*
Electric stitches extending into ankle—*Kreos.*
Emetic, he had taken an—*Thea*
Empty, stomach were—*All. c., Mill., Verb., Vib., Zing.*
  –epigastrium were—*Podo.*
  –after an emetic, stomach were—*Euph.*
  -from hunger, stomach were—*Coca, Nat. m., Petr.*
  -after a meal, stomach were—*Ptel.*
  –from smoking, stomach were—*Phos.*
  –not satisfied, stomach were—*Tub.*
  –stomach, to raise mucus would—*Chlor.*
  –sinking in stomach—*Calc. p.*
Emptiness of stomach, would faint from—*Bufo*
Enlarged, pit of stomach were—*Mang.*
Eructate, he would—*Spig.*
Eructation would occur—*Tell.*
Eructations were of rancid grease—*Thuj.*
Eviscerated, stomach were—*Ol. an.*
Excoriated, stomach were—*Cit. v., Cupr. ac., Sal. ac.*
Exhalation rising from stomach, acrid, pungent—*Phel.*
  -fatty, from stomach—*Sulph.*
Expanded, stomach were—*Calc. ar.*
Faint from emptiness of stomach, one would—*Bufo*
Faintness, she must not eat because of—*Colch.*
Fall out, stomach would—*Hall*
  –down, stomach would—*Lyc.*
Fallen out of stomach, bottom had—*Ox. ac.*
Falling in pit of stomach—*Cact.*
Falls into stomach like a stone, food—*Crot. c.*
  –into stomach heavily, food—*Elaps*
Fastened to pharynx, stomach were—*Agar.*
Fasting in stomach—*Anac., Aran. s., Bov., Caust., Dign., Fago.,
    Ign., Indg., Laur., Lyc., Mag. m., Merl., Mez., Mill., Nat. c.,
    Nat. s., Nicc., Ol. an., Phos., Rhus g., Scroph.*

Fasting—*Continued*
  –she had been—*Tarent.*
  –in pit of stomach—*Anac.*
  –but without hunger—*Chin. s., Cocc., Lach., Lyc.*
  –yet stomach full—*Am. m., Card. b.*
Fat, he had eaten too much—*Cyc.*
Feeling in epigastrium, she had no—*Ign.*
Fell, stomach rose and—*Xanth.*
Fermentation of contents of stomach—*Acet. ac., Croc., Ferr. s.,
    Nux v.*
Fiber were torn out of stomach—*Kreos.*
Filled with air, stomach were—*Cob.*
  –with food, stomach were—*Rheum*
  –with food, stomach and œsophagus were—*Arg. n.*
  –with heart beat, pit of stomach were—*Jac.*
Filling up to the top with food, stomach were—*Graph.*
Fire, stomach were on—*Tart. ac.*
  –in stomach, coals of—*Ars., Ars. s. r.*
  –were rushing from stomach to eyes, a spark of—*Stram.*
Fist were forcibly pressing against stomach—*Rhod.*
Flame were rushing out of throat and stomach—*Euph.*
Flames were rising from stomach—*Manc.*
Flowing through stomach, warm water were—*Sumb.*
Fluid pouring into stomach—*Hell.*
Fluttering in pit of stomach—*Æsc.*
  –in stomach, a bird were—*Calad.*
  –in pit of stomach, heart were—*Nux v.*
Folded together, epigastrium were—*Tell.*
Food until hunger were gone, one had been without—*Cocc.*
  –collected into a ball while sitting—*Merc.*
  –would come up—*Manc.*
  –undigested, stomach contained—*Cob., Lob., Phys., Rumx.*
  –did not digest properly—*Phos.*
  –stomach were filled with—*Rheum*
  –stomach and œsophagus were filled with—*Arg. n.*
  –stomach were filling up to the top with—*Graph.*
  –formed into lumps with hard angular surfaces—*Nux m.*
  –had frozen—*Berb.*
  –lay dry in stomach—*Calad.*
  –lay heavy in—*Hydrs.*
  –lay at bottom of cardia and would not pass, morsel of—*Tus. f.*

Food—*Continued*

—lying in stomach—*Abies n., Bell., Bry., Chin.*

—lying above the cardiac orifice—*Ign.*

—had lodged behind stomach—*All. c.*

—had lodged in cardiac region—*Acon.*

—lodged over orifice of stomach—*Ign., Puls.*

—stomach were overloaded with—*Meny.*

—were pressing upon and bursting stomach—*Chin.*

—were pushed to the left side of stomach with a snapping noise —*Bry.*

—remained above the stomach—*Nux v.*

—remained in stomach, undigested—*Dios.*

—remained in stomach, lump of hard undigested—*Abies n.*

—remained a long time in stomach—*Mez.*

—were settled too little in stomach—*Thuj.*

—sticking in stomach—*Ign.*

—stopped midway in stomach—*Rhus v.*

—had been swallowed too hastily—*Ter.*

—had swallowed a morsel of hot; followed by cold water— *Gent. c.*

—were suddenly swallowed, large pieces of—*Phys.*

Forced through too small an opening, bolus were—*Tab.*

Forcing its way through stomach, air were—*Bar. c.*

—passage through pit of stomach, something were—*Valer.*

—through from stomach to flesh, pins were—*Med.*

Foreign body in stomach—*Agar., Cupr., Fago., Grat., Nat. m., Thuj.*

—body pressed stomach—*Cahin.*

—body sticking in cardiac orifice and behind sternum—*Nat. m.*

—body, round, difficult of digestion—*Raph.*

—body, round, rising to stomach—*Pip. n.*

Freezing in stomach—*Phos.*

Frozen, food had—*Berb.*

Fruit then drank water, he had taken much—*Prun.*

Fruits lie like ice in stomach—*Elaps*

Full, stomach were—*Phys.*

—even though fasting, stomach were—*Am. m.*

—stomach were too—*Bar. c., Lob.*

—up to neck—*Sanic.*

—of bile, stomach were—*Kali i.*

—of gas in stomach—*Carb. ac.*

Full—_Continued_
   —as after a hearty meal—_Myric._
   —of water, stomach were—_Grat._
Fullness in the pit of stomach—_Alumn._
Furred over, mucous membranes of stomach were—_Pip. m._
Gangrene in stomach—_Linar._
Gas in stomach, full of—_Carb. ac._
   —stomach would burst with—_Arg. n._
Gases collected in a ball in—_Hydrc._
Glass were cutting in stomach—_Calad._
Gnawed, stomach were—_Saba._
Gnawing of acid in stomach to throat—_Hep._
   —in stomach were caused by something alive—_Anan._
   —burning in stomach—_Ox. ac._
   —hunger in stomach—_Colch., Mill., Ox. ac._
   —in stomach, something were—_Lach._
   —of worms in stomach—_Am. m._
Gone in stomach. all—_Dub., Tub._
   —feeling in pit of stomach at 11 a. m., all—_Nat. m., Phos._
   —in stomach, everything were—_Stram._
   —stomach were quite—_Gels., Murx._
Grasping inside of stomach, a hand were—_Nux v._
Grinding of worms in stomach—_Am. m._
Griping of a worm in stomach—_Nat. c._
Gripped by a hand, stomach were—_Tub._
Growing together, stomach were—_Spong._
Hammers were beating in stomach—_Graph._
   —beating in an ulcerated spot in stomach—_Lachn._
Hand were grasping inside of stomach—_Nux v._
Hanging down, stomach were—_Carb. v., Staph._
   —down like a bag, stomach were too large and—_Rhus t._
   —down by a thread, stomach were—_Nat. m._
   —down by a thread which would break, stomach were—_Agar. em._
   —heavily in stomach—_Carb. v._
   —loose when walking, stomach were—_Hep._
   —relaxed, stomach were—_Bar. c., Ip., Lob., Staph., Tab._
   —in water, stomach were—_Abrot._
Hangs in the body like an empty bag, stomach—_Thea_
Hank in stomach and pharynx—_Coloc._

Hard ball of potato in epigastrium—*Ovi g. p.*

 –undigested food remained in stomach—*Abies n., Phys.*

 –lump in pit of stomach—*Rumx.*

 –pieces were lying in stomach—*Manc.*

 –potato, he had swallowed—*Ovi g. p.*

 –like stone, everything in stomach were—*Hep.*

 –angular surfaces, food formed into lumps with—*Nux m.*

 –substance in stomach—*Bapt., Ferr., Mos., Rumx., Sang., Tab.*

Hardness rolling around in stomach—*Lil. t.*

Hastily, food had been swallowed too—*Ter.*

Heart palpitated in pit of stomach—*Med.*

 –beat filled pit of stomach—*Jac.*

Heat, gentle, passed from stomach through arms to fingers—*Con.*

Heaved up and down, stomach—*Cocc.*

Heaviness in stomach would be > by food—*Sep.*

 –from stone in stomach—*Æsc., Lach.*

Heavy in stomach, food lay—*Hydrs.*

 –lump in stomach—*Arg. n.*

Hole in epigastrium through to back and air were passing through—*Med., Rhus t.*

Hollow, stomach were—*Calad., Chin. a.*

Hot coal lay in stomach, red—*Ars., Ars. s. r., Tep.*

 –in small spot beneath ensiform cartilage, something—*Spire.*

Hung down relaxed, stomach—*Ip.*

 –down relaxed, stomach and intestines—*Ign.*

 –down heavily, stomach—*Merc.*

 –loose, stomach—*Hep.*

Hunger, gnawing, in stomach—*Colch.*

 –in stomach, ravenous—*Verat. a.*

Hungry, satiety if he eats a little yet—*Rhus t.*

 –in stomach—*Abies c., Ant. t., Apoc., Magnol.*

Ice were in stomach—*Kreos.*

 –were in stomach, after cold drinks or fruit—*Elaps*

 –were lodged in stomach, lump of—*Bov., Crot. h.*

Imprisoned at epigastrium, air became—*Rhus t.*

Indigestible, he had eaten something—*Chin. s., Wye.*

Indigestion in stomach—*Æth., Cob., Ferr., Iber., Mez., Phys., Wild.*

Inflammation in stomach—*Bell., Ferr.*

Inflated, stomach were—*Card. m.*

 –pit of stomach were—*Dulc.*

Instrument had made wound in stomach, some sharp, with cough—*Tab.*

Iron, he had swallowed a ball of lead or cold—*Samars.*

Jerked up, stomach were—*Kali bi.*

Jumping about in pit of stomach, something alive were—*Croc., Sang.*

Knife, cutting with a sharp—*Paraf.*

  —epigastrium were pierced with a—*Colch.*

  —were running into her stomach—*Sil.*

  —stomach were being split open with a—*Rhus t.*

  —stabbed in pit of stomach—*Nicc.*

  —were stabbing in stomach—*Phos.*

  —passed through and transfixed, with cutting in pit of stomach—*Cupr.*

Knives cutting in region of stomach—*Bry., Lepi.*

  —were cutting in stomach after eating—*Kali bi.*

  —were sticking in stomach when sitting bent—*Indg.*

Laced, acute pain in stomach—*Nux m.*

  —tightly, lower part of stomach were—*Ign.*

  —tightly, region of stomach were—*Plat.*

Lameness of stomach—*Am. br.*

Large and hanging down, stomach were too—*Rhus t.*

  —he had swallowed something too—*Tab.*

Lead were in stomach—*Hep., Sil.*

  —he had drunk melted—*Ip.*

  —or cold iron, he had swallowed a ball of—*Samars.*

Lime burned in stomach with rising of air—*Caust.*

  —bubbling in stomach from—*Caust.*

Liquid moving from stomach into intestines—*Mill.*

Liquor, burning in stomach caused by—*Chim. umb.*

Living in stomach, something—*Croc., Manc., Saba., Sabin., Sang., Thuj., Verat. a.*

  —jumping about in pit of stomach, something—*Croc.*

Loaded—see also OVERLOADED

Load in stomach—*Am. m., Bism., Calc. c., Kali ox., Lob. c., Plb., Samars., Sin.*

  —after cold drinks, lies like—*Acet. ac.*

  —in stomach after eating—*Tub.*

  —in stomach heavy—*Gels., Phos. ac.*

  —of stone in stomach—*Calc. c.*

ᴸodged behind stomach, food had—*All. c.*

–in cardiac region, food had—*Acon.*

–in cardiac end of stomach, something were—*Form.*

–over the orifice of stomach, food had—*Ign.*

–in stomach, lump of ice were—*Bov., Crot. h.*

–in stomach that would not pass off, something remained—
  Sep.

ᴸoose when vomiting, something would tear—*Sep.*

–in pit of stomach, something were—*Staph.*

ᴸump in stomach—*Arg. n., Bar. c., Bry., Dirc., Graph., Hydr.
  ac., Lil. t., Lob., Med., Naja, Nat. c., Nux v., Plb., Polyp.
  o., Rhus t., Sàmars., Sanic., Sep., Sil.*

–in epigastrium—*Agar., Sulph.*

–burning in stomach—*Lob.*

–hard, in pit of stomach—*Rumx.*

–of hard undigested food remained—*Abies n.*

–of undigested food in stomach—*Lob.*

–or hard ball in epigastrium like a potato—*Ovi g. p.*

–heavy, in stomach—*Arg. n.*

–of ice were lodged in stomach—*Bov., Crot. h.*

–as large as fist in stomach—*Kali c.*

–and then suddenly opened, stomach drew together in—*Manc.*

ᴸumps with hard angular surfaces, food formed into—*Nux m.*

ᴸying in stomach, a ball were—*Coc. c.*

Marble were pressing from epigastrium to heart—*Kalm.*

Meat would not digest—*Pyrus*

Medicine, he had taken—*Linar.*

Mental acts were performed in the stomach—*Acon.*

Missed his regular meal, he had—*Scroph.*

Motion, nerves in stomach were in (causing convulsion)—*Bell.*

Moved up and down in stomach and bowels, something—*Lyc.*

Moving in stomach toward throat, something alive were—*Tarent.*

–from stomach into intestines, liquid were—*Mill.*

Nausea, sudden, from pit of stomach—*Mosch.*

–would set in—*Fl. ac.*

Nauseated, he would become—*Malar.*

–from smoking strong tobacco—*Zinc.*

Needles pressing in stomach—*Puls. n.*

–or shocks from a battery between end of sternum and umbilicus
  —*Thlaspi*

Nerve were quivering in stomach—*Ferr.*
Nerves in stomach were in motion causing convulsion—*Bell.*
Nervous in stomach—*Phys.*
Nothing, he had eaten—*Sars.*
   –for some time, he had eaten—*Bruc., Sol*
Obstructed in epigastrium—*Eup. per.*
Open, stomach were standing—*Spong.*
Opened suddenly, stomach drew together in a lump and—*Manc.*
Opening in the stomach through which air passed—*Crot. c.*
Overloaded, stomach were—*Am. c., Ant. c., Ant. t., Ars., Carb ac., Cimic., Coff., Cyc., Dig., Eucal., Euph., Ign., Kali bi, Ptel., Puls., Rhus t., Sacc., Sulph., Tax., Til.*
   –with food, stomach were—*Meny.*
Palpitated in pit of stomach, heart—*Med.*
Passed through an opening in stomach, air—*Crot. c.*
   –from stomach through arms to fingers, gentle heat—*Con.*
Passes up right side of throat, hot air; although stomach feel cold—*Am. br.*
Passing into stomach, something were—*Cupr.*
   –into chest, contents of epigastrium were—*Cham.*
Pebbles, sharp, in stomach—*Anan.*
Pepper, burning in stomach were from—*Caust.*
   –he had swallowed—*Euph.*
Peppermint lozenges, he had eaten—*Camph.*
Perforated, boring, stomach would be—*Kali i., Nat. s.*
Peristaltic motion were driven toward throat—*Asaf.*
Pieces, stomach were cut to—*Kali c., Mag. m., Rat.*
   –hard, were lying in the stomach—*Manc.*
Pierced with a knife, epigastrium were—*Colch.*
Piercing through flesh, paper of pins were—*Med.*
Pincers, stomach were torn with—*Sulph.*
Pins were sticking in stomach—*Ign.*
   –in stomach were piercing through flesh, paper of—*Med.*
Plug were pressing in stomach—*Mill.*
   –reaching from stomach to spine—*Lob.*
Poisoned, stomach were—*Aur. m., Hæm., Lach.*
Potato, he had swallowed a hard—*Ovi g. p.*
Pouring into stomach, fluid were—*Hell.*
Pressed off below pit of stomach, something would be—*Kalm.*
   –out, everything in stomach would be—*Sul. ac.*
   –together from both sides, stomach were—*Lyc.*

Pressed—*Continued*
 –toward spine, walls of stomach would be forcibly—*Arn.*
Pressing forcibly with fist against stomach, someone were—*Rhod.*
 –upon and hurting stomach, food were—*Chin.*
 –in stomach, dull instrument were—*Nit. s. d.*
 –heavily on stomach, something were—*Phos.*
 –from epigastrium to heart, marble were—*Kalm.*
 –into scrobiculum, stone were—*Cham.*
 –at pit of stomach, stone were—*Ptel., Rob.*
Pressure came from stomach and compressed heart—*Nat. m.*
 –of a bar in stomach—*Bell.*
 –from dull instrument in stomach—*Nit. s. d.*
 –from a foreign body, following burning—*Agar.*
 –from eating too much—*Bov., Hyper., Lyc., Rheum, Sil.*
 –from a plug in stomach—*Mill.*
 –from a dull point in stomach—*Asar.*
 –from a stone in stomach—*All. s., Calc. c., Sep.*
 –from mineral water in stomach—*Coc. c.*
 –where xiphoid cartilage were pressed inward—*Arn.*
Puckered, rugæ of stomach were—*Jab.*
Pulled down, dragging three hours after eating, stomach were—*Bism.*
 –up on coughing, loose flesh at pit of stomach were—*Staph.*
Pulling from adherent diaphragm—*Mez.*
Purring like a cat in region of stomach—*Ferr. s.*
Pushed to the left side of stomach with a snapping noise, food were—*Bry.*
Quivering in stomach, a nerve were—*Ferr.*
Ragged and full of sores, stomach smarted and felt—*Stram.*
Rancid, stomach were—*Bry., Com., Crot. h.*
Raw, inside of stomach were—*Mez.*
 –inside on pressure, stomach were—*Ign.*
 –by acrid substance, stomach and œsophagus were—*Ars.*
Re-echoed in stomach, cough—*Cupr.*
Relaxed, stomach were—*Ign., Ip., Tab.*
Remained above the stomach, food—*Nux v.*
 –a long time in stomach, food—*Mez.*
 –in stomach that would not pass off, something lodged and—*Sep.*
 –in stomach, a lump of hard undigested food—*Abies n.*

Removed, stomach had been—*Phos.*
Retained in stomach, breath were—*Eupi.*
Retracted, muscles of stomach were—*Verat. v.*
Reversed, peristaltic motion were—*Asaf.*
Rice water were apple cores—*Stram.*
Rising from stomach to throat, ball were—*Asaf., Kali ar., Lyc.,
    Lyss., Mag. m., Senec.*
    –from stomach, a ball were; spreading cool air over vertex and
        occiput—*Arn.*
    –from stomach, acrid, pungent exhalation were—*Phel.*
    –from stomach into throat, living body were—*Tarent.*
    –from stomach, flames were—*Manc.*
    –from stomach, something warm were—*Valer.*
    –from stomach, she would suffocate from—*Solid.*
Rolled up into a ball, stomach were—*Bry.*
    –into a ball in stomach, thread were—*Arn.*
Rolling up into a ball, something in stomach were—*Arn.*
    –about during menses, a ball in stomach were—*Tong.*
    –to side lain on when turning in bed, weight in stomach were
        —*Nast.*
Rose in pit of stomach, ball—*Con.*
    –into throat, contents of stomach—*Dign.*
    –and fell, stomach—*Xanth.*
    –from stomach to chest, waves—*Verat. a.*
Rugæ of stomach were puckered—*Jab.*
Running into her stomach, a knife were—*Sil.*
Rushing from stomach to eyes, a spark of fire were—*Stram.*
    –out of throat and stomach, flame were—*Euph.*
Sand in stomach—*Ptel.*
Satiety, he had eaten to—*Colch., Con., Cyc., Eucal., Ferr. i.,
    Paraf., Puls., Rheum, Sabin., Sil., Staph., Sulph.*
    –as soon as he has eaten anything—*Ruta*
    –if he eats a little; yet hungry—*Rhus t.*
Scalded, stomach were—*Kali ox., Rob.*
Scarified, stomach were—*Merc.*
Scraped, stomach were being—*Sep.*
Screwed together in stomach—*Canth., Kali c., Phel., Sil.*
Screwing feeling in stomach—*Uran.*
    –together in stomach—*Zinc.*
    –together in epigastrium—*Sil.*

Sensation, stomach were without—*Sars.*

Settled too little, food were—*Thuj.*

Shocks from battery from stomach to epigastric region—*Iris*
 —from a battery between end of sternum and umbilicus, or needles—*Thlaspi*

Shook when walking, stomach had to be held up—*Merc.*

Shortened, stomach were—*Ign.*

Sink down with pain in stomach, she must—*Elaps*
 —into abdomen, stomach would—*Agar., Dig.*

Sinking in stomach—*Acon., Alumn., Apoc., Calad., Chlol., Croc., Dig., Ery. m., Jatr., Saponin., Sulph., Tab., Thea*
 —empty, in stomach—*Calc. p.*
 —in pit of—*Chlol., Verat. a.*

Sitting bent, he had been—*Lact.*

Sleep, stomach would go to—*Castor.*

Slipping toward epigastrium, something in œsophagus were—*Ther.*

Smarted and felt ragged, stomach were full of sores and—*Stram.*

Smoking strong tobacco, nauseated from—*Zinc.*

Something in stomach that ought to come up—*Eup. per.*

Sore in pit of stomach—*Glon.*
 —internally, stomach were—*Sep.*
 —spot were pressed below pit of stomach—*Saba.*

Soured and disordered by grapes, stomach were—*Lipp.*

Spark of fire rushed from stomach to eyes—*Stram.*

Spice, one had eaten—*Rumx.*

Spirits, he had swallowed—*Euph.*

Splashed about when walking, stomach full of water—*Tep.*

Split open with a knife, stomach were closed and being—*Rhus t.*

Spoiled in stomach—*Ambr., Graph.*

Sprained in stomach—*Ign., Thuj.*

Spree, he had been on—*Æth.*

Squeezed by a hand, stomach were—*Tarent.*

Stabbed in pit of stomach with a knife—*Nicc.*

Stabbing in stomach, knife were—*Phos.*

Steam rising from stomach into head—*Lyc.*

Sticking in cardiac orifice, a foreign body were—*Nat. m.*
 —in stomach, pins were—*Ign., Med.*

Stitches, electric, from stomach into ankle—*Kreos.*

Stone in stomach—*Acon., Æsc., Agar., Ars., Ars. s. f., Bar. c., Brom., Bry., Calc. c., Cedr., Cham., Coc. c., Coloc., Cupr., Dios., Gent. c., Grat., Herac., Ign., Kali c., Lac c., Lach., Merc., Merl., Naja, Nat. c., Nat. m., Nux v., Op., Osm., Paull., Par., Puls., Rhus t., Rob., Saba., Sep., Sil., Squill., Sul. ac., Zing.*

–in pit of stomach—*Æsc., Ptel.*

–heavy, in stomach—*Bry.*

–or ball lying in stomach—*Coc. c.*

–in stomach on early waking—*Puls.*

–cold, were in stomach—*Acon., Ars., Sil.*

–were buried deep in stomach while talking—*Paull.*

–food falls into stomach like—*Crot. c.*

–in stomach goes off with eructations—*Bry.*

–everything in stomach were hard like—*Hep.*

–in stomach, load of—*Calc. c.*

–on stomach—*Cedr., Paraf.*

–pressing at pit of stomach—*Ptel., Rob.*

–pressing into scrobiculum—*Cham.*

–in stomach, pressure of—*All. s., Calc. c., Sep.*

–rolling from side to side in stomach—*Grat.*

–causing nightly pressure on stomach—*Sep.*

–rose up from stomach—*Sul. ac.*

Stones, he had swallowed a lot of broken—*Osm.*

Stool were felt in stomach, urging to—*Vichy*

Stopped, pit of stomach were—*Rhus t.*

–midway in stomach—*Rhus v.*

Stiff straight tube extending from stomach to throat—*Abies n.*

Strapped together, stomach were—*Tell.*

Stretched, stomach were—*Tarent.*

Struck by blows in epigastrium—*Lac c.*

Substance, a hard, in stomach—*Bapt., Rumx., Sang., Tab.*

–indigestible, in stomach—*Ostrya*

Suffocate from rising from stomach, she would—*Solid.*

Suffocation, ball in stomach caused—*Pana.*

–and constriction in stomach—*Sang.*

Swallowed too much air, he had—*Plat.*

–a ball, he had—*Ter.*

–a ball of lead or cold iron, he had—*Samars.*

–a bullet which lodged in pit of stomach, he had—*Ter.*

–too hastily, food had been—*Ter.*

wallowed—*Continued*
  –food without chewing, he had—*Magnol. gl.*
  –large pieces of food were suddenly—*Phys.*
  –a morsel of hot food followed by cold water—*Gent. c.*
  –too large a morsel, one had—*Ol. an.*
  –something too large, he had—*Tab.*
  –pepper, he had—*Euph.*
  –a hard potato, he had—*Ovi g. p.*
  –spirits, he had—*Euph.*
  –a lot of broken stones, he had—*Osm.*

Swelling, stomach were—*Bry.*

Swimming or hanging in water, stomach were—*Abrot.*

Swinging back and forth in stomach, something were—*Lyc.*

Swollen, pit of stomach were—*Bry., Juncus, Rhus t.*

Tallow, he had eaten—*Saba.*

Tear loose during eructations or when vomiting, something
    would—*Sep.*

Tearing off in stomach, something were—*Petr.*

Thickened after eating, walls of stomach were—*Æsc.*

Thread were drawn through stomach—*Kreos.*
  –were being rolled in a ball, in stomach—*Arn.*

Tied together, stomach were—*Carb. s.*

Tight about stomach, clothes were too—*Caust., Crot. h., Gins.,*
    Lyc., Spong., Tub.
  –in stomach, everything were too—*Lyc.*

Tobacco, nauseated from smoking strong—*Zinc.*

Torn, stomach were about to be—*Ars.*
  –apart during eructations, stomach would be—*Phos.*
  –away in stomach, something would be—*Petr.*
  –loose in stomach, something were—*Ars., Puls.*
  –with pincers, stomach were—*Sulph.*
  –out of stomach, fiber were—*Kreos.*
  –out when yawning, stomach were being—*Ars.*

Tough, stomach were—*Chim. rotund.*

Trembling in stomach—*Ham.*

Tube extending from stomach to throat, a stiff straight—*Abies n.*

Tumor in pylorus, a hard—*Anan.*

Turn over, stomach would—*Tab.*
  –about on coughing, stomach would—*Kali c.*

Turned to air in the stomach, every particle of food he ate—*Iod.*
  –over, stomach—*Ruta*
  –quite over with a sudden desire to vomit, stomach—*Ol. an.*

Turning inside out, stomach were—*Saba.*
  –inside out, viscera were—*Sep.*
Turns as she turns over in bed, stomach were a bag of water which—*Ornith.*
Twisted, stomach were—*Tub.*
  –stomach were being—*Paraf.*
  –about, stomach were—*Con.*
  –about in stomach, something were—*Nux v.*
  –in epigastrium, ball were—*Inul.*
Twisting about in stomach, a large round body were—*Phel.*
  –in stomach rising to throat, something were—*Sep.*
  –in stomach as of thread being rolled into a ball—*Arn.*
  –in epigastrium, a ball were—*Inul.*
Twitching of a worm in stomach—*Nat. c.*
Ulcer in stomach—*Acet. ac., Carb. ac., Ill., Kali i., Lach.*
Ulcerated in stomach and abdomen—*Rhus t.*
Undigested in stomach, food remained a long time—*Mez.*
Unsatisfied, stomach is (nausea)—*Tab.*
Urging to stool were felt in stomach—*Vichy*
Vanished forever, appetite had—*Rhus t.*
Vitriol, burning in stomach were from—*Iris fœ.*
Vomit, he would—*Aloe, Bism., Corn., Crot. t., Eup. pur., Ign., Laur., Stram., Verat. a.*
  –about to, > eating—*Æsc.*
  –without nausea, he would—*Bapt., Ferr.*
  –he had taken an emetic and would—*Laur.*
  –when drinking water, he would—*Ars. h.*
  –it would be a relief to—*Bapt.*
Vomited, stomach itself would be—*Pip. n.*
  –up, blood were—*Ip.*
Vomiting would come on—*Sabin.*
  –would relieve stomach—*Ind.*
Vapor, hot, were rising from stomach—*Merc.*
Vapors, hot, rose from stomach to shoulder—*Laur.*
Warm were rising from stomach, something—*Valer.*
Water, region of stomach were bathed in hot—*Coc. c., Phos.*
  –cold, were in stomach—*Ant. t., Caps., Kreos., Pyrus*
  –cold, or ice in epigastrium—*Kreos.*
  –lukewarm, he had drunk a great deal of—*Spong.*
  –he had drunk too much warm—*Spong.*
  –warm, flowing through stomach—*Sumb.*

Water—*Continued*
  –stomach were full of—*Coc. c., Grat., Kali c., Laur., Mag. c., Mill., Ol. an., Phel., Tep.*
  –stomach were full of cold—*Ant. t., Grat., Pyrus*
  –stomach were constantly full of—*Kali c.*
  –stomach full of hot—*Quass.*
  –stomach were hanging down and swimming in—*Abrot.*
  –quarts of, were in stomach and bowels—*Tub.*
  –and splashed about when walking, stomach were full of—*Tep.*
  –he had swallowed a morsel of hot food followed by cold—*Gent. c.*
  –he had taken too much fruit and then drank—*Prun.*
  –turns as she turns over in bed, a bag of—*Ornith.*
  –in stomach, warm—*Æsc., Cic., Coc. c., Quass.*
Waves rose from stomach to chest—*Verat. a.*
Weakness came from stomach—*Mag. m.*
  –in stomach seems to come from head—*Calc. s.*
Weight in stomach—*Ars. s. r., Pic. ac., Rob.*
  –in epigastrium—*Ferr. i.*
  –attached to stomach—*Dig.*
  –in stomach with burning—*Ovi g. p.*
  –heavy, in stomach—*Agar., Ox. ac., Phos., Pip. n., Plb., Nit. ac., Sec.*
  –heavy, on stomach—*Con.*
  –heavy, were lying on stomach—*Staph.*
  –in stomach rolling to side lain on when turning in bed—*Nast.*
Weighted down, everything in epigastrium were—*Plb.*
Whiskey, stomach were burnt up with—*Pyrus*
Wind, stomach would burst with—*Arg. n.*
  –on stomach, belching were caused by—*Lyc.*
  –stomach were full of—*Carb. v.*
Wine, water contained—*Tab.*
Worm rising from stomach—*Valer.*
  –in stomach, formication from—*Cocc.*
  –were griping in stomach—*Nat. c.*
Worms in stomach—*Grat.*
  –biting in stomach—*Hell.*
  –burning in stomach were from—*Hell.*
  –burrowing in stomach—*Lach.*
  –crawling in stomach—*Alum.*
  –numberless, crawling in epigastrium and stomach—*Cina*

19

Worms—*Continued*

  —gnawing in stomach—*Am. m.*

  —were moving in stomach—*Cocc.*

Wound in stomach from some sharp instrument, with cough—*Tab.*

Wriggling in epigastrium, an animal were—*Chel.*

Wrinkled and dry, stomach were—*Pyrus*

Writhing in stomach—*Am. m., Bar. c.*

Yeast, stomach were full of—*Stict.*

ABDOMEN

Abscess were forming near umbilicus—*Plb.*

Abortion, pain in abdomen as before—*Tarent.*

Accumulation of wind in abdomen—*Graph.*

Aching as before menses—*Nat. c.*

Acid in intestines, he had dissolved—*Linar.*

Adhere to chest, abdomen would—*Mez.*

Adhered to anterior abdominal walls and were torn away, intestines had—*Verb.*

Adherent to walls and torn off, right side of abdomen were—*X-ray*

  –in abdomen, something were—*Sep.*

  –to wall of abdomen, intestines about umbilicus were—*Verb.*

Air, abdomen were distended with—*Saba.*

  –abdomen were filled with—*Raph.*

  –were bursting in abdomen, small bladder of—*Lyc.*

  –bubbles along colon—*Dig.*

  –bubbles were passing through water from symphysis pubis to right side—*Conv.*

  –bubbles were pressed forcibly through intestines and passed upward—*Pall.*

  –bubbles were running transversely over abdomen—*Merc. i. f.*

  –diagonally across above umbilicus, a draft of—*Sulph.*

  –hot, blowing over lower abdomen and thighs—*Trom.*

  –hot, were in hernia—*Amph.*

Alive in abdomen, something were—*Calc. p., Cann. s., Croc., Cyc., Kali i., Kali n., Nux v., Saba., Sabin., Sep., Sil., Stram., Thuj.*

  –in upper abdomen, something were—*Phos.*

  –in right abdomen, something were—*Croc.*

  –were pushing out in ileus, something—*Thuj.*

  –and quivering in abdomen like fœtal movement—*Sabin.*

  –were running and crawling in intestines, something—*Cyc.*

  –beneath skin of abdomen, something—*Spong.*

  –in muscles, something were—*Hyos.*

Animal, living, were in abdomen—*Stram., Thuj.*

  –were snapping and tearing portions of intestines and insides—*Pall.*

  –were wriggling about above umbilicus—*Chel.*

Appear, a hernia would—*Berb., Calc. ar., Camph., Cham., Clem., Coff., Dig., Gran., Nux v., Phos., Plan.; Prun., Raph., Rheum, Rhus t., Sil., Stann., Sulph., Sul. ac., Ter., Verat. a., Wies., Zinc.*

Arrows, two, drawn through abdomen in opposite directions—*Plb.*

Ascending from abdomen to throat, ball were—*Arg. n., Raph.*

Asleep—*Calc. p., Ferr. i., Merc.*

  —muscles were—*Petr.*

  —left side of abdomen were—*Sulph.*

Astringent in abdomen, extending to stomach—*Gal. ac.*

Backwards, blood in abdomen were flowing—*Elaps*

Bag not quite filled with fluid lay in bowels—*Plb.*

Ball in abdomen—*Bell., Delph., Tub.*

  —or lump at umbilicus—*Anac., Kali bi., Nat. m., Nit. ac., Nux v., Plb., Ran. s., Spig.*

  —ascended from abdomen to throat—*Arg. n., Raph.*

  —and abdomen empty, bowels were drawn up into a—*Cham.*

  —intestines were pressed like a rubber—*Ferr. i.*

  —of fire in abdomen—*Kreos.*

  —hard, or hen's egg in right lower abdomen—*Merc.*

  —hard, in right iliac region—*Hydrs.*

  —of gas were rolling in abdomen—*Aur. s., Lach.*

  —were rolling from right side of abdomen toward stomach—*Lach.*

  —of thread were turning and moving rapidly through abdomen—*Saba.*

  —were turning over in abdomen—*Lach.*

  —were lying in umbilical region, a hard twisted—*Kreos.*

Balls of gas were rolling together in abdomen—*Coloc., Jatr., Ornith.*

Band around abdomen—*Con., Crot. c., Zinc.*

  —tight around lower abdomen—*Nat. m.*

  —tight around lower abdomen as if laced—*Ign.*

  —drawn tightly from crest of one ilium to other—*Eug.*

  —tightly drawn about abdomen—*Arg. n.*

  —around hypogastrium—*Con.*

Bandage, cold, were over lower part of abdomen—*Lac f.*

  —tight, were in uterine region—*Hyper.*

Bar in abdomen—*Gins.*

  —around abdomen—*Ars.*

Battery drawn upward to epigastric region, a galvanic—*Iris*

   —or needles between end of sternum and umbilicus, electric shock from a—*Thlaspi*

Bearing down from inactivity of rectum—*Podo.*

   —down and passing out, something were—*Cimic.*

Beaten, had been—*Calad.*

   —in right side—*Ang., Pall.*

   —above pelvis—*Verat. a.*

   —in hip joint—*Zinc.*

   —intestines were—*Ferr., Nux v.*

   —together, intestines would be—*Sep.*

Bile were deficient—*Abies n.*

Biting in abdomen, worms were—*Am. c., Nat. ac.*

   —on right side of abdomen, fleas were—*Grat.*

Bitten by something on lower part of abdomen (itching)—*Carb. ac.*

Bladder of air, small, were bursting in abdomen—*Lyc.*

Blood in abdomen were flowing backward—*Elaps*

Blowing over lower abdomen and thighs, hot air were—*Trom.*

Body, foreign, in right side of pelvis—*Thuj.*

   —from waist to lower pelvis would collapse—*Vib.*

   —foreign, as large as walnut lodged in left inguinal region—*Myris.*

   —foreign, drawing in abdomen when walking—*Seneg.*

   —hard biconvex, were in abdomen—*Med.*

   —hard, were lying in groin—*Carb. an.*

   —hard, were opposing pressure from pharynx into abdomen—*Zinc.*

   —hard, pressed from within outward at right inguinal ring—*Bell.*

   —hard, pressing in spot left of umbilicus—*Par.*

   —hard, rolled up in intestines—*Op.*

   —hard, rolled or fell from umbilicus when turning from one side to other—*Lyc.*

   —resistant, on deep pressure at umbilicus—*Hydr. ac.*

   —or plug, stiff, inside of abdomen—*Sep.*

   —soft, were lying in abdomen—*Nat. s.*

   —weight were too great for pelvis—*Sulph.*

Boiler were working in abdomen—*Nit. ac.*

   —abdomen were—*Lachn.*

Boiling water were poured over small of back and through pelvis
   —*Verat. v.*
Bound across, hypogastrium were—*Ox. ac.*
  –tightly in groins and pelvic region—*Sulph.*
  –by lead poison—*Ostrya*
  –up and would burst, he were—*Lyc.*
Bounding in body, child were—*Ther.*
Brandy, he had been drinking (in abdomen)—*Eug.*
Break in pelvis, something would—*Ars. h.*
Broke in left lower abdomen, bubbles formed and—*Cupr.*
Broken, hip and pelvis were—*Pimp.*
Bruised in abdomen—*Ang., Arg. m., Caust., Camph., Mag. m.
   Merc. c., Nux v., Sulph.*
  –everything in abdomen were sore and—*Ran. b.*
  –on every step, everything were sore and—*Nux v.*
  –intestines were—*Apis, Ferr., Picrot., Verat. a.*
  –in abdominal walls—*Manc.*
  –in abdominal muscles—*Nux v.*
  –below umbilicus—*Form.*
  –and weary in loins, belly and thighs—*Bov.*
Bubbles of air in abdomen—*Lyc., Merc., Nat. m., Pall., Phos.
   Puls., Stann., Sulph., Sumb.*
  –of air along colon—*Dig.*
  –of air running transversely over abdomen—*Merc. i. f.*
  –of air were passing through water from symphysis pubis to
    right side—*Conv.*
  –of air were pressed forcibly through intestines and passed up
    ward—*Pall.*
  –were bursting in abdomen—*Ant. c., Coloc.*
  –forming and bursting in abdomen—*Arg. m., Cupr., Tarax.*
  –were forming and wanted to burst in right lower abdomen—
    X-ray
  –formed and broke in left lower abdomen—*Cupr.*
  –formed and burst in hypogastrium—*Tarax.*
  –rising up in abdomen—*Gent. l.*
  –great, were rumbling in upper abdomen—*Sulph.*
Bubbling in abdomen—*Puls.*
  –water under walls of abdomen were—*Rhus t.*
  –as of wind in abdomen—*Com.*
  –or gurgling in abdomen, extending back to left side of spine
    when lying on left side—*Pyrog.*

Burnt or scraped in abdomen—*Bell.*

　–him internally, something—*Cact.*

Burning in abdomen, hot iron were—*Bell.*

　–in abdomen, electric sparks were—*Phel.*

Burrowing in inguinal region—*Coc. c.*

Burst, abdomen would—*Am. m., Bar. c., Carb. v., Chim. mac., Cop., Hyos., Lyc., Nit. ac., Sanic., Spig., Valer.*

　–when coughing, abdomen would—*Anac.*

　–by flatus, abdomen would be—*Coff.*

　–intestines would—*Coloc., Lyc., Pip. n.*

　–from load, abdomen would—*Am. m., Lac c.*

　–he were bound up and would—*Lyc.*

　–at menses, abdomen would—*Ovi g. p.*

　–in abdomen, ulcer would—*Laur.*

　–before stool, abdomen would—*Ars.*

　–when walking, abdomen would—*Lac c., Lyc.*

　–in hypogastrium, bubbles formed and—*Tarax.*

　–out through abdomen, intestines would—*Squill.*

　–in right lower abdomen, bubbles were forming and wanted to —*X-ray*

　–if pressed, a distended sac in abdomen would—*Med.*

Bursting in abdomen—*Anac., Carb. v., Caust., Coff., Dulc., Hyos., Ign., Lyc., Phos., Puls., Sulph., Tub.*

　–in abdomen, bubbles were—*Ant. c., Coloc.*

　–upward as though everything in abdomen were coming out at mouth—*Asaf.*

　–in abdomen, bubbles of air were forming and—*Tarax.*

　–from waist down, she must hold herself up—*X-ray*

Button were pressing above umbilicus—*Am. c.*

Caved in, abdomen were—*Coloc., Ptel.*

Cavity or large hole in region of spleen—*Chin.*

Cement, lower abdomen were filled with hardened—*Pyrog.*

\Child in uterus, thrust in left abdomen as from a—*Stann.*

　–were bounding in her body—*Ther.*

　–in abdomen, first movement of—*Carl.*

Child-birth, in throes of—*Verat. a.*

Child's knee were pushed against anterior wall from within— *Thuj.*

　–fist moved in abdomen—*Sulph.*

　––arm moved in abdomen—*Conv.*

Chill spread from abdomen—*Mar.*

Chisel were thrust deep into upper abdomen, thence passing in a curve backward and downward into pelvis, then cutting its way upward again—*Coloc.*

Choke from swelling of abdomen, she would—*Raph.*

Close together, abdomen and back were too—*Plb.*

Closed suddenly, water were poured through tube which—*Elaps*

Cloth, hot dry, on abdomen—*Nit. ac.*

   —hot wet, on a spot over left ovarian region—*Lach.*

Clothes about abdomen were too tight—*Op., Tub.*

Clothing about abdomen, he must unfasten—*Dios.*

Clutched by hand in abdomen and stomach—*Bell.*

   —with fingers, right side of abdomen were—*Sanic.*

Coal, red-hot, flying about in abdomen—*Samars.*

Coals, hot, in abdomen—*Verat. a.*

   —hot, at umbilicus < when inspiring—*Merc. p.*

   —of fire in abdomen—*Tub.*

   —red-hot, deep in pelvis—*Kreos.*

Cobweb, abdomen were covered with a—*Rhus t.*

Cold bandage were over lower part of abdomen—*Lac f.*

   —in abdomen, taking—*Coloc.*

   —he had taken—*Aloe, Carb. v., Coloc., Croc., Dulc., Ign., Juncus, Lyc., Merc., Nit. ac., Nux v., Op., Petr., Sabin.*

   —abdomen were exposed and—*Ter.*

   —round plate, abdomen were covered by a—*Ter.*

   —extreme, passing in a fine line from center of pubis to point two inches above—*Sac. lac.*

   —fluid passed through intestines during menses—*Kali c.*

   —water, shivering in abdomen from movement of—*Cann. s.*

   —water passed through intestines—*Kali c.*

   —water as far as abdomen, seated in—*Plb.*

Coldness in abdomen—*Æth., Ambr., Camph.*

   —would become colic—*Hell.*

   —icy, in abdomen—*Ambr.*

   —rising from abdomen to throat—*Carb. ac.*

   —as if piece of ice were in abdomen—*Crot. h.*

   —and emptiness and hollowness in abdomen—*Agar.*

Colic, coldness in abdomen would become—*Hell.*

Collapse, body from waist to lower pelvis would—*Vib.*

Coming out at mouth, bursting upward as though everything in abdomen were—*Asaf.*

Commotion, whole intestinal contents were in fluid state and in violent—*Polyg.*

Congestion were rising from abdomen to head—*Crot. t.*

Constricted, abdomen were—*Ferr. ma., Plat.*

  –by a string, abdomen were—*Caust., Chel.*

  –everything in abdomen were—*Mosch.*

  –one-third of abdomen were—*Lipp.*

  –intestines were—*Plb., Spig.*

Contents, intestinal, would issue through genital organs—*Sep.*

Contracted, abdomen were—*Chel.*

  –to spinal column, abdomen were—*Quass.*

  –near umbilicus—*Cocc.*

Contracting, spleen were—*All. c.*

Contused in abdomen—*Arn., Guare.*

Cord around abdomen—*Paraf.*

  –connected anus and umbilicus with pain on straightening—*Ferr. i.*

  –constricted hypogastrium—*Chel.*

  –about hips, tight—*Sil.*

  –tightly drawn across lower part of loins—*Arn.*

  –extended to inguinal region, a large—*Conv.*

Corsets pinched umbilicus—*Phys.*

Cough came from abdomen—*Con.*

Coughing rising from abdomen—*Ant. c.*

  –two knives going toward each other in abdomen, when—*Kali c.*

Cramps would set in—*Opun., Sel.*

Crawling in abdomen—*Calc. ar., Pall., Stann.*

  –worms were—*Arund., Calc. c., Dulc., Saba.*

  –up and down in abdomen and biting and gnawing parts, worms were—*Dulc.*

  –in abdominal muscles—*Oxyt.*

  –in intestines, something alive were running and—*Cyc.*

  –in lower abdomen to beginning of urethra—*Zinc.*

Creeping things, abdomen were full of—*Stann.*

  –in abdomen, mouse were—*Plb.*

  –under skin near umbilicus—*Slag*

Crushed, abdomen were—*Apis, Led.*

Cut, intestines were being—*Coff., Coloc.*

  –into a wound in abdomen, someone would—*Arn., Phys.*

Cut—*Continued*

    –with a knife, intestines were being—*Alet., Coloc., Sol. n.*

    –to pieces, intestines were—*Laur.*

    –to pieces, intestines would be—*Ant. t., Op.*

    –in pieces, bowels were—*Laur., Merc.*

    –intestines were torn out or—*Asaf.*

    –to pieces, abdomen would be—*Jalap.*

    –with knives, abdomen were—*Alet., Lach.*

    –with knives, intestines settled in lower abdomen and were—*Alet.*

    –off under ribs, would be—*Euon.*

Cutting from knives in abdomen—*Chel., Kali bi., Saba., Verat. a.*

    –in toward center of abdomen, thread were—*All. c.*

    –with knives in pelvic region—*Med.*

    –small knives were—*All. c.*

    –into wounds in abdomen when touched—*Arn.*

    –toward each other, two knives were—*Crot. t.*

    –in abdomen, hard, sharp, movable pieces were—*Bov.*

Darting in abdomen, needles were—*Acon., Apoc., Iris, Still., Trom.*

    –through abdomen to anus, electric shocks were—*Coloc.*

Debauch, he had been on a—*Aral.*

Develop, appear or protrude, hernia would—*Berb., Calc. ar., Camph., Cham., Clem., Coff., Dig., Gran., Nux v., Phos., Plan., Prun., Raph., Rheum, Rhus t., Sil., Stann., Sulph., Sul. ac., Ter., Verat. a., Wies., Zinc.*

Digging fingers into intestines, someone were—*Bry.*

Dilated, inguinal ring were—*Mag. p. Aust.*

Discharge itself into region of duodenum, some fluid in lower part of right lung wanted to—*Chen. v.*

Discharged, flatus were about to be—*Mag. p. Aust.*

    –but neither occurs, pain would arise and flatus would be—*Fl. ac.*

Disemboweled—*Paraf., Sars.*

Diseased, spot in lower part of abdomen were—*Zinc.*

Distended, abdomen were—*Cocc., Lith.*

    –with air, abdomen were—*Sabin.*

    –abdomen were greatly—*Tub.*

    –to extremest degree, abdomen were—*Stram.*

    –upper abdomen were—*Cinnb.*

    –bowels were—*Nat. s.*

Distended—*Continued*

  –with gas, intestines were—*Plb.*

  –right abdomen were—*Nat. s.*

  –below umbilicus—*Laur.*

  –from eating too much—*Nat. m., Tax.*

Distension of sac which would burst if pressed upon—*Med.*

Draft of air diagonally across above umbilicus—*Sulph.*

Dragging when walking, abdominal viscera were—*Nat. m.*

  –down contents of abdomen—*Sabal*

Drawing on abdomen, leeches were—*Coc. c.*

  –in from abdomen to back—*Plb.*

  –something were loose and—*Mag. m.*

  –and gnawing in region of appendix—*X-ray*

  –in abdomen when walking, foreign body were—*Seneg.*

Drawn in, abdomen were—*Verat. v.*

  –in, umbilicus were—*Nux v.*

  –into a lump, intestines were—*Inul., Sep.*

  –together, bowels were—*Mang.*

  –together, all intestines were violently—*Ricin.*

  –tightly from crest of one ilium to other—*Eug.*

  –up, contents of chest and abdomen were—*Antip.*

  –up into a ball and abdomen were empty, bowels were—*Cham.*

  –upward to epigastric region, galvanic battery were—*Iris*

  –out and downward, abdomen were—*Thlaspi*

  –tightly about—*Arg. n.*

  –toward spine, intestines were being—*Ter.*

  –to spine by string—*Plb.*

  –back against vertebral column, abdominal contents were—*Tril.*

  –together by stitches, abdomen were—*Nat. s.*

  –up and backward to spine, colon were forcibly—*Dios.*

  –through abdomen in opposite directions, two arrows were—*Plb.*

  –through abdomen, a hundred knives were—*Sec.*

  –around waist, strap as wide as hand—*Sep.*

  –suddenly tight and then gradually loosened, string were tied around intestines in umbilical region—*Chion.*

  –transversely across from ilium to ilium—*Paraf.*

  –across lower part of loins, cord were—*Arn.*

  –over region of uterus, abdominal muscles were all being—*Aml. n.*

Drawn—*Continued*

    —connecting anus and umbilicus, with pain on straightening, a cord were—*Ferr. i.*

    —down and relaxed, skin of abdomen were greatly—*Psor.*

    —to spine, anterior wall were—*Ptel.*

Drinking brandy (in abdomen), he had been—*Eug.*

Drop when walking, belly would—*Asc. t.*

    —intestines would—*Cann. s.*

    —they are so relaxed, whole abdomen, contents and walls would —*Staph.*

    —on walking, viscera of abdomen would—*Ferr.*

    —through pelvis, everything would—*Podo.*

Dropped in left abdomen while at stool, marble were—*Nat. p.*

Dropping in left groin, fluid were—*Zing.*

Dropsy in abdomen—*Chim. mac.*

Drunk and enraged, in violent colic—*Alum.*

Dug in abdomen, an oblong hole were—*Tong.*

Eaten too much, in abdomen—*Carb. v., Clem., Coc. c., Graph., Meny., Nux m., Staph., Ter.*

    —unripe fruit, she had—*Ox. ac.*

Eating in bowels, something were—*Kali bi.*

Ebullition, everything in abdomen were in—*Pip. n.*

Electric shocks darted through abdomen to anus—*Coloc.*

    —shocks from abdomen to vagina—*Kreos.*

    —shock from battery or needles, between end of sternum and umbilicus—*Thlaspi*

    —sparks burning in abdomen—*Phel.*

Emetic in morning, she had taken (in bowels)—*Euph.*

Emptied out, all bowels would be—*Schinus*

Emptiness in abdomen—*Merc., Phos.*

    —and hollowness and coldness in abdomen—*Agar.*

Empty, whole abdomen were—*Cham., Cocc., Dulc., Quass., Saba., Sulph.*

    —after stool, abdomen were—*Podo.*

    —bowels were drawn up into a ball and abdomen were—*Cham.*

    —feeling in groins—*Pall.*

Enraged and drunk, in violent colic—*Alum.*

Entrails were hanging loose and flabby when walking—*Ictod.*

Eruption would make its appearance across abdomen—*Com.*

Evacuate fæces, intestines had no power to—*Hell.*

Everything would fall out at groins—*Ars. h.*

Eviscerated, he were—*Gamb., Lach., Olnd., Sars.*

Evisceration would relieve—*Merc. d.*

Excoriated on pressure, abdomen were—*Coloc.*

Expanded, abdomen were—*Calc. ar.*

 —to utmost limit, abdomen were—*Stram.*

 —throat and abdomen were—*Hyper.*

Exposed and cold, abdomen were—*Ter.*

Fall down, everything in abdomen would—*Nux v.*

 —out at groin, everything would—*Ars. h.*

 —out, everything in abdomen would—*Alum., Asc. t., Nat. c.*

 —out over pubes, bladder were full and contents of abdomen would—*Sep.*

 —out of abdomen when coughing, everything would—*Carb. an.*

 —from pit of chest to pit of abdomen, weight seems to—*Nat. h.*

 —out at umbilicus, bowels would—*Ran. b.*

 —out if diarrhœa followed, whole abdomen would—*Ars. h.*

 —out of pelvis, everything would—*Hydrs., Til.*

Fallen upon abdominal muscles, he had—*Hyos.*

 —in abdomen, something had—*Plb.*

 —and settled into lower abdomen, bowels were—*Opun.*

Falling out, anterior wall were wanting and bowels were in danger of—*Coloc.*

 —intestines were—*Podo.*

 —down in abdomen, something large were—*Laur.*

 —out, abdomen were—*Alum., Aur. s., Ferr., Nat. m., Nux v., Ran. b.*

 —out, bowels were—*Kali br.*

 —from above umbilicus to small of back, lump were—*Laur.*

 —apart, bones of pelvis were—*Tril.*

 —in abdomen, drops of water were—*Lyc.*

 —in right iliac and lumbar region, lump size of hen's egg were rising and—*Hydrs.*

False labor pains in abdomen—*Kali c.*

Fasting—*Lach., Puls.*

Feather, abdomen were tickled with a—*Morph.*

Fell down in abdomen, something—*Laur.*

 —down, something were torn off and—*Plb.*

 —from umbilicus to either side when turning to that side, hard body—*Lyc.*

 —from one side to other, intestines—*Bar. c.*

Fell—*Continued*

    –from one side to other when turning in bed, intestines—*Bar. c., Merc.*

    –to side on which one were lying, bowels—*Merc.*

Fermenting, bowels were—*Agar., Aran., Rhus t.*

Festering in abdominal walls—*Coloc.*

Filled with stones, abdomen were—*Ant. t., Calc. c., Cocc.*

    –with air, abdomen were—*Raph.*

    –with pins, bowels were—*Helod.*

    –with water, intestines were—*Cench., Kali c.*

    –up in abdomen—*Conv.*

    –with hot water, pelvis were—*Aloe*

    –with flatus, abdomen were—*Zinc.*

    –with hardened cement, lower abdomen were—*Pyrog.*

Fingertips were pressed upward and backward at umbilicus—*Dios.*

Fire were in intestines—*Manc.*

    –in abdomen, ball of—*Kreos.*

    –in abdomen, coals of—*Tub.*

    –passed through abdomen with stool, streams of—*Asc. t.*

Fish were turning over each other in abdomen—*Podo.*

Flabby when walking, entrails were hanging loose and—*Ictod.*

Flatus passed down left side of abdomen to rectum but seemed to turn and go upward to bladder or uterus—*Pulx.*

    –be discharged but neither occurs, pain would arise and—*Fl. ac.*

    –were pressing against coccyx—*Zinc.*

    –lay like a sausage from left to right above umbilicus—*Sulph.*

    –incarcerated—*Meny., Nat. c., Nux v., Sil., Staph., Sulph., Trom.*

    –incarcerated in hypochondria—*Rhod.*

Flea bites on abdomen—*Zinc.*

Fleas biting on right side—*Grat.*

Flowing backward, blood in abdomen were—*Elaps*

    –through abdomen, hot water were—*Sumb.*

Fluctuation in groin—*Bad.*

Fluid from taking a cathartic, full of—*Tanac.*

    –state and in violent commotion, whole intestinal contents were in a—*Polyg.*

    –were poured from one intestine into another—*Arg. m.*

    –were pouring into abdomen—*Rhod.*

Fluid—*Continued*

    –rolled from one side to other in abdomen—*Plb.*

    –were running in intestines—*Jatr.*

    –were washing about in abdomen—*Crot. t.*

    –in lower part of right lung wanted to discharge itself into region of duodenum—*Chen. v.*

    –were forcing its way through left iliac region, to groin and half-way down thigh—*Coc. c.*

    –cold, passed through intestines during menses—*Kali c.*

    –dropping in left groin—*Zing.*

Fœtus, living, in abdomen—*Arn., Conv., Croc., Lyc., Nux v., Op., Plb., Sulph., Tarent., Thuj.*

    –were kicking in left abdomen—*Croc.*

Forced out, contents of abdomen would be—*Lac c.*

    –out, bowels would be—*Merc.*

    –out on standing, everything would be—*Sul. ac.*

    –through a narrow space in abdomen, something were—*Op.*

    –out in both groins, hernia would be—*Calc. ar.*

    –up through intestines, something were—*Sulph.*

    –out of pelvis, everything would be—*Xanth.*

    –asunder, symphysis pubis were suddenly—*Ter.*

Forcing its way through left iliac region and half-way down thigh, fluid were—*Coc. c.*

    –itself through abdomen, something were—*Dig.*

Foreign body in right side of pelvis—*Thuj.*

    –body drawing in abdomen when walking—*Seneg.*

    –body as large as a walnut lodged in left inguinal region—*Myris.*

Formed and burst in hypogastrium—*Tarax.*

    –and broke in left lower abdomen, bubbles—*Cupr.*

Forming and wanted to burst in right lower abdomen, bubbles were—*X-ray*

Fruit, she had eaten unripe—*Ox. ac.*

Full, abdomen were—*Dor.*

    –abdomen were too—*Linar.*

    –of stones, abdomen were—*Ant. t., Calc. c., Cocc.*

    –and contents of abdomen would fall out over pubes, bladder were—*Sep.*

    –of water, bowels were—*Acon., Apoc., Hell., Urt. u.*

    –of creeping things, abdomen were—*Stann.*

Gave way in groin, something—*Ovi g. p.*

—way with him, everything in pelvis—*Sanic.*

Girdle on abdomen—*Gins.*

—on abdomen, from a tight—*Raph.*

Give way, everything in abdomen would—*Cocc.*

—way in left groin, always < from any exertion, something would—*Ovi g. p.*

Giving way in hypogastrium—*Pic. ac.*

Glow within beat against one—*All. c.*

Glued to spine, walls of abdomen were—*Plb.*

Gnawing in abdomen, worms were—*Cyc., Dulc.*

—about umbilicus, worms were—*Grat.*

--the parts, worms were crawling up and down in abdomen and were biting and—*Dulc.*

—and drawing in region of appendix—*X-ray*

Grasped, abdomen were—*Ip.*

—by hand in right side of abdomen—*Caust.*

Grasping intestines and each finger were sharply pressing in, hand were—*Ip.*

Griping with a hand in intestines—*Ip.*

—in abdomen, worms were—*Dulc., Nat. m., Nux v.*

Gripped at side of umbilicus—*Jac.*

Gurgling like distant thunder in abdomen—*Sanic.*

—and moving about in abdomen—*Pip. n.*

—in abdomen as if it would be heard—*Rheum*

—or bubbling in abdomen, extending back to left side, when lying on left side—*Pyrog.*

Hair were pulled up in abdomen—*Chin.*

Hanging heavily, abdomen were—*Alum., Carb. v.*

—across pelvis and bladder, weight were—*Nat. m.*

—down and must hold it up, abdomen were—*Staph.*

—down and relaxed, stomach and intestines were—*Ign.*

—down, intestines were—*Psor.*

—loose and flabby, entrails were—*Ictod.*

Hard as a rock, bowels were—*Eup. pur.*

—lying in abdomen, pressing; something—*Sin. a.*

—pieces in abdomen—*Bor.*

—sharp movable pieces cutting in abdomen—*Bov.*

—tumor near umbilicus with griping pains—*Zinc.*

—twisted ball were lying in umbilical region—*Kreos.*

Hardened cement, lower abdomen were filled with—*Pyrog.*

Heaviness of a stone in abdomen—*Cinch., Op., Puls., Sin. a.*
  —as from a stone, causing great fatigue on walking—*Lac d.*
  —while sitting and walking, tension in lower abdomen—*Kali c.*

Heavy, abdomen were—*Dor.*
  —load resting on abdomen—*Acon.*
  —weight in pelvis pressing downward and backward—*Kali p.*
  —were lying on left side of abdomen, something—*Lyc.*
  —as lead, all viscera were—*Ery. m.*
  —lump were falling from above umbilicus to small of back—*Laur.*
  —weight in lower abdomen—*Med.*
  —lump pressed in abdomen—*Rhus t.*
  —weight came into pelvis low down—*Kali c.*

Held up, bowels shook when walking and had to be—*Merc.*
  —up, intestines had to be—*Merc.*
  —up by strings which might tear, intestines were—*Coloc.*

Hernia were present—*Spong.*
  —umbilical, after strain—*Gran.*
  —would protrude, develop or appear—*Berb., Calc. ar., Camph., Cham., Clem., Coff., Dig., Gran., Nux v., Phos., Plan., Prun., Raph., Rheum, Rhus t., Sil., Stann., Sulph., Sul. ac., Ter., Verat. a., Weis., Zinc.*
  —would be forced out through both groins—*Calc. ar.*
  —in groin—*Coloc.*
  —were pressing out in left side—*Sil.*
  —hot air were in—*Amph.*
  —were receding—*Coloc.*
  —would become incarcerated—*Nux v.*

Hold it up, abdomen were hanging down and must—*Staph.*
  —abdomen up, she had to—*Merc.*

Hole or large cavity in region of spleen—*Chin.*
  —in his side, there were a—*Stann.*
  —oblong, were dug in abdomen—*Tong.*

Hollow, abdomen were—*Cham., Merc., Phos.*

Hollowness, emptiness and coldness in abdomen—*Agar.*

Horseback ride, he had been on a long (groins)—*Spig.*

Hot air were in hernia—*Amph.*
  —dry cloth on abdomen—*Nit. ac.*
  —iron burning in abdomen—*Bell.*
  —wet cloth on a spot over left ovarian region—*Lach.*
  —water running down into abdomen—*Chin.*

Hot—*Continued*
   —water undulated in abdomen when moving—*Casc.*
   —water filled pelvis—*Aloe*
   —water flowing through abdomen—*Sumb.*
   —water were being poured into bowels—*Ip.*
   —water poured from chest into abdomen—*Sang.*
   —wavelike steam moving in abdomen, chest and throat—*Lyss.*
Hung on easily tearing threads, bowels were—*Coloc.*
Hungry, abdomen were—*Squill.*
Ice, abdomen were full of—*Calc. c.*
   —coldness in abdomen as if a piece of ice were in—*Crot. h.*
   —water in lower abdomen—*Onos.*
   —skin over pelvis were touched with—*Arg. m.*
Icy coldness in abdomen—*Agar.*
Immovable, abdomen were—*Puls.*
Impediment below diaphragm—*Linar.*
Incarcerated flatus—*Meny., Nat. c., Nux v., Sil., Staph., Sulph., Trom.*
   —flatus in hypochondria—*Rhod.*
   —hernia would become—*Nux v.*
Inflamed, diaphragm were—*Paraf.*
Inflated, abdomen were—*Apis, Merl.*
   —umbilical region were—*Coloc.*
Insect stinging on abdomen—*Chlor.*
Instrument, bowels, bladder and rectum pressed by a sharp—*Nux v.*
   —going through right groin into abdomen—*Sul. ac.*
Iron, hot, in abdomen—*Bell.*
Issue through genital organs, intestinal contents would—*Sep.*
Jelly, abdomen quivering like—*Cob.*
Kicking in left abdomen, fœtus were—*Croc.*
   —over os pubis—*Calc. p.*
Knife drawn transversely across from ilium to ilium—*Paraf.*
   —in abdomen, pierced by—*Coloc.*
   —sticking in abdomen—*Con., Cast.*
   —thrust through—*Ip., Lach.*
   —transfixed through abdomen from left to right—*Ip.*
   —thrust from umbilical region to back—*Cupr.*
   —in right abdomen on walking—*Rhus t.*
   —through from left to right side of abdomen when breathing—*Stann.*

Knife—*Continued*
  –stabbed with a—*Op.*
  –were sticking between umbilicus and right groin—*Inul.*
  –like sticking in right side of abdomen—*Verb.*
Knives cutting in abdomen—*Chel., Kali bi., Saba., Verat. a.*
  –small, cutting in abdomen—*All. c.*
  –cutting in pelvic region—*Med.*
  –two, were cutting toward each other in abdomen—*Crot. t.*
  –two, going toward each other in abdomen when coughing—
    Kali c.
  –a hundred, were drawn through abdomen—*Sec.*
  –were plunged into abdomen—*Con.*
  –stabbing in abdomen—*Merc.*
Knotted by thread, intestines were—*Sulph.*
  –string were shooting down through and across upper abdomen
    —*Merc. i. f.*
Knots, intestines were strung in—*Sulph.*
  –intestines were being tied in—*Bol.*
  –small intestines were being tied in—*Polyp.*
  –intestines were being twisted into—*Verat. a.*
Labor pain in lower abdomen—*Ther.*
Laced, abdomen were—*Aur.*
  –abdomen were tightly—*Ign.*
Larger than usual, abdomen were—*Conv.*
Lay like a sausage from left to right above umbilicus, flatus—
  Sulph.
Lead poison, abdomen were bound by—*Ostrya*
  –all viscera were heavy as—*Ery. m.*
Leeches were drawing on abdomen—*Coc. c.*
Liquid, abdomen were full of—*Rheum*
  –gurgling and moving about in abdomen—*Pip. n.*
  –from stomach into intestines—*Mill.*
Live things were moving about in abdomen, a thousand—*Podo.*
Living in abdomen, something were—*Cann. s., Croc., Rat., Sabin.,*
  Spong., Ther., Thuj.
  –thing causing movement in—*Arund., Arum t., Calc. p.*
  –fœtus in abdomen—*Arn., Conv., Croc., Lyc., Op., Plb., Sulph.,*
  Tarent., Thuj.
Load in epigastrium—*Sil.*
  –heavy, resting on abdomen—*Acon.*
  –were resting in pelvis—*Kreos.*

Lodged behind umbilicus, plug were—*Ran. s.*

—in left inguinal region, foreign body as large as a walnut—*Myris.*

Loose, abdomen were—*Ail., Aran., Coloc., Coca, Nux v., Phys.*

—in abdomen, something were torn—*Rhus t.*

—in abdomen, something were coming—*Ruta*

—intestines had lost their hold and were—*Mag. m.*

—part of intestines were—*Cyc.*

—and dragging, something were—*Mag. m.*

—and dragging when walking, abdominal viscera were—*Nat. m.*

—and shaking about on walking, bowels were—*Mang.*

—and flabby when walking, entrails were hanging—*Ictod.*

—bones of pelvis were getting—*Murx.*

Loosened in abdomen, everything were—*Sulph.*

—something would become—*Caust.*

—from bone in hip joint, flesh were—*Zinc.*

—string tied around intestines in umbilical region, suddenly drawn tight and then gradually—*Chion.*

Lost their hold and were loose, intestines had—*Mag. m.*

Lump in abdomen—*Bell., Bry., Rhus t.*

—in center of abdomen—*Sep.*

—or ball at umbilicus—*Anac., Kali bi., Nat. m., Nit. ac., Nux v., Plb., Ran. s., Spig.*

—in lower abdomen—*Nux m.*

—heavy, were falling from just above umbilicus to small of back—*Laur.*

—heavy, pressed in abdomen—*Rhus t.*

—intestines were drawn up into a—*Inul., Sep.*

—size of a hen's egg rising and falling in right iliac and lumbar region—*Hydrs.*

—rolling over and over when coughing, rising from abdomen to throat and falling back again—*Kali c.*

—turning and twisting in whole abdomen—*Saba.*

Lying in abdomen, pressing, something were—*Sin. a.*

—in umbilical region, a hard twisted ball were—*Kreos.*

—in abdomen, soft body were—*Nat. s.*

—in groin, hard body were—*Carb. an.*

—crosswise and being pressed out at menses, a piece of wood were—*Nux m.*

—something were rolling over from right side when—*Lach.*

—in abdomen, stone were—*Aloe, Aran.*

Lying—*Continued*

 –on back, abdomen were sunken when—*Acet. ac.*

 –on left side of abdomen, something heavy were—*Lyc.*

Machine working in abdomen—*Nit. ac.*

Marble were dropped in left abdomen while at stool—*Nat. p.*

Medicine, she had taken—*Æth.*

Menses—see FEMALE SEXUAL ORGANS

Motion, all organs were in—*Hydrc.*

 –bowels were all in—*Corn.*

 –of intestines were lessened, peristaltic—*Camph.*

Mouse were in abdomen—*Plb.*

Movable pieces were cutting in abdomen, hard sharp—*Bov.*

Moved in abdomen, child's arm—*Conv.*

 –in abdomen, fist of child—*Sulph.*

Movement, first, of child—*Carl.*

 –in bowels caused by a living thing—*Arund., Arum t., Calc. p.*

Moving in abdomen, chest and throat, hot wavelike steam—*Lyss.*

 –in abdomen, worm were—*Rhus t.*

 –and gurgling in abdomen—*Pip. n.*

 –and turning rapidly through abdomen, a ball of thread were —*Saba.*

 –living thing were—*Arum t., Arund., Calc. p.*

 –about in abdomen, a thousand live things were—*Podo.*

Muscles of abdomen below short ribs, needles in—*Calc. c.*

 –were seized by pincers—*Caust.*

 –by arm of child, without pain, pushing of—*Thuj.*

Muscular fibers were tense—*Carb. v.*

Nails, spot in abdomen were seized with—*Bell.*

 –pushing in abdomen—*Eupi.*

Naked, abdomen were—*Ter.*

Needle were thrust in abdomen—*Lyc.*

Needles in abdomen—*Thuj., Verb.*

 –darting in abdomen—*Acon., Apoc., Iris, Still., Trom.*

 –pricking in sides of abdomen—*Ferr. i.*

 –intestines were pierced with fine—*Zinc.*

 –many, about umbilicus—*Verb.*

 –in muscles of abdomen below short ribs—*Calc. c.*

 –or shocks from a battery between end of sternum and umbilicus—*Thlaspi*

 –sticking in abdomen—*Thuj.*

Needles—*Continued*

    –dull, sticking in right abdomen by umbilicus—*Verb.*

    –in abdominal muscles on inspiration, tearing or stitching of—
      Calc. c.

    –stitches in abdomen—*Nux v.*

    –in abdomen above hips on taking a deep breath, being stuck
      with—*Cast.*

Opposing pressure from pharynx into abdomen, hard body were
    —*Zinc.*

Pain would give her a twist—*Verb.*

    –in abdomen as before abortion—*Tarent.*

    –would arise and flatus be discharged, but neither occurs—
      Fl. ac.

    –labor, in lower abdomen—*Ther.*

Pains in abdomen, false labor—*Kali c.*

Pass involuntarily with anxiety in abdomen, stool would—*Sep.*

Passed down left side of abdomen to rectum but seemed to turn
    and go upward to bladder or uterus, flatus—*Pulx.*

    –through abdomen with stool, streams of fire—*Asc. t.*

Passing through water from symphysis pubis to right side, bub-
    bles of air were—*Conv.*

Perforated, intestines were—*Kali i.*

Pieces, hard, were in abdomen—*Bor.*

    –were cutting in abdomen, hard sharp movable—*Bov.*

Pierced with fine needles, intestines were—*Zinc.*

    –by a knife in abdomen—*Coloc.*

Pimples in bowels, with tenderness—*Sulph.*

    –covered abdomen on being rubbed by clothes—*Meny.*

Pinched with corsets, umbilicus were—*Phys.*

Pincers pinching in abdomen—*Verat. a.*

    –muscles were seized by—*Caust.*

Pins, two, pricking to right of umbilicus—*Inul.*

    –extending downward from right side of chest to scrotum,
      pricking of—*Antip.*

    –bowels were filled with—*Helod.*

    –pricking in pubic region—*Cinch. b.*

Plate, abdomen were covered by a cold round—*Ter.*

Plucking in abdomen—*Nux m.*

Plug were wedged in between symphysis pubis and os coccygis—
    Aloe

    –in abdomen, stiff body or—*Sep.*

Plug—*Continued*
  –blunt, were squeezed into intestines with pain about umbilicus —*Anac.*
  –were lodged behind umbilicus—*Ran. s.*
Plugged, bowels were—*Spig.*
Plunged into abdomen, knives were—*Con.*
Poured from one intestine to another, fluid were—*Arg.*
  –through tube which closed suddenly, water were—*Elaps*
  –out of bottle from throat to abdomen, water were—*Cina*
  –hot water from chest into abdomen—*Sang.*
  –boiling water over small of back and pelvis—*Verat. v.*
Pouring hot water into bowels—*Ip.*
  –into intestines, fluid were—*Rhod.*
Power to evacuate fæces, intestines had no—*Hell.*
Press out in small spot, something would—*Nit. ac.*
  –through Poupart's ligament, the part would—*Laur.*
Pressed out, intestines were—*Bell., Sars.*
  –out, intestines were sinking down and would be—*Cann. s.*
  –by a sharp instrument in bowels, bladder and rectum—*Nux v.*
  –out at menses, piece of wood lying crosswise and being—*Nux m.*
  –asunder, abdomen were—*Euph.*
  –him, clothes—*Sil.*
  –forcibly through intestines, everything—*Sulph.*
  –in intestines—*Merc.*
  –inward, bowels were—*Coloc.*
  –forcibly through intestines and passed upward, bubbles of air were—*Pall.*
  –downward, intestines were—*Ang.*
  –upward and backward at umbilicus, fingertips were—*Dios.*
  –outward immediately below umbilicus, intestines were—*Bell.*
  –from within out in right inguinal region, hard body were—*Bell.*
  –in abdomen, heavy lump—*Rhus t.*
  –between two millstones, front to back—*Ip.*
  –off below stomach, something would be—*Kalm.*
  –like a rubber ball, intestines were—*Ferr. i.*
  –distended sac which would burst if—*Med.*
Pressing down in abdomen and small of back, stone were—*Puls.*
  –on umbilicus, stone were—*Cocc., Verb.*
  –against coccyx, flatus were—*Zinc.*

Pressing—*Continued*

   —out left side, hernia were—*Sil.*

   —above umbilicus, button were—*Am. c.*

   —against sharp edge of table, abdomen were—*Ran. b.*

   —in right side of pelvis—*Both. a.*

   —in spot left of umbilicus, hard body were—*Par.*

   —in sore spot in pelvis, something were—*Murx.*

   —something were lying in abdomen and—*Sin. a.*

   —in pelvic region, tip of thumb were—*Rheum*

   —downward and backward, heavy weight were in pelvis— *Kali p.*

   —in abdomen, heavy weight were—*Rhus t.*

   —in abdomen, stone were—*Ant. t., Bell., Merc., Op.*

Pressure would > pain in abdomen but it does not—*Dios.*

   —of a sharp stone at menses—*Cocc.*

   —from pharynx into abdomen, hard body were opposing—*Zinc.*

   —at umbilicus, resistant body on deep—*Hydr. ac*

   —abdomen were excoriated on—*Coloc.*

Pricking of pins in pubic region—*Cinch. b.*

   —in sides of abdomen, needles were—*Ferr. i.*

   —of pins extending downward from right side of chest to scrotum—*Antip.*

Prolapse from their own weight, bowels would—*Trif. p.*

Protrude, develop or appear, hernia would—*Berb., Calc. ar., Camph., Cham., Clem., Coff., Dig., Gran., Nux v., Phos., Plan., Prun., Raph., Rheum, Rhus t., Sil., Stann., Sulph., Sul. ac., Ter., Verat. a., Wies., Zinc.*

   —in abdomen, bunch would—*Con.*

   —gut would—*Plan.*

   —in left side, hernia would—*Stann.*

   —at left side of inguinal ring, bowels would—*Picrot.*

   —in pelvic organs, everything would—*Nit. ac.*

Puffed up, abdomen were—*Stram., Sulph.*

Pulled up in abdomen, hair were—*Chin.*

   —inward, abdominal walls were—*Plb.*

   —behind umbilicus, all bowels were—*Thuj.*

Pulse in abdomen—*Med.*

Purgative, bowels had been acted upon by a—*Ferr.*

Pushed out against anterior walls in morning, a child's knee were —*Thuj.*

   —out from abdomen—*Linum*

Pushed—*Continued*
 –into a funnel, contents of abdomen were—*Lil. t.*
 –toward heart, intestines were—*Rhus t.*
 –forward, diaphragm were—*Anthox.*
Pushing of nails in abdomen—*Eupi.*
 –of muscles by arm of child, without pain—*Thuj.*
 –out in ileus, something alive were—*Thuj.*
Quivering over os pubis—*Calc. p.*
 –in abdomen like jelly—*Cob.*
 –in abdomen like fœtal movement, alive and—*Sabin.*
Raising leg, someone tapped her on groin when—*Ther.*
Raw in abdomen—*Sulph.*
 –as after child-birth, everything were—*Sulph.*
 –and sore, abdomen were—*Bell.*
Receding, hernia were—*Coloc.*
Relaxed, weak and if diarrhœa followed, the whole would fall
   out—*Ars. h.*
 –and drawn down, skin of abdomen were—*Psor.*
 –the whole abdomen, contents and walls would drop, they are
   so—*Staph.*
 –and hanging down, stomach and intestines were—*Ign.*
Resting in pelvis, load were—*Kreos.*
 –on abdomen, heavy load were—*Acon.*
Resisted passage in bowels, sphincter—*Gels.*
Retracted, abdomen were—*Abrot., Acet. ac., Carb. ac., Dios.,
   Graph., Phos., Quass., Sulph.*
 –against spine, abdominal walls were—*Zinc.*
Ride, he had been on a long horseback (groins)—*Spig.*
Rigid, abdomen would become—*Mez.*
Ring stretched around abdomen—*Carl., Lyc.*
Rising from abdomen to head, congestion were—*Crot. t.*
 –from abdomen, coughing—*Ant. c.*
 –up in abdomen, bubbles were—*Gent. l.*
 –and falling in right iliac and lumbar region, lump size of hen's
   egg—*Hydrs.*
 –from abdomen to throat and back again, lump were rolling
   over and over when coughing—*Kali c.*
Rock, bowels were as hard as—*Eup. pur.*
Rolled up into a ball, parts in abdomen were—*Cham.*
 –up in intestines, hard body were—*Op.*
 –from one side to other in abdomen, fluid—*Plb.*

Rolled—*Continued*

–over and over in abdomen with pain in lower abdomen, something—*Ovi g. p.*

–from umbilicus when turning from left to right side, a hard body—*Lyc.*

Rolling in abdomen, ball of gas were—*Aur. s., Lach.*

–in abdomen, balls of gas were—*Coloc., Jatr., Ornith.*

–of thread were—*Saba.*

–over from right side when lying, something were—*Lach.*

–over and over when coughing, lump were rising from abdomen to throat and falling back again—*Kali c.*

Room in abdomen, there were not enough—*Plb.*

–in hypogastrium, there were not enough—*Tarent.*

Rubbed together with every movement, sharp stones—*Cocc.*

Rumbling in upper abdomen, great bubbles were—*Sulph.*

Running down into abdomen, hot water were—*Chin.*

–and crawling in intestines, something alive were—*Cyc.*

–in intestines, fluid were—*Jatr.*

–transversely over abdomen, air bubbles were—*Merc. i. f.*

Rupture, inguinal ring would—*Mag. p. Arct.*

Sausage from left to right above umbilicus, flatus lay like a—*Sulph.*

Scraped in abdomen, burnt or—*Bell.*

Scratched in right abdomen—*All. c.*

Screwed together, left inguinal region were being—*Zinc.*

–together, pelvis were—*Caust.*

Seated in cold water as far as abdomen—*Plb.*

Seized by pincers, muscles were—*Caust.*

–by nails, spot in abdomen were—*Bell.*

–one by one, intestines were—*Mez.*

Separated, pelvic bones were—*Sulph.*

Serpent were turning around in abdomen—*Cact.*

Settled down in lower abdomen, bowels were—*Opun.*

–in lower abdomen and were cut with knives, intestines were—*Alet.*

Shaken up, intestines were—*Sil.*

Shaking about when walking, bowels were loose and—*Mang.*

Sharp edge of table, abdomen were pressing against—*Ran. b.*

–stones rubbed together with every movement—*Cocc.*

Shattered and torn, everything in umbilical region were being—*Nux v.*

Shivering in abdomen from movement of cold water—*Cann. s.*

Shocks from a battery between end of sternum and umbilicus, needles or—*Thlaspi*

–electric, darting through abdomen to anus—*Coloc.*

–electric, from abdomen to vagina—*Kreos.*

Shook, bowels—*Asaf.*

–when walking and had to be held up, bowels—*Merc.*

Shooting down through and across upper abdomen, knotted string were—*Merc. i. f.*

Shrunk together, abdomen were—*Lipp.*

Sink down, abdomen would—*Staph.*

–down of their own weight, intestines would—*Pimp.*

Sinking down, bowels had been—*Abrot.*

–down and would be pressed out, intestines were—*Cann. s.*

Snapping and tearing portions of insides and intestines, an animal were—*Pall.*

Sore, everything in abdomen were—*Nux v.*

–and bruised on every step—*Nux v.*

–and bruised, everything in abdomen were—*Ran. b.*

–and raw, abdomen were—*Bell.*

Soreness between abdominal rings extending downward—*Am. be.*

Space in abdomen, something were forced out through a narrow —*Op.*

–in hypogastrium, there were not sufficient—*Tarent.*

Sparkling in abdomen—*Veratn.*

Sparks, electric, burning in abdomen—*Phel.*

Spot in abdomen were seized with nails—*Bell.*

–in lower part were diseased—*Zinc.*

Sprain in ovarian region—*Apis*

Sprained in left abdomen—*Am. m.*

–in left groin—*Am. m.*

–in right groin—*Ars., Sol. t. æ.*

Squeezed to pieces, bowels were—*Apis*

–between two stones, intestines were—*Coloc.*

–into intestines, blunt plug were, with pain about umbilicus—*Anac.*

–through abdomen, something would be—*Carb. an.*

Stabbed in right pelvic region—*Coloc.*

–with a knife—*Op.*

Stabbing in abdomen, knives were—*Merc.*

Steam moving through abdomen, chest and throat, hot wave-like
    —*Lyss.*

Stick with a ball on each end extending from throat to left side
    of abdomen—*Kali c.*

  –abdomen were struck by a pointed—*Manc.*

Sticking in right side of abdomen, knife-like—*Verb.*

  –in abdomen, needles were—*Thuj.*

  –to right side of umbilicus, two pins were—*Inul.*

  –in sides—*Ferr. i.*

  –in abdomen, knife were—*Cast., Con.*

  –dull needles in right side of abdomen—*Verb.*

  –with needles in abdomen above hips on taking a deep breath
    —*Cast.*

  –between umbilicus and right groin, knife were—*Inul.*

Stinging of insect in abdomen—*Chlor.*

Stitches of needle in abdomen—*Nux v.*

  –drew abdomen together—*Nat. s.*

Stitching of needles, or tearing, in abdominal muscles on inspira-
    tion—*Calc. c.*

Stone in abdomen—*Ars. h., Bell., Lac d., Merc., Op., Puls.,
    Saba., Sil.*

  –heavy, in abdomen, causing great fatigue on walking—*Lac d.*

  –just below umbilicus—*Nux v.*

  –in lower abdomen—*Cupr.*

  –heavy, in hypogastric region—*Cocc.*

  –heavy, in abdomen—*Chim. mac., Cinch., Op., Puls., Sin. a.*

  –pressing in abdomen—*Ant. t., Bell., Merc., Op.*

  –pressing down in abdomen and small of back—*Puls.*

  –pressing on umbilicus—*Cocc., Verb.*

  –at menses, pressure of a sharp—*Cocc.*

  –rolled from umbilicus to groin when lying on left side—*Lyc.*

  –contents of abdomen changed to—*Ars. h.*

  –lying in abdomen—*Aloe, Aran.*

Stones, abdomen were full of—*Ant. t., Calc. c., Cocc.*

  –sharp, rubbed together with every movement—*Cocc.*

  –intestines were squeezed between two—*Coloc.*

  –abdomen were stuffed full of—*Ant. c., Ant. t.*

Stool would pass involuntarily, with anxiety in abdomen—*Sep.*

Strained himself in groins, he had—*Hydrs.*

  –sides were stiff—*Ferr. i.*

Strangulated, intestines were—*Pall., Spong.*

Strap as wide as hand drawn around waist—*Sep.*

Stretch violently in every direction, she must—*Plb.*

Stretched around abdomen, ring were—*Carl., Lyc.*

  —ligaments from stomach were—*Lach.*

  —skin were—*Lil. t.*

String, abdomen were constricted by a—*Chel.*

  —when breathing abdomen were constricted by—*Caust.*

  —tied around intestines in umbilical region, suddenly drawn tight and then gradually loosened—*Chion.*

  —abdomen were strung upward by a—*Plb.*

  —knotted, were shooting down through and across upper abdomen—*Merc. i. f.*

Strings which might tear, intestines were held up by—*Coloc.*

Struck in abdomen—*Cupr.*

  —by a pointed stick—*Manc.*

Strung in knots, intestines were—*Sulph.*

  —upward by a string, abdomen were—*Plb.*

  —together as a knot in intestines, twisted together as by a cord and—*Elaps*

Stuck with needles in abdomen above hips on taking a deep breath—*Cast.*

Stuffed, abdomen were—*Laur.*

  —with stones—*Ant. c., Ant. t.*

Sunken, abdomen were—*Saba.*

  —when lying on back, abdomen were—*Acet. ac.*

Support, abdomen needed—*Trom.*

  —abdomen when coughing, he must—*Con.*

Supported by hands, abdomen must constantly be—*Agn.*

Suppurate, parts of abdomen would—*Cann. s.*

Suppurating in abdomen—*Bov., Cinnb., Con., Juncus, Kreos.*

  —in groin—*Bad.*

  —in swelling of inguinal gland—*Lyc.*

Swashing about in abdomen, water were—*Acon., Crot. t., Kali c., Mag. c., Nat. m., Phos. ac.*

Swelling, abdomen were—*Pall.*

  —of inguinal gland, suppurating in—*Lyc.*

  —from lower abdomen to throat—*Sec.*

  —of abdomen would cause her to choke—*Raph.*

Swollen, abdomen were—*Com.*

  —from both sides forward nearly meeting in middle line during menses—*Cinnb.*

Swollen—*Continued*

–inguinal rings were—*Thuj.*

–in groin—*Am. m.*

–in left groin—*Con.*

Taken an emetic, he had (in abdomen)—*Euph.*

Tapped her on groin when raising leg, someone—*Ther.*

Tear, intestines were held up by strings which might—*Coloc.*

–had occurred in abdomen—*Coloc.*

Tearing or stitching of needles in abdominal muscles on inspiration—*Calc. c.*

–and snapping in insides and intestines, an animal were—*Pall.*

Tense, muscular fibers were—*Carb. v.*

Tension in lower abdomen and sense of heaviness while sitting or walking—*Kali c.*

Thickened, walls of abdomen were—*Pen.*

Thread cutting in toward center of abdomen—*All. c.*

–at right side of umbilicus, there were—*Tong.*

–from œsophagus to abdomen, there were—*Valer.*

–were moving, turning and twisting rapidly through abdomen, ball of—*Saba.*

Threads, intestines were knotted by—*Sulph.*

–bowels were hanging on easily tearing—*Coloc.*

Thumb, tip of, were pressing in pelvic region—*Rheum*

Thrust deep into upper abdomen, thence passing in a curve backward and downward into pelvis, then cutting its way upward again, a chisel were—*Coloc.*

–into abdomen, knife were—*Ip., Lach.*

–into abdomen, needle were—*Lyc.*

–from umbilical region to back—*Cupr.*

–in left abdomen as from a child in uterus—*Stann.*

Tickled with a feather, abdomen were—*Morph.*

Tied up, intestines were—*Ars.*

–in knots, intestines were being—*Bol.*

–tightly, with a band around bowels—*Arg. n.*

–in knots, small intestines were being—*Polyp.*

Tight and then gradually loosened, string tied around intestines in umbilical region, suddenly drawn—*Chion.*

–band around abdomen—*Arg. n.*

–band around lower abdomen—*Nat. m.*

–band around lower abdomen, as if laced—*Ign.*

–about abdomen, clothes were too—*Op., Tub.*

Tight—*Continued*
   –girdle on abdomen, from a—*Raph.*
   –on abdomen, skin were too—*Calc. s., Rhus t.*
   –cord about hips—*Sil.*
   –across lower part of abdomen, skin were too—*Calc. s.*
   –bandage in uterine region—*Hyper.*
   –in right side of pelvis—*Both. a.*
Tightly laced, abdomen were—*Ign.*
   –tied with a band across bowels—*Arg. n.*
   –from crest of one ilium to other, drawn—*Eug.*
   –bound in groins and pelvic regions—*Sulph.*
   –drawn across lower part of loins, cord were—*Arn.*
Torn open, abdomen would be—*Cupr. ac., Verat. a.*
   –to pieces, abdomen were—*Kali c.*
   –to pieces in abdomen, everything would be—*Graph.*
   –apart when walking, intestines would be—*All. s.*
   –loose in abdomen, something were—*Rhus t.*
   –out, intestines were—*Sep.*
   –or cut, intestines were—*Asaf.*
   –everything under false ribs were—*Dig.*
   –off from right side of abdominal wall, abdomen were being—
     X-ray
   –off and fell down, something were—*Plb.*
   –out, umbilicus were about to be—*Stram.*
   –out of groin, something would be—*Sil.*
   –and shattered on coughing, everything in umbilical region
     were being—*Nux v.*
   –away, intestines adhered to anterior abdominal wall and were
     —*Verb.*
   –when menstruating, parts would be—*Caust., Graph.*
   –parts of groin would be—*Pall.*
Tossed about, intestines were—*Sil.*
Touched with ice over pelvis, skin were—*Arg. m.*
Transfixed through abdomen from left to right—*Ip.*
Tumor in right side of abdomen—*Med.*
   –hard, in region of umbilicus, with griping pains—*Zinc.*
Tube which closed suddenly, water were poured through—*Elaps*
Turn inside out, bowels would—*Sep.*
Turned around, everything in abdomen were—*Sep.*
   –over or rolled over in abdomen with pain, something were—
     Ovi g. p.

Turning over in abdomen, ball were—*Lach.*

—over each other in abdomen, fish were—*Podo.*

—like wheel, bowels were—*Saba.*

—upside down, pelvic organs were—*Vib.*

—in bed, intestines fell from one side to the other when—*Bar. c., Merc.*

—twisting and moving rapidly through abdomen, ball of thread or lump were—*Saba.*

—around in abdomen, serpent were—*Cact.*

Twist about umbilicus—*Verb.*

—pain would give her a—*Verb.*

Twisting, turning and moving rapidly through abdomen, lump or ball of thread were—*Saba.*

Twisted ball, hard, were lying in umbilical region—*Kreos.*

—intestines were—*Plb.*

—out, intestines would be—*Merc.*

—together, bowels became—*Sol. t. æ.*

—into a knot, intestines were—*Verat. a.*

—in different directions, intestines were—*Pall.*

—by a cord and strung in knots, intestines were—*Elaps*

Undulated in abdomen when moving, hot water—*Casc.*

Undulating in abdomen—*Lyss., Rhod.*

Unfasten clothing about abdomen, he must—*Dios.*

Ulcer were forming in ileocœcal region—*Iris t.*

—in abdomen—*Cocc., Hell.*

—would burst in abdomen—*Laur.*

Ulcerated in abdomen—*Alum., Arg. m., Eupi., Puls., Valer.*

—in abdomen and stomach—*Rhus t.*

—in hypogastrium—*Asc. t.*

Ulceration, subcutaneous, in abdomen—*Ran. b., Til.*

Uncovered, abdomen were—*Ter.*

Viscera were gone in flanks—*Pall.*

Vise, bowels were in a—*Coloc.*

Vomit, about to—*Dios.*

Wall, anterior, were wanting and bowels were in danger of falling out—*Coloc.*

Walls were pulled inward, abdominal—*Plb.*

Wanting and bowels were in danger of falling out, anterior walls were—*Coloc.*

Washing about in abdomen, fluid were—*Crot. t.*

Water, bowels were full of—*Acon., Apoc., Hell., Urt. u.*

–intestines were filled with—*Cench., Kali c.*

–in intestines, nothing but—*Crot. t.*

–in stomach and bowels, quarts of—*Tub.*

–bubbling under walls of abdomen—*Rhus t.*

–falling in abdomen, drops of—*Lyc.*

–swashing about in abdomen—*Acon., Crot. t., Kali c., Mag. c., Nat. m., Phos. ac.*

–were poured through tube which closed suddenly—*Elaps*

–poured out of bottle from throat to abdomen—*Cina*

–boiling, poured over small of back and through pelvis—*Verat. v.*

–hot, poured from chest into abdomen—*Sang.*

–hot, were being poured into bowels—*Ip.*

–hot, flowing through abdomen—*Sumb.*

–hot, filled pelvis—*Aloe*

–hot, running down in abdomen—*Chin.*

–in abdomen, shivering from movement of cold—*Cann. s.*

–cold, passed through intestines—*Kali c.*

–hot, undulated in abdomen when moving—*Casc.*

–ice, in lower abdomen—*Onos.*

–as far as abdomen, seated in cold—*Plb.*

Wave, hot, like steam moving through abdomen and chest—*Lyss.*

Weak, relaxed, and if diarrhœa followed, whole abdomen would fall out—*Ars. h.*

–abdominal rings were too—*Cham.*

Weary and bruised in loins, belly and thighs—*Bov.*

Wedged in between symphysis pubis and os coccygis, plug were—*Aloe*

Weight in abdomen—*Op.*

–fell on abdomen—*Spig.*

–seems to fall from pit of chest to pit of abdomen—*Nat. h.*

–heavy, pressing in abdomen—*Rhus t.*

–rolled over from umbilicus to loins—*Lyc.*

–heavy, in lower abdomen—*Med.*

–hanging across pelvis and bladder—*Nat. m.*

–of body were too great for pelvis—*Sulph.*

–heavy, came into pelvis low down—*Kali c.*

–intestines would sink down of their own—*Pimp.*

Weight—*Continued*

   –heavy, in pelvis pressing downward and backward—*Kali p.*

   –bowels would prolapse from their own—*Trif. p.*

Wheel, bowels were turning like a—*Saba.*

Whirled around like a wheel in abdomen—*Saba.*

Wind, abdomen were full of—*Carb. ac.*

   –in abdomen, accumulation of—*Graph.*

   –in bowels and uterine region—*Hydrs.*

Wood, abdomen were made of—*Crot. h.*

   –parts of abdomen were made of—*Kali n.*

   –lying crosswise and being pressed out at menses, a piece of—*Nux m.*

Working in abdomen, boiler were—*Nit. ac.*

Worm moving in abdomen—*Rhus t.*

   –he had a tape—*Anan.*

   –long, were writhing in transverse colon—*Calad., Euph.*

   –were biting in abdomen—*Am. c., Nat. ac.*

Worms were crawling in abdomen—*Calc. c., Dulc., Saba.*

   –crawling up and down in abdomen and were biting and gnawing the parts—*Dulc.*

   –crawling in right abdomen—*Arund.*

   –were gnawing in abdomen—*Cyc., Dulc.*

   –griping in abdomen—*Dulc., Nat. m., Nux v.*

   –gnawing about umbilicus—*Grat.*

Wound, there were an internal—*Arn.*

   –in abdomen, someone cut into—*Arn., Phys.*

Wrenched in groins—*Agar.*

Wriggling about above umbilicus, animal were—*Chel.*

Writhing in abdomen—*Agar., Aloe, Alum., Berb., Stram.*

   –in transverse colon, long worm were—*Calad., Euph.*

HYPOCHONDRIUM

Abscess were forming in spleen—*Lyss.*
Ache, spleen would—*Malar.*
Air, hypochondrium were filled with—*Phos.*
Alive in right hypochondrium, something were—*Inul., Phos.*
Ants were crawling around waist—*Tab.*
Asleep in left hypochondrium—*Any.*
Ball were in liver—*Bar. c.*
  –in left hypochondrium—*Bov., Brom.*
  –going to and fro under ribs—*Cupr.*
  –beneath the liver, great—*Cyc.*
Band about waist—*Lepi., Nux v.*
  –of discomfort around waist, broad—*Dulc.*
  –were drawn tightly around body at stomach—*Mag. p.*
  –constricting about hypochondrium—*Con.*
  –around waist, iron—*Paull., Raph.*
  –around hypochondrium—*Arg. m., Arg. n.*
  –around waist, tight—*Cench., Cocc., Con., Helod., Lyss., Nux v., Paull., Phys., Pyrus, Raph., Sep.*
  –around waist, tight, unbearable—*Cench.*
  –around waist as wide as hand were drawn tightly—*Sep.*
Beaten in hypochondrium—*Asaf., Carb. v., Cocc., Rhus t.*
Beating in liver—*Laur.*
Blistered inside hepatic region—*Tell.*
Blow in liver, pain from—*Lyc.*
Body, hard, rolling in right hypochondrium—*Op.*
  –size of a pea moved in narrow channel in back of liver—*Card. m.*
Bottle of water in left hypochondrium, shaking up and down—*Cench.*
Break in two at waist, she would—*Corn.*
Broken in both ribs and sticking in the flesh—*Sep.*
Bruised, liver were—*Alum.*
  –hypochondria were—*Carb. v., Cocc., Cupr. s., Kali n., Ox. ac., Ran. b., Stront., Sulph.*
  –left hypochondrium were—*Chel., Ox. ac., Acon.*
  –right hypochondrium were—*Acon. l., Clem., Fago., Lact., Lyc., Mur. ac., Paull.*
Bubbling in liver—*Laur.*
  –and gurgling in hypochondrium when lying on side—*Pyrog.*
  –in right hypochondrium—*Lil. t.*

Eurst open, liver would—*Nat. s.*

   –gall bladder would—*Chlor.*

Bending, liver had been strained by—*Cimx.*

Chopped in half, waist were—*Stry.*

Claws of ice cold insects in liver—*Med.*

Constricted about the waist—*Cench., Helod., Lyss., Nux v., Paull., Phys., Pyrus, Raph., Sep.*

   –by a band—*Ars. s. f., Cocc.*

Cord around the waist, ligated with—*Arg. n.*

   –around hypochondria, tight—*Paull.*

   –drawn tight around the body at diaphragm—*Lycpr.*

   –drawn tight around the left side of hypochondria—*Lach.*

   –making attachments to diaphragm—*Lyc.*

Crawling around the waist, ants were—*Tab.*

Creeping over whole region of left short ribs, snake were—*Murx.*

Crookedness, great, in left side, < left leg—*Ovi g. p.*

Distended, spleen were—*Helon.*

Dogs were gnawing in region of liver—*Lycpr.*

Dragging her down at the waist, someone were—*Visc.*

   –over to the left side when lying upon it, something were—*Mag. m.*

Drawn tightly around the body at stomach, band were—*Mag. p.*

Drop down, spleen would—*Cob.*

Fallen out in region of spleen, something had, or as of a large hole—*Chin.*

Flatus in right hypochondrium—*Rhod.*

Fluid bubbling in right hypochondrium—*Pyrog.*

   –hot, running through the splenic vessels—*Vib.*

Full, liver were—*Arg. n., Pin. s.*

Gliding from right to left hypochondrium, something smooth were—*Daph. o.*

Gnawing in left side over the tenth rib and must press hard for >—*Seneg.*

   –in region of liver, dogs were—*Lycpr.*

Grasping with hand in right hypochondrium, just above the ilium—*Caust.*

Grown fast in region of left lower ribs, something had—*Thuj.*

Gurgling passing downward, in left hypochondrium—*Sanic.*

   –and bubbling in hypochondrium, when lying on side—*Pyrog.*

Hard and small, liver were—*Abies c.*

   –body in right hypochondrium—*Brom., Mag. c.*

Hernia would appear in right hypochondrium—*Cham.*

Hole in side, there were—*Stann.*

  –large, in region of spleen as if something had fallen out—*Chin.*

Hoop in hypochondria—*Lyc.*

  –iron, around the waist—*Upas*

Insects, ice cold, with claws in—*Med.*

Iron hoop around the waist—*Upas*

Knife stabbed in—*Nicc.*

Laced below hypochondria—*Calc. c.*

Large for the body, liver were too—*Stel.*

Ligated with a cord around waist—*Arg. n.*

Living were moving about in right hypochondrium during menses, something—*Inul.*

Lodged in right hypochondrium, something were—*Lach.*

Loose in left hypochondrium, something were torn—*Berb.*

Needles pricking in the side—*Ferr. i.*

Passing through liver, something were—*Apoc.*

Peg were sticking in liver—*Crot. c.*

Pin were sticking into liver—*Crot. c.*

Plucking in liver—*Nux m.*

Pressed out, hypochondria were—*Bell.*

Pressure from sharp stones in—*Nux m.*

Pulled from region of spleen into chest—*Bor.*

Pulling in right hypochondrium, when lying on left side—*Nat. s.*

Ribs broken in hypochondria and pressing into flesh—*Sep.*

Rising from right hypochondrium into chest, something were—*Glon.*

Scorched, liver were being—*Nux m.*

Screwing in hypochondrium—*Alumn., Nat. c.*

Shock in region of liver—*Lyc.*

Short in right hypochondrium, something were too—*Ang.*

  –in region of liver, too—*Carb. v.*

Small and hard, liver were—*Abies c.*

Smaller than usual, liver were—*Kali c.*

Smooth gliding from right to left hypochondrium, something were—*Daph. o.*

  –liver were—*Phos.*

Snake creeping over whole region of left short ribs—*Murx.*

Sore spot inside left hypochondrium and iliac region—*Brom.*

Spring were unrolled in left hypochondrium—*Sol. t. æ.*

Squeezed and gradually let go, waist were—*Phys.*
Stabbed in hypochondria by knives—*Nicc.*
Sticking into liver, pin were—*Crot. c.*
Stitches in middle of liver—*Merc. c.*
 –in right side of diaphragm—*Asaf.*
Stone in liver when walking—*Thuj.*
 –heavy, in region of hypochondria—*Arn., Cocc.*
Stones in liver, pressure from—*Nux m.*
Strained by bending, liver had been—*Cimx.*
Strap as wide as hand drawn tightly around waist—*Sep.*
Suppurating in hypochondrium—*Chin. s., Laur.*
Swollen, spleen were—*Gymn.*
Tape tied around waist—*Sil.*
Thick, liver were—*Absin.*
Tight around body at diaphragm, cord were drawn—*Lycpr.*
 –around hypochondrium, something were—*Ars. s. f., Luna*
 –around waist, clothes were too—*Rumx.*
 –waist were—*Lyc.*
 –around left side of hypochondrium—*Lach.*
Torn away in spleen, something were—*Ambr.*
 –loose in left hypochondrium, something were—*Berb.*
Touched him gently on both sides, something had—*Bapt.*
Tuberosities, liver were full of painful—*Anan.*
Tumor in liver—*Pip. n.*
Ulcer would form in hypochondrium—*Laur., Nux v.*
 –in hypochondria—*Stann.*
Ulcerated in—*Lach.*
Warmth over region of liver, extending to heart—*Cench.*
Water, bottle of, shaking up and down in left hypochondrium—
      Cench.
Wave, hot, like steam moving through abdomen and chest—
      Lyss.
Weight, liver had increased in, and had dragged out its ligaments
      —*Agar.*
 –heavy, in hypochondrium—*Zinc.*
 –round, were lying in right—*Tab.*
Worms extending from hypochondria to umbilicus—*Rhus t.*
Wringing in left hypochondrium—*Dios.*

RECTUM, ANUS AND STOOL

Acrid were in anus, something—*Chin., Lil. t., Merc.*
  –biting liquid were in rectum—*Nux m.*
Air escaping from anus, bubbles of—*Arg. m.*
  –escaping from anus one by one, bubbles of—*Nat. m.*
Alive were moving in anus, something—*Gran.*
Ants were crawling in rectum—*Sec.*
Appear if attempted, stool would—*Cocc.*
Arrested by hard body in anus, stool were—*Gamb.*
Ascended to chest, fæces had—*Lach.*
Ball in rectum, there were a great—*Sac. lac.*
  –in rectum before stool—*Merc.*
  –pressing on perineum when sitting—*Cann. i., Chim. umb.*
  –were in anus—*Sep.*
  –in anus, sitting on a—*Cann. i.*
Beating of hammers in rectum—*Lach.*
Biting of salt in rectum—*Dulc.*
Blood would pass from rectum while sitting—*Lipp.*
Body will pass away with stool—*Rob.*
  –had been pressed into rectum, an angular—*Prun.*
  –foreign, or lump in rectum—*Cann. i., Caust., Crot. t., Kali bi., Lach., Nat. m., Phos., Plat., Sep., Sil., Syph.*
  –hard, were pressing down and back against rectum—*Lil. t.*
  –rough, passing through rectum during stool—*Plb.*
  –anus and part of urethra were filled up by a hard round—*Cann. i.*
  –foreign, in anus—*Der., Hell., Rumx., Sulph.*
  –hard, in anus arresting stool—*Gamb.*
  –hard, in anus before stool—*Sin. a.*
Boiling lead passed through rectum during stool—*Thuj.*
  –water, stools were—*Merc.*
Bored upward and downward in rectum, screw—*Ferr. i.*
Boring in rectum, worm were—*Thuj.*
  –in anus—*Calad.*
Break in two if effort were made at stool, something would—*Apis*
Broken in anus—*Puls.*
Bruised in anus—*Urt. u.*

Bubbles of air escaping from anus—*Arg. m.*
  –of air escaping from anus one by one—*Nat. m.*
  –of air, oblong, were passing through anus—*Arg. m.*
  –slippery, escaping from anus—*Coloc.*
Bug were creeping out of rectum—*Æsc.*
Burning in wound in rectum or anus, salt were—*Prun.*
  –in anus—*Verat. a.*
Burnt, stool were—*Mag. m.*
Burst at stool, head would—*Sanic.*
  –even after stool, rectum would—*Agar.*
Bursting during stool, rectum were—*Nat. m.*
Carved square with knife, stool were—*Sanic.*
Chafed when riding, rectum were—*Psor.*
Circle in rectum, something turned in—*Ferr. i.*
Closed on making exertion at stool, rectum were—*Op.*
  –anus were—*Hell., Lach., Op., Sumb.*
  –during stool, anus were—*Spire.*
  –anus were completely—*Agar.*
Cocklebur were in grasp of sphincter ani—*Coll.*
Cold, stool were—*Con.*
Come out, bowels would—*Asc. t.*
  –out of rectum, everything would—*Rhus t.*
  –out of anus, everything would—*Sulph.*
Coming out at anus after stool, everything were—*Trom.*
Compressed, anus were—*Ferr. i.*
Constipated in anus—*Hell.*
Constricted, rectum were—*Alum., Staph.*
  –lower rectum were—*Benz. ac.*
  –in anus—*Lyss., Sil., Staph.*
Contracted and drawn, rectum were—*Pulx.*
  –in anus—*Chel., Nux v., Sol. t. æ.*
Contractibility, anus had lost its—*Graph.*
Contractive power of anus were lost—*Rhod.*
Cracked, skin of anus were—*Thuj.*
Crawling—see also WORMS
Crawling in rectum—*Croc., Ign., Spig., Spong.*
  –in rectum, ants were—*Sec.*
  –in rectum, worms were—*Bov., Calc. c., Oxyt., Ter.*
  –in rectum, little worms were—*Hep., Oxyt., Sulph.*
  –in anus—*Mar., Plat., Sac. lac.*
  –out of anus, insects were—*Nat. m.*

Crawling—*Continued*
   –in anus, worms were—*Calc. c.*
   –in anus, thread worms were—*Anan., Croc., Hell., Iod., Merc., Nux v., Plat., Sin. a.*
Creeping out of rectum, bug were—*Æsc.*
   –about in rectum, worm were—*Sulph.*
   –of cool worm in anus and protruding hæmorrhoids—*All. c.*
   –out of anus, worm were—*Ferr.*
   –in anus—*Sac. lac.*
Cut in rectum some hours after stool—*Nux v.*
Darting through abdomen to anus with gurgling in rectum, electric shocks were—*Stry.*
Diarrhœa, he had—*Carl., Colch.*
   –would set in—*Agn., Aloe, Ang., Ant. c., Ars. s. f., Bor., Calc. ar., Carb. ac., Carb. an., Carb. s., Caust., Cham., Chin. a., Cimic., Cob., Colch., Con., Crot. t., Dios., Dulc., Eucal., Form., Gran., Grat., Hell., Helon., Ind., Kali bi., Led., Lil. t., Meph., Merc. sul., Mez., Myric., Nat. c., Nux m., Nux v., Onos., Opun., Phel., Phos., Plan., Ran. b., Ran. s., Rhod., Rumx., Sang. n., Sars., Sel., Seneg., Spong., Squill., Staph., Sulph., Tab., Ter., Vichy, Zinc.*
   –if he drank anything, he would have—*Caps.*
   –would set in after smoking tobacco—*Bor.*
   –would come on following heat and colic—*Acet. ac.*
   –would come on, constantly—*Onos.*
   –after—*Rheum*
Discharged, more stool would be—*Sin.*
   –flatus were about to be—*Mag. p. Aust.*
Dislocated, anus were—*Puls.*
Distended, anus were—*Hell., Kali bi.*
   –with gas, rectum were—*Ign.*
Distending rectum, wind were forcibly—*Iris*
Done with stool, he were not—*Merc., Sanic.*
Dragging in rectum, weight were—*Til.*
Drawing anus up into rectum, string were—*Plb.*
Drawn upward, rectum were—*Plb.*
   –and contracted, rectum were—*Pulx.*
   –up into rectum, anus were—*Iodof., Spire.*
   –into bowel, anus were—*Sin. a.*
Dried up, rectum were—*Alum.*
   –up and shrunken, rectum were—*Pyrus*

Drops were running from rectum into bladder—*Thuj.*
 —of water flowed down—*Ferr. i.*
 —of cold water were falling out from anus—*Cann. s.*
Dry, anus were—*Agar., Calc. c., Carb. v.*
Dysentery were coming on—*Euph.*
Electric darts through abdomen to rectum with gurgling—*Stry.*
 —shocks darting through abdomen to anus—*Coloc.*
Emissions of flatus were the last, then renewal of—*Fl. ac.*
Escape from rectum, worm tried to—*Pen.*
 —while passing flatus, stool would—*Aloe*
Escaping from anus, bubbles of air were—*Arg. m.*
 —from anus one by one, bubbles of air were—*Nat. m.*
 —from anus, slippery bubbles were—*Coloc.*
 —from anus, warm fluid were—*Acon.*
Evacuate stool, unable to—*Linar.*
Everything would fall out of abdomen with relaxation after
    stool—*Ars. h.*
 —would come out of rectum—*Rhus t.*
 —had been pressed out of rectum—*Sulph.*
 —would come out of anus—*Sulph.*
Excoriated, anus were—*Ant. c., Calc. s., Carb. ac., Mag. m.*
 —around anus—*Sep.*
 —interior of anus were—*Polyg.*
 —after tenesmus, anus were—*Trom.*
 —hæmorrhoids were—*Ign.*
Expel stool, insufficient power to—*Stann.*
Expelled, stool stayed in rectum and could not be—*Nit. ac.*
Fæces would ascend to chest—*Lach.*
 —were lodged in rectum and would not come away—*Caust.*
 —remained after stool—*Equis., Nat. n., Nit. ac., Nux v., Sulph.*
 —were retained—*Tab.*
Fall out from weakness and relaxation if diarrhœa followed, ab-
    domen would—*Ars. h.*
 —out, rectum would—*Aloe, Eug.*
 —involuntary stool would—*Sep.*
Falling down during stool, intestines were—*Podo.*
 —out during stool, bowels were—*Kali br.*
Fermented, stools were—*Ip.*
Filled up by a hard round body, anus and part of urethra were
    —*Cann. i.*
 —with wind, anus were—*Sarr.*

Finished at stool, he were not—*Nux v., Stann.*

Fire while passing diarrhœic stool, it were a stream of—*Asc. t.*
–in anus, it were on—*Iris*

Fissured, anus were—*Kali c., Nit. ac.*

Flatus—see also GAS and WIND

Flatus would pass—*Conv., Staph.*
–passed down left side of abdomen to rectum but then turned and went upward to bladder or uterus—*Pulx.*
–but it did not; thin stool passed during emission of—*Spig.*
–he could pass neither stool nor—*Puls.*
–were pressing against coccyx by which it were retained—*Zinc.*
–were retained in anus—*Fl. ac.*
–went back—*Mur. ac.*
–were the last, then renewal of emissions—*Fl. ac.*

Flowed down rectum, drops of water—*Ferr. i.*

Flowing along rectum, hot water were—*Ox. ac.*

Fluid, rectum were full of—*Aloe*
–warm, escaping from anus—*Acon.*

Forced outward in rectum, plug were—*Crot. t.*
–into rectum, rough stick were—*Rumx.*
–into anus by blows, plug were—*Apoc.*

Forcibly distending rectum, wind were—*Iris*

Forcing passage of stool—*Alet.*
–out in rectum premonitory of hæmorrhoids—*Ran. s.*
–out of anus, worm were—*Arg. m.*

Foreign substance in rectum—*Caust., Nat. m., Sin. a.*

Form, hæmorrhoids would—*Nit. ac.*

Formication from worms in anus—*Croc., Elaps, Nat. c., Nux v., Ox. ac., Sin. a., Spig., Zinc.*

Full around anus—*Musa, Sulph.*

Gas, rectum were full of—*Conv.*
–rectum were distended with—*Ign.*

Glass in anus, splinter of—*Rat.*

Gnawing in anus, worm were—*Elaps*

Gravel in rectum—*Coll.*

Grown up, one side of rectum had—*Rhus t.*

Gun went off with every movement, a pop-—*Tub.*

Gurgling in rectum with electric darts—*Stry.*

Hammered into anus, wedge were being—*Apoc.*

Hammers, little, throbbing in anus—*Lach.*

Hanging upon rectum, ten-pound weight were—*Eug.*
–from anus, thread worm were—*Arg. m.*

Hard body were pressing down and back against rectum—*Lil. t.*
  —round body filled anus and part of urethra—*Cann. i.*
  —substance in rectum—*Caust., Sin. a.*
  —body in anus arrested stool—*Gamb.*
Hæmorrhoid were there but there is not—*Sulph.*
Hæmorrhoids were coming on—*Linum*
  —were split with a knife on taking step or sitting—*Graph.*
Hard remained in anus during and after stool, something—*Sin. a.*
Head grew large during stool—*Cob.*
Hold herself up in region of vulva when at stool, she must—
  Lil. t.
Hot, fæces were—*Dios.*
Inactive, rectum were—*Thuj.*
Inactivity of bowels—*Nux v.*
Insects were crawling out of anus—*Nat. m.*
Itching in anus—*Sac. lac.*
Iron, hot, were moving up and down in anus—*Merc. p. r.*
  —red-hot, were in anus—*Kali ar.*
Jagged with sticks, lower rectum were—*Coll.*
  —particles, stool were full of—*Sanic.*
Jerk, something passed out of rectum with—*Sars.*
Knife lancinating in anus, < washing any part of body with cold
  water—*Crot. c.*
  —stabbing in anus—*Rat.*
  —sawing back and forth through anus—*Æsc.*
  —hæmorrhoids were split with—*Graph.*
  —stool were carved with—*Sanic.*
Knives in rectum—*Calad.*
  —in anus—*Nat. h.*
Lacerated, anus were—*Kali c.*
Large during stool, head grew—*Cob.*
  —stool but passed away without, he would have—*Malar.*
Lead, boiling, passed through rectum during stool—*Thuj.*
Ligated, rectum were—*Paraf.*
Liquid, acrid, were biting in rectum—*Nux m.*
  —which feels heavy and would fall out, rectum were full of—
  Aloe
Locked up, anus were—*Corn.*
Lodged in rectum and would not come away, fæces were—*Caust.*
Loose, rectum were—*Aloe*
  —stool, she would have—*Malar.*

Lump or plug six inches in rectum, immovable—*Aloe*
  –or foreign body in rectum—*Cann. i., Caust., Crot. t., Kali bi.,*
    Lach., Nat. m., Phos., Plat., Sep., Sil., Syph.
  –in uterine region pressing against rectum when lying—*Ars. i.*
  –lying in perineal region—*Ther.*
  –heavy, in anus—*Sil.*
  –large, on posterior surface of sphincter ani—*Med.*
Lumps in rectum during stool—*Nat. c.*
  –in rectum which obstruct passage and make stool agonizing,
    two large—*Syph.*
Lying close to anus, hard stool were—*Sin. a.*
Marble were dropped in left abdomen while at stool—*Nat. p.*
Mass in lower part of rectum—*Sang.*
  thick, in rectum—*Samb.*
Moisture came from anus—*Agar., Coloc., Sulph.*
Move, bowels would—*Ferr., Hydrs., Lachn., Phys., Puls.*
  –stool, she could not—*Con.*
  –bowels, unable to—*Sulph.*
Moved when breathing, bowels were—*Card. m.*
  –immediately without being able to do so, bowels must be—
    Eup. pur.
Moving in rectum, something were—*Gran., Sumb.*
  –in anus, something alive were—*Gran.*
  –up and down in anus, hot iron were—*Merc. p. r.*
Needles in rectum—*Carb. v., Med.*
  –rectum were pierced by—*Mag. c.*
  –rectum were pricked with hot—*Ars.*
  –fine, stitching in rectum—*Thuj.*
  –sitting on—*Guaj.*
Nothing were there on attempting to evacuate bowels—*Vib.*
Obstructed, rectum were—*Phos.*
  –by folds of mucous membrane, rectum were—*Æsc.*
Occur, stool would—*Gran., Puls., Raph., Rat., Sul. ac., Zinc.*
Open, anus were—*Apis, Phos., Sec.*
  –wide, anus were—*Apoc., Sumb.*
Out at anus after stool, everything were coming—*Trom.*
Paralyzed, rectum were—*Sil.*
  –anus were—*Coca, Sabin.*
Particles, stool were full of jagged—*Sanic.*
Pass out of rectum, something would—*Æsc., Asc. t.*
  –from rectum while sitting, blood would—*Lipp.*

Pass—*Continued*

    —away with stool, whole body would—*Rob.*

    —loose stool would—*Sulph.*

    —more stool would—*Form., Laur., Lil. t., Nux m., Tanac.*

    —out with urine, stool would—*Aloe*

    —flatus would surely—*Conv., Staph.*

    —neither stool nor flatus, he could—*Puls.*

    —wind would—*Sulph.*

Passed out of rectum with a jerk, something—*Sars.*

    —through rectum during stool, boiling lead—*Thuj.*

    —in pieces, a thin stool—*Carl.*

    —during emission of flatus but it did not, a thin stool—*Spig.*

    —down left side of abdomen to rectum then turned and went upward to bladder or uterus, flatus—*Pulx.*

    —down rectum, stick thick as thumb—*Asim.*

Passage of bowels, he would have—*Lil. t.*

    —of stool, forcing—*Alet.*

    —of stool were obstructed by two large lumps which make stool agonizing—*Syph.*

Passing out of rectum, something were—*Lept.*

    —through rectum during stool, rough body were—*Plb.*

    —from rectum, sand were—*Ars.*

    —sticks in stool—*Sanic.*

    —sharp stones at stool—*Coloc.*

    —through anus, oblong bubbles of air were—*Arg. m.*

Pepper were in anus—*Dulc.*

    —were smarting in anus—*Grat.*

    —were sprinkled on hæmorrhoids—*Caps.*

Pieces during stool, anus would fly to—*Thuj.*

    —thin stool were passed in—*Carl.*

Pierced by needles at 4 a.m., rectum were—*Mag. c.*

Pin, hot, in rectum—*Carb. v.*

Plug in rectum—*Anac., Sep.*

    —six inches in rectum, immovable lump or—*Aloe*

    —were forced outward in rectum—*Crot. t.*

    —were wedged between pubes and os coccygis—*Aloe*

    —in anus—*Aloe, Anac., Bry., Crot. t., Kali bi., Lach., Nat. m., Sarr.*

    —were forced in anus by blows—*Apoc.*

    —were in anus, rough pointed—*Nat. m.*

Poker, red-hot, in rectum—*Lob. d.*

    –red-hot, were thrust up rectum—*Kali c.*

Pop-gun went off with movement—*Tub.*

Power in rectum to expel stool, there were no—*Carb. an., Sep., Sil., Stann.*

Pressed out, bowels were—*Sars.*

    –out of rectum, everything had been—*Sulph.*

    –out after stool, mucous membranes were—*Sulph.*

    –out, rectum would be—*Sars.*

    –into rectum, angular body had been—*Prun.*

    –in rectum, a sharp instrument—*Nux v.*

    –into rectum or anus, sharp sticks were—*Nit. ac.*

Pressing on perineum when sitting, ball were—*Cann. i., Chim. umb.*

    –out in perineum, something dull were—*Asaf.*

    –backward and downward against rectum and anus at stool, hard body were—*Lil. t.*

    –out of rectum, something were—*Cann. s., Sep.*

    –in rectum, flatus were—*Kreos., Sil., Zinc.*

    –against coccyx by which it were retained, flatus were—*Zinc.*

Pricked with hot needles, rectum were—*Ars.*

Pricking in anus, thorn were—*Lyss.*

Prolapse, rectum would—*Sulph.*

    –during stool, uterus would—*Dirc.*

Prolapsus of rectum during menses—*Ovi g. p.*

Protrude with stool, bowels would—*Asc. t.*

    –rectum would—*Equis.*

    –during stool, rectum would—*Sulph.*

    –if effort to stool were continued, rectum would—*Æsc.*

    –hæmorrhoids would—*Ham.*

Protruded and gone back with a jerk, rectum had—*Rat.*

Protruding, rectum were—*Sumb.*

Puckering string were pulled at both ends of rectum—*Benz. ac.*

Purgative, bowels had been acted on by—*Ferr.*

Pushed out, mucous membrane of anus were swollen and—*Bell.*

Rasped after stool, rectum were—*Lil. t.*

Raw in rectum—*Uran.*

    –anus were—*Æsc., Apis, Ham., Nat. p., Nux v., Sep., Sulph., Sumb.*

    –around anus when sitting—*Berb.*

Recovered from pain in anus, one had just—*Berb.*

Remained in rectum, part of fæces had—*Equis., Nat. n., Nit. ac.*
–in rectum after stool, something—*Sulph.*
–to be passed, more fæces—*Nux v.*

Retained in rectum or anus, wind were—*Fl. ac.*
–fæces were—*Tab.*

Retracted, anus were—*Camph.*

Rough body were traversing rectum during stool—*Plb.*
–pointed plug were in anus—*Nat. m.*

Rubbed together in rectum, sharp stones—*Cocc.*
–off anus, skin were—*Carb. ac.*

Running from rectum into bladder, drops were—*Thuj.*

Salt were biting in rectum—*Dulc.*
–in wound in rectum—*Prun.*

Sand, sticks or gravel in rectum—*Coll.*
–were passing from rectum—*Ars.*

Sawing back and forth through anus, knife were—*Æsc.*

Screw were boring upward and downward in anus and rectum—*Ferr. i.*

Sharp, one were sitting on something—*Lach.*

Shocks, electric, darting through abdomen to anus—*Coloc.*
–electric, in rectum—*Apis*

Shrunken and dried up, rectum were—*Pyrus*

Sitting on something sharp—*Lach.*
–on needles in rectum—*Guaj.*
–on a ball in anus—*Cann. i.*

Smarting in anus, pepper were—*Grat.*

Splinter in rectum—*Arg. n., Form., Lach., Nit. ac.*
–in anus—*Nat. p.*

Splinters of glass in rectum and anus—*Rat.*

Split, anus would—*Staph.*
–anus, stool would—*Mez.*
–with knife, hæmorrhoids were—*Graph.*

Sprained after stool, anus were—*Sin. a.*

Spurted on him, stool were—*Jat.*

Square, stool had been carved—*Sanic.*

Stabbing in anus, knife were—*Rat.*

Stick, rough, were forced into rectum—*Rumx.*
–thick as thumb passed down rectum—*Asim.*

Sticks, rectum were filled with small—*Æsc.*
–sand or gravel in rectum—*Coll.*

Sticks—*Continued*

    –sharp, were being pressed into rectum or anus—*Nit. ac.*

    –in stool, one were passing—*Sanic.*

Sticking in rectum, sharp points were—*Iris*

Stiff and thick, mucous membranes were—*Æsc., Form.*

Stitch, very painful, extends along rectum—*All. c.*

Stitching from fine needles in rectum—*Thuj.*

    –with knives in rectum—*Calad.*

    –with an awl in rectum—*Laur.*

Stones, sharp, rubbed together in rectum—*Cocc.*

    –at stool, he were passing—*Coloc.*

Stool, about to have—*Gran., Puls., Quass., Raph., Rat., Sul. ac., Zinc.*

    –at once, he must go to—*Bism., Puls. n., Spig.*

    –would have a loose—*Malar., Sulph.*

    –would have a large (but passed away without)—*Malar.*

    –would pass, more—*Aloe, Form., Laur., Lil. t., Nux m., Tanac.*

    –would pass out with urine—*Aloe*

    –as after (before stool)—*Phys.*

    –one had been to—*Berb.*

    –forcing passage of—*Alet.*

    –thin, passed during emission of flatus, but it did not—*Spig.*

    –went back—*Mur. ac.*

    –were shaped like bullets—*Helon.*

    –nor flatus, he could pass neither—*Puls.*

Stream of fire while passing diarrhœic stool—*Asc. t.*

String were pulled at both ends of rectum, puckering—*Benz. ac.*

    –were drawing anus up into rectum—*Plb.*

Stuffed, rectum were—*Colch.*

    –full, anus were—*Apis*

Substance would come out of rectum—*Inul.*

    –foreign, lying in rectum—*Nat. m.*

Suppurating about anus—*Arg. n., Cyc.*

Swelling in perineum—*Chim. umb.*

Swollen, rectum were—*Cact., Crot. t., Linum*

    –and pushed out, mucous membrane of anus were—*Bell.*

Thick and stiff, mucous membrane were—*Æsc., Form.*

Thorn were pricking in anus—*Lyss.*

    –large, were lancinating in anus—*Jac.*

Tickling in rectum, pin worms were—*Cupr.*

Tied up with strictures, rectum were—*Syph.*

22

Torn, rectum were—*Erig.*

   —open during stool, rectum were—*Grat.*

   —open during soft stool, rectum were—*Calc. c.*

   —to pieces during stool, rectum were—*Sul. ac.*

   —out when coughing, rectum would be—*Tub.*

   —from bones of perineum after stool, flesh and rectal membranes were—*Grat.*

   —anus were—*Erig.*

   —anus would be—*Sulph.*

   —by stool, sphincter would be—*Colch.*

Trickling from anus, something cold were—*Cann. s.*

Turned inside out in hæmorrhoid or gut were overturned—*Æsc.*

   —in a circle in rectum, something—*Ferr. i.*

Twinging extending from anus into rectum, stitches were—*Zinc.*

Twisted up, rectum and anus were—*Rat.*

   —and turned about in circle in anus, something; and drops of water flowed down—*Ferr. i.*

Ulcers in anus—*Mag. c., Sulph.*

Warm fluid were escaping from anus—*Acon.*

Water flowed down, drops of—*Ferr. i.*

   —hot, were flowing along rectum—*Ox. ac.*

   —stools were boiling—*Merc.*

   —cold, were trickling in or falling from anus—*Cann. s.*

Weak to hold their contents, bowels were too—*Sulph.*

   —to expel stool, rectum were too—*Kali c.*

Weakened by long diarrhœa, anus were—*Coloc.*

   —sphincter ani were—*Alum.*

Wedge in rectum—*Carl.*

   —were being hammered into anus—*Apoc.*

Wedged between pubes and os coccygis, plug were—*Aloe*

Weight were dragging in rectum—*Til.*

   —of ten pounds were hanging upon rectum—*Eug.*

   —like a ball in anus—*Sep.*

Wind would pass—*Sulph.*

   —were forcibly distending rectum—*Iris*

   —were retained in rectum and anus—*Fl. ac.*

   —anus were filled with—*Sarr.*

Worm were boring in rectum—*Thuj.*

   —large, in anus—*Ail., Cinnb., Ferr. i.*

   —cool, in anus and protruding hæmorrhoids—*All. c.*

   —were creeping about with escape of slimy fluid—*Sulph.*

Worm—*Continued*

  –were creeping out of anus—*Ferr.*

  –were forcing out of anus—*Arg. m.*

  –were gnawing in anus—*Elaps*

  –thread, were hanging from anus—*Arg. m.*

  –tried to escape from rectum—*Pen.*

Worms were in rectum—*Colch., Ferr. i.*

  –little, in rectum—*Oxyt.*

  –were crawling in rectum—*Bov., Calc. c., Oxyt., Ter.*

  –pin, tickling in rectum—*Cupr.*

  –thread, in rectum—*Cocc., Mur. ac., Nit. ac., Nux v.*

  –thread, crawling in rectum—*Calc. c., Chin., Cocc., Hep., Jat., Laur., Nux v., Rhus t., Spig.*

  –in rectum and anus—*Agar.*

  –in anus—*Agar., Cinch. b., Croc., Elaps, Ferr. i., Nat. c., Nux v., Ox. ac., Sin. a., Spig., Zinc.*

  –were crawling in anus—*Calc. c., Calc. ox., Ter., Verat. v., Zinc.*

  –thread, crawling in anus—*Anan., Croc., Iod., Hell., Merc., Nux v., Plat., Sin. a.*

  –would extrude from anus—*Ip.*

  –about anus—*Fago.*

  –round, in anus—*Sil.*

Wound in rectum were burning—*Prun.*

URINARY ORGANS

Acid at close of urination, urine were—*Sulph.*
Acrid urine would pass from urethra, a drop of—*Berb., Ox. ac.*
  —urine would pass during coition, a drop of—*Merc.*
Affected, bladder were—*Lith.*
Air in bladder, distended from—*Staph.*
Alive in urethra, something were—*Juncus*
Bags of water, kidneys were—*Helon.*
Ball were rolling in bladder—*Bell., Lach.*
  —were rolling in bladder or abdomen when turning—*Lach.*
  —urethra were filled with hard—*Cann. i.*
Band across bladder during urination—*Thuj.*
Bent forward while sitting, bladder were—*Sars.*
Biting passing urethra, something were—*Guaj.*
  —drop forcing its way out at tip of urethra—*Sel.*
Blocked up in passage of bladder, something were—*Clem.*
Blood rushed to bladder—*Fl. ac.*
Blunt instrument big as thumb were pressing in kidney—*Gels.*
Body, cylindrical, were being forced through urethra—*Stram.*
  —hard round, filled up anus and part of urethra—*Cann. i.*
  —hard, like pencil lead were being forced upward and backward from bladder to kidney—*Sanic.*
Bruised in region of kidney—*Manc.*
  —or crushed in loins and kidneys—*Berb.*
Bubbles of water were in right kidney—*Med.*
Bubbling in right kidney, something were—*Med.*
Bullets or something similar fill in bladder at its outlet—*Pulx.*
Burning drops ran along urethra after urination—*Arg. n.*
Burnt, urethra were—*Pic. ac.*
Burst, bladder were going to—*Elect., Zinc.*
Coals, live, in—*Pip. n.*
Cold drop of urine were passing—*Agar.*
  —feeling in renal region—*Med.*
  —when urine passed—*Nit. ac.*
Constricted, urethra were—*Clem., Dig.*
  —in urethra when urinating—*Bry.*
Contract, muscles did not—*Mag. p.*
Contracted, urethra were—*Graph.*

Contracting, muscles of bladder were—*Oxyt.*
Crawling in urethra—*Tus. p.*
 –insects in urethra—*Phos. ac.*
Creeping in region of right kidney, insects with cold claws were
 —*Med.*
Crushed or bruised in loins and kidneys—*Berb.*
Cutting instrument were pressing in forepart of urethra—*Nux v.*
Cylinder were passed through urethra—*Stram.*
Desire, urine were in meatus with sudden—*Sanic.*
Discharge from the urethra—*Helod.*
 –gonorrhœal, in urethra—*Cann. i.*
Distended from air in bladder—*Staph.*
 –bladder were—*Pareir.*
 –after urinating, bladder were—*Conv.*
 –bladder were over—*Sep.*
Drawn together in right kidney—*Helod.*
 –up into knots, urethra were—*Cann. s.*
Dribbling continually down urethra, urine were—*Kali bi., Lact.,
 Petr., Thuj.*
Drop of urine remained behind—*Kali bi.*
 –were in urethra—*Cedr.*
 –of water flowing through urethra—*Laur.*
 –biting, forcing its way out at tip of urethra—*Sel.*
 –of urine were passing, a cold—*Agar.*
 –of viscid fluid pressing forward in urethra while sitting—
 Thuj.
Drops were passing out—*Sel.*
 –remained behind on urinating, last—*Arg. n.*
 –of urine remained in the urethra, a few—*Alum.*
 –ran down after urinating, a few—*Thuj.*
 –of urine had passed through urethra, a few—*Ambr., Sel.,
 Thuj.*
 –ran along urethra after urination, burning—*Arg. n.*
 –of urine were in urethra—*Cedr.*
 –were running though urethra from behind—*Thuj.*
 –came out of bladder during rest—*Sep.*
Dropping of urine from urethra—*Ambr., Cedr., Lact., Sel.,
 Thuj.*
 –from urethra constantly—*Cedr.*
Emptied, bladder were—*Brach.*
 –bladder could not be—*Hep.*

Empty, bladder were nearly—*Dig., Sumb.*

  —bladder were not—*Brach., Bry., Calc. c., Gins., Staph.*

Entered the urethra, urine had not—*Rumx.*

Expulsive force, bladder had lost its—*Eucal.*

Fall to side on which one lay, bladder would—*Puls.*

  —out over os pubis, bladder would—*Sep.*

Fell from side to side and were enlarged, bladder—*Sep.*

Filled, bladder were—*Pall.*

  —with a hard ball, urethra were—*Cann. i.*

Flapping back and forth in urethra with soreness and cutting, after urination—*Arg. n.*

Flatulence were pressing on bladder—*Prun.*

Flow after urinating, urine continued to—*Vib.*

Fluid were running down the urethra—*Arg. n.*

Fluttering in region of kidney, something were—*Chim. umb.*

Force its way through a narrow space, something had to—*Op.*

Forced upon the groins, bladder were—*Sulph.*

  —from bladder along urethra, shot were—*Kali br.*

  —through a narrow meatus, urine were—*Sabal*

Full, bladder were—*Pip. n.*

  —bladder were, when not—*Calad., Kali br.*

  —bladder were too—*Dig., Sabal*

  —bladder were, after urinating—*Calc. c., Con., Equis., Lac c., Ruta*

  —bladder were too, without call—*Sulph.*

  —bladder were constantly—*Ruta*

  —bladder were, and contents of abdomen would fall out over pubes—*Sep.*

Gonorrhœal discharge in urethra—*Cann. i.*

Gush away, urine would—*Puls.*

Hand were placed in region of bladder—*All. c.*

Hard round body filled anus and part of urethra—*Cann. i.*

Hot, red-hot iron passed along urethra—*Canth., Ox. ac.*

  —urine were—*Ferr.*

  —urine were too—*Aur. m.*

  —water passed over parts when urinating—*Lac d.*

Inflamed, neck of bladder were—*Still.*

Injured at urethral orifice—*Cop.*

Insects crawling in urethra—*Phos. ac.*

Instrument, blunt, were pressed into region of kidney—*Gels.*

Iron, red-hot, passed along the urethra—*Canth., Ox. ac.*

Knife were entering urethra—*Fago.*
Knives were plunged into kidneys—*Arn.*
    –a hundred, were drawn from abdomen to uterus, ovaries, urethra and vulva—*Sec.*
Knotty, urethra were—*Arg. n.*
Metallic in region of urethra—*Alum.*
Motion in bladder after urination—*Ruta*
Narrow, middle of urethra were too—*Dig.*
Needle sticking in right kidney—*Staph.*
    –sticking in forepart of urethra—*Caps.*
Needles at orifice of urethra—*Nit. ac.*
    –pricking in urethra—*Cann. i.*
    –dull, suddenly thrust into urethra—*Coc. c.*
Obstructed by calculus, flow of urine were—*Helod.*
    –on urination, urethra were—*Coc. c.*
Obstruction were being overcome—*Asim.*
Open a passage in the morning, urine had to—*Seneg.*
Openings, urethra had two—*Prun.*
Paralyzed, bladder were—*Agar., Atrop., Bar. ac., Canth., Cod., Stram., Thuj.*
    –muscles of urethra were partially—*Scut.*
Pass, calculus would (with craving for ice)—*Med.*
    –urine constantly, he would—*Cact.*
    –more urine would—*Colch., Stann.*
    –more urine would, but it does not—*Ruta*
    –out with the urine, stool would—*Aloe*
Passage in morning, urine had to open a—*Seneg.*
Passed through urethra, a cylinder were—*Stram.*
    –through urethra, few drops—*Ambr., Sel., Thuj.*
    –all urine had not—*Cean., Sin.*
    –enough urine, she had not—*Samars.*
    –urine were not—*Nym.*
Passing urethra, something biting were—*Guaj.*
    –ureters, calculus were—*Med.*
    –some urine were—*Aspar.*
    –drops of urine were—*Sel.*
    –after urinating, urine were still—*Aspar., Vib.*
    –over parts when urinating, very hot water were—*Lac d.*
Pencil, hard body like lead, were being forced upward and backward from bladder to kidneys—*Sanic.*
Pierced, urethra were—*Sulph.*

Power to close the neck of the bladder, he had none—*Stram.*
  –to retain urine, he had none—*Stram.*
Pressed against right kidney, something were—*Am. br.*
  –upon the bladder, something were—*Sulph.*
  –upon by a sharp instrument in bladder—*Nux v.*
  –out, bladder and urinary organs would be—*Sep.*
Pressing in kidney, blunt instrument big as thumb were—*Gels.*
  –on bladder, flatulence were—*Prun.*
  –in forepart of urethra, cutting instrument were—*Nux v.*
  –forward in urethra while sitting, a drop of viscid fluid were
    —*Thuj.*
Prevented passage of water, tape—*Thuj.*
Pricking in urethra, needles were—*Cann. i.*
Prolapsed, bladder were—*Pyrus*
Push some rough article down to spot in urethra and rub it, he
    must—*Petros.*
Pushed through urethra, cylindrical body were—*Stram.*
Raw, urethra were—*Colch.*
Remained in urethra, urine—*Agar., Aspar., Cedr., Ery. a.*
  –in urethra, something more—*Med.*
  –behind on urinating, something—*Berb., Gels.*
  –in fossa navicularis, urine had—*Ferr. i.*
Retain urine, could not—*Brach.*
  –urine, could not long—*Rumx.*
Retained by contraction of sphincter, urine were—*Sulph.*
  –at orifice during urination, urine were—*Canth.*
Rub it, he must push some rough article down to spot in urethra
  and—*Petros.*
Run out of urethra, something would—*Carb. s.*
Running out of urethra, after emission, something were—*Dig.*
Rushed to bladder, blood—*Fl. ac.*
Scalded, urethra were—*Apis*
  –from urine, raw surfaces were—*Merc.*
Sensation in the bladder, there were none—*Stann.*
Shot were forced from bladder along urethra—*Kali br.*
Sore were in urethra when urinating—*Cinnb.*
Sound were being turned in urethra—*Bell.*
Splinter in urethra—*Nit. ac.*
  –in middle of urethra—*Arg. n.*
Squeezed, bladder were—*Tarent.*
Started and then went back, urine—*Ip., Prun.*

Sticking in urethra, something were—*Aspar.*
   –in right kidney, needle were—*Staph.*
   –in forepart of urethra, needle were—*Caps.*
Sticks in urethra—*Nit. ac.*
   –in urine while urinating—*Clem.*
Stone in bladder—*Puls., Sars.*
   –in urethra during urination—*Coc. c.*
   –impacted in left ureter—*Cere. b.*
   –passing ureters—*Med.*
   –flow of urine were being obstructed by—*Helod.*
Stool would pass with urine—*Aloe*
Strangulated in bladder—*Bell., Polyg.*
Stretch during coition, urethra were put on—*Arg. n.*
Stricture about two inches in urethra—*Sabal*
Stuffed up, urethra were—*Syph.*
Suppurated, urethra were—*Rhod.*
Suppurating in region of kidney—*Berb.*
Swelling retarded passage of urine—*Hipp.*
   –in urethra—*Til.*
Swollen preventing last few drops passing, urethra were—*Arg. n.*
Tape prevented passage of water—*Thuj.*
Thorn were twitching in urethra—*Berb.*
Thrust into urethra, dull needles were suddenly—*Coc. c.*
Torn in kidney—*Mez.*
Turned in urethra, sound were being—*Bell.*
Twinging in urethra from drops passing out—*Sel.*
Twisting in bladder, large worms were—*Bell., Sep.*
Urge, sudden, as from urine—*Sanic.*
Urinate, he had constantly waked to—*Chim. umb.*
   –as soon as the thought comes to mind, he must—*Sanic.*
   –he were constantly obliged to—*Sulph.*
Urinated for hours, he had not—*Equis.*
Urine were obliged to open passage through urethra—*Seneg.*
   –remained in urethra—*Agar., Aspar., Cedr., Ery. a.*
Voided, more urine would be—*Sin.*
Warm, urine were very—*Colch.*
Water in right kidney, bubbles of—*Med.*
   –bladder contained—*Cub.*
   –bubbling in right renal region—*Med.*
   –flowing through urethra, drop of—*Laur.*

Water—*Continued*

  –very hot, passing over parts when urinating—*Lac d.*

  –in urethra, cold—*Agar.*

Wire, red-hot, passed along urethra—*Canth., Ox. ac.*

Worms in bladder—*Bell.*

  –large, twisting in bladder—*Bell., Sep.*

MALE SEXUAL ORGANS

Absent with cold relaxed feeling, penis were—*Coca*

Air or water, prepuce were distended with—*Merc.*

Asleep when going upstairs, organs were—*Form.*

   –penis were—*Merc.*

Blood, spermatic cord and testes were filled with—*Psor.*

Blow on testicles—*Nat. a.*

   –on left testicle—*Nat. a.*

Body were being forced out, a rough jagged—*Asim.*

Break in penis from waving sensation, it would—*Ars. h.*

Bruised, testicles were—*Clem., Pall.*

   –on touching testicles—*Clem.*

   –one testicle, he had—*Chim. umb.*

   –in scrotum—*Kali c.*

   –penis were—*Caps.*

   –while seated, penis were—*Thuj.*

Bubbling in scrotum—*Staph.*

   –in penis—*Graph.*

   –in penis during erection—*Kali c.*

Burnt in penis—*Cann. s.*

Clogged about one inch from orifice, urethra were—*Syph.*

Coition had been oft repeated—*Glon.*

Compressed and drawn up, testicle were—*Zinc.*

   –testicles were, particularly the right—*Staph.*

   –penis were—*Alum.*

Cord were tied around penis—*Plb.*

Corroded, penis were—*Narz.*

Cough were felt in testicles—*Zinc.*

Crawling or creeping in scrotum—*Clem.*

   –over back of scrotum, insects were—*Staph.*

   –on prepuce, worms were—*Petr.*

Creeping downward in left spermatic cord—*Osm.*

Crushed, testicles were—*Caust.*

   –left testicle were—*Colch.*

   –testicles were being—*Rhod.*

   –testicles would be—*Thuj.*

   –in end of penis after urinating—*Coloc.*

Denuded, glans penis were—*Sil.*
  —genitals were—*Plat.*
Distended with air or water, prepuce were—*Merc.*
Drawing in spermatic cord into testicle—*Staph.*
  —from spermatic cords and extending to hollow between thighs
     and scrotum—*Saba.*
Drawn up into abdomen, testicle were—*Bell.*
  —up into ring, testicles were being—*Sec.*
  —up, testicles were compressed and—*Zinc.*
  —through swollen testicle, a knife were—*Aur. m.*
  —up into knots, urethra were—*Cann. s.*
Drop of viscid fluid extended from urethra—*Thuj.*
Drops passing from penis—*Ced., Sumb.*
Emission, he were having—*Am. c., Cere. s., Mez.*
  —had been surpressed—*Clem.*
Empty, organs were—*Lyss.*
Excoriated, penis were—*Cann. s.*
Filled with blood, spermatic cord and testes were—*Psor.*
Fluid, viscid, extended from urethra—*Thuj.*
Forced out, a rough jagged body were being—*Asim.*
  —out, scrotum would be—*Sec.*
Gurgling in prostate—*Phyt.*
Insects crawling over back of scrotum—*Staph.*
Knife were drawn through testicles—*Aur. m.*
  —were drawn through swollen testicle—*Aur. m.*
Knots, urethra were drawn up into—*Cann. s.*
Larger, genitals were—*Calad.*
Moved, testicles—*Thuj.*
Needles pricked in frænum of penis—*Cor. r.*
Overstrained, organs were—*Sal. ac.*
Pin, penis were punctured with—*Syph.*
Pricked with needles in frænum of penis—*Cor. r.*
Pricking of needles extending downward from right side of
    chest to scrotum—*Antip.*
Puffed, organs were—*Calad.*
Pulled up, testicle were—*Ol. an.*
  —severely, testicles were seized by hand and—*Ol. an.*
Punctured with a pin, penis were—*Syph.*
Revolving in left testicle—*Saba.*
Rough and rubbed penis when walking, shirt were—*Zinc.*
Scalded on glans penis—*Rhus t.*

Seized, a small bundle of fibers in prepuce were—*Jac.*
–by a hand and pulled severely, testicles were—*Ol. an.*
Shriveled, genitals were—*Chlf.*
Sleep, organs had gone to—*Form.*
–penis had gone to—*Sulph.*
Small, genitals were—*Cere. b., Cere. s.*
Splinters sticking in ulcer or chancre—*Nit. ac.*
Squeezed, testicles had been—*Bapt., Nux v.*
–testicles had been, especially the left—*Bapt.*
Sticking in ulcer or chancre, splinters were—*Nit. ac.*
Sticks were jagging into ulcers on glans—*Nit. ac.*
Stretch, urethra were put on, during coition—*Arg. n.*
Stretched from root of penis with hard erection and slight chordee—*Saba.*
Swollen, testicles were—*Helod.*
–prostate gland were—*Aloe*
Thick as hog's hide, scrotum were—*Rhus t.*
Thrill, tingling, were running down dorsum of penis—*Canth.*
Tied around with a cord, penis were—*Plb.*
Tight, testicles were too—*Zinc.*
–too, at orifice of urethra—*Thuj.*
Torn away, some fiber of penis were—*Mag. p. Aust.*
–to pieces, spermatic cord would be—*Nat. m.*
–on coughing, spermatic cord would be—*Nat. m.*
Twisting in seminal cord—*Iod.*
Ulcerating, glans were—*Thuj.*
Water, prepuce were distended with air or—*Merc.*
Weakness in the penis—*Alum.*
Wet, external genitals were—*Eup. pur.*
Worms crawling on prepuce—*Petr.*

FEMALE SEXUAL ORGANS

Abscesses in mammæ—*Crot. c., Sil.*

Acrid on genitals, urine were—*Eupi.*

Air streamed from nipples—*Cyc.*

Arrows were forced through breasts—*Calc. c.*

Astringent in vagina, after menses—*Dirc.*

Ball of fire in pelvic region—*Kreos.*

  –of cotton in vagina—*Pulx.*

Balls, hot, dropped from each breast through to back, rolling down back, along each limb and dropping off at heels, followed by balls of ice—*Lyc.*

Bandage, tight, in uterine region—*Hyper.*

  –with menses—*Hyper.*

Bear the least touch of the uterus, she could not—*Cham.*

Beating against right ovary, uterus were—*Ang.*

Biting and sore, vagina were—*Thuj.*

Bitten off, nipple were—*Tab.*

Bladder were pressing outward in mammæ—*Lact.*

Blood might rush out in torrents from uterus—*Ovi g. p.*

  –all genital organs were filling with—*Calc. p.*

Body, foreign, rising from uterus to chest—*Raph.*

Boiling water were running from vulva up to mouth—*Sec.*

Boils were in labia—*Chim. mac.*

Boring in tumor in ovarian region, something were—*Zinc.*

Bounding in her body, child were—*Ther.*

Breath would leave body and heart would cease (during menstrual period)—*Vib.*

Bruised in left breast—*Arum t.*

  –in neck of uterus—*Nux v.*

  –in uterus, extending to vulva—*Tarent.*

  –in region of uterus—*Ether.*

  –parts were, in menstruating—*Caust.*

  –vagina were—*Cimic.*

Bubbling in right ovary, something were—*Med.*

Bullet or rivet in region of breast—*Lil. t.*

Burning in breast, a fire were—*Cast.*

  –and swollen, uterus were—*Pyrus*

  –in the vagina, hot coals were—*Tarent.*

Burnt, uterus were—*Sec.*

Burst in uterus, something were—*Elaps*

   –ovary would—*Med.*

   –right ovary would—*Graph.*

   –abdomen would, at menses—*Ovi g. p.*

Cease, breath would leave the body and heart would (during menstrual period)—*Vib.*

Child were bounding in her body—*Ther.*

Child-birth, she were in the throes of—*Verat. a.*

   –as after—*Sol*

Cloth on left ovarian region, hot, wet, and very sensitive to touch—*Lach.*

Clutched then suddenly released, uterus were—*Sep.*

Coals, hot, were burning in vagina—*Tarent.*

Coition, after (on waking)—*Am. m.*

Cold fluid passed through intestines during menses—*Kali c.*

Come out of vulva, parts would—*Tub.*

Coming out of vagina, something were—*Kreos.*

   –away with bearing down, something were—*Ferr. i.*

Compressed in uterus—*Hura*

Conception, as at—*Sol*

Congested, uterus were—*Caul.*

Consciousness of uterus—*Murx.*

Contents of pelvis would pass through genitals—*Sep.*

Contracted by strong electric currents, uterus were—*Luna*

Cord around right mamma—*Lepi.*

Corkscrew pains in left uterus and appendages—*Sumb.*

Cotton in vagina, small ball of—*Pulx.*

Crawling in the female sexual organs—*Apis, Coff., Petr., Plat., Staph., Tarent.*

   –insects, above the left mamma—*Ant. t.*

   –up the legs under skin from feet to uterus, something were—*Tarent.*

Crossed to prevent protrusion from vagina, limbs must be—*Sep.*

Crosswise, fœtus were lying—*Arn.*

Crushed, breast were being—*Spig.*

Cutting as from knives in uterus—*Coloc.*

   –instrument in uterus, wounded by—*Murx.*

   –sharp, with a knife in left ovary—*Syph.*

Cysts, uterus were full of—*Sarr.*

Darting upward in uterus, needles were—*Lac c.*

Descended and retroverted, uterus were—*Conv.*

Deranged by bladder, uterus were—*Tarent.*

Dilate, os uteri would not—*Gels.*

Dilating, os uteri were—*Sanic.*

Dislocation of hip joint with pain in uterus—*Sol. t. æ.*

Distended in left ovary, sac were—*Med.*

  –uterus were—*Lact.*

Down, uterus were—*Lac. ac.*

Drawn through breasts with oppression, something painful were —*Eupi.*

  –up together, heart and ovaries were—*Naja*

  –up into pelvis, whole external genitals were—*Puls.*

  –over region of uterus, abdominal muscles were—*Aml. n.*

Drop off, breasts would—*Cast. eq., Iod.*

  –nipples would—*Sulph.*

Dry, uterus were—*Murx.*

Electric currents contracted uterus—*Luna*

Empty feeling in breasts after being emptied—*Bor.*

Enlarged, mammary glands were—*Sep.*

  –left ovary were—*Med.*

  –uterus were, in order to keep all the pain within its walls—*Wye.*

  –vulva were—*Sep., Sil., Zinc.*

Enter uterus, something were about to—*Pip. n.*

Escape from vulva, everything would—*Alst.*

Everything would come into the world through vagina—*Lil. t.*

Excoriated in vagina—*Berb.*

Expanding, uterus were—*Wye.*

Fall off, breasts would—*Cast. eq., Hall, Iod.*

Fall out, genital organs would—*Podo.*

  –out during stool, genitals would—*Podo.*

  –out of genitals, everything would—*Bell.*

  –out of pelvis, everything would—*Til.*

  –out of vagina, everything would—*Lac c., Sep.*

  –out, uterus would—*Bell.*

  –from dragging in lower abdomen, uterus would—*Frax.*

  –forward, contents of uterus would—*Sec.*

Falling over, uterus were—*Ang.*

  –apart in hæmorrhage, bones of pelvis were—*Tril.*

Fell from right to left, uterus—*Lil. t.*

Filled with wind, uterus were—*Phos. ac.*

Filling up with blood, all female parts were—*Calc. p.*

Finger pressing on cervix uteri—*Cast.*

Fire were burning in breast—*Cast.*

—were running out of her vagina—*Gua.*

Flatus passed down left side of abdomen to rectum but seemed to turn and go upward to bladder or uterus—*Pulx.*

Flea-bites on left mamma—*Am. m.*

—biting labial fissures—*Culx.*

Fluid, cold, passed through intestine during menses—*Kali c.*

Fœtal movement in abdomen, quivering—*Sabin.*

Fœtus were kicking in left abdomen—*Croc.*

—were knocking—*Conv.*

—living, in abdomen—*Croc., Nux v., Op., Sulph., Thuj.*

—were lying crosswise—*Arn.*

—were moving in uterus—*Nat. c., Tarent.*

—were turning somersaults in uterus—*Lyc.*

—there were not room enough in uterus for the—*Plb.*

Force itself out of vagina, something heavy would—*Sep.*

Forced through breasts, arrows were—*Calc. c.*

—out, everything would be—*Tep.*

—out, a rough jagged body were being—*Asim.*

—out of pelvis, everything were being—*Xanth.*

—into vulva, uterus would be—*Con.*

—from vulva, uterus would be—*Con.*

—through vulva, parts would be, and she must support the part—*Vib.*

Full within and below, breasts were—*Fl. ac.*

—of hard lumps, breasts were—*Lac c.*

—of cysts, uterus were—*Sarr.*

Fuller than usual, breasts were—*Clem.*

Gave way in pelvis, everything—*Sanic.*

Gnawing in left ovary—*Arg. m.*

—over surface of ulcer on uterus, mice were—*Cur.*

Grasped by a hand, uterus were—*Gels.*

Grasping or holding, something were—*Oxyt.*

Hæmorrhage, she were having—*Phos.*

Heaviness in breasts—*Iod.*

Hold herself up in region of vulva when at stool, she must—*Lil. t.*

Hot water were pouring from breast into abdomen—*Sang.*

Ice, balls of ice dropped from each breast through to back and rolling down back along legs and off heels, preceded by hot balls—*Lyc.*

Inflamed, labia were—*Chim. mac.*

Insects were crawling over left breast—*Ant. t.*

Instrument, sharp, were thrust into uterus—*Hura*

Irons, torn with red hot, in left breast—*Chin. a.*

Issue from vulva, everything would—*Bell., Lach., Lil. t., Nat. c., Sep.*

–through the vulva, uterus would—*Sep.*

Knife thrust into left nipple—*Paull.*

–were stabbing in uterus—*Crot. c.*

–suddenly thrust from pudendum into right thigh—*Croc.*

–cutting into ovary—*Saba.*

Knives were thrust into breast—*Hydrs.*

–a hundred, were drawn from abdomen to uterus, ovaries, urethra and vulva—*Sec.*

Knocking, a fœtus at eight months were—*Conv.*

Knot, uterus were drawn up into—*Ust.*

Labor pains in lower abdomen—*Ther.*

Lacerated, organs were—*Aloe*

Large left ovary were gnawing—*Arg. m.*

–vagina were—*Sanic.*

Larger, breasts were—*Calc. p., Cyc.*

Lay on clitoris, urethra—*Alumn.*

Lump in uterine region which pressed against rectum when lying —*Ars. i.*

Lumps, breasts were full of hard—*Lac c.*

Lying crosswise, fœtus were—*Arn.*

Menses were coming on—*Med., Ovi g. p., Phys., Puls. n., Vib., Visc.*

–were on—*Pip. n.*

–would come on—*Apis, Calc. p., Croc., Lil. t., Mag. c., Med., Mosch., Mur. ac., Onos., Phyt., Plat., Puls., Rhus t., Ruta, Saba., Sang., Senec., Sep., Sul. ac., Sulph., Ter., Til.*

Mice were gnawing over surface of uterine ulcer—*Cur.*

Milk would appear in breast—*Kreos., Puls.*

–would rush in as when child nurses—*Sol. t. æ.*

–were coming into right breast—*Conv.*

–reached into breasts—*Sulph.*

Motion in uterus as of fœtus—*Tarent.*

Movement in uterus of fœtus—*Nat. c.*

Muscles and tendons were too short—*Merc.*

Narrow, uterus were growing—*Bell.*

Needle sticking into left thigh and vulva—*Goss.*
Needles sticking in left breast—*Con.*
　–stitches with, in small spot between left nipple and axilla, deep in—*Calad.*
　–darted upward in uterus—*Lac c.*
　–in cervix—*Caul.*
　–sticking in ovaries—*Coloc.*
Open, os uteri were—*Lach.*
Opened and closed, uterus were—*Nat. h., Sec.*
Pass out the vagina, internal organs would—*Lil. t.*
　–out of uterus on going to stool, child would—*Nux v.*
Passing out of uterus, something were—*Aster.*
　–out from bearing down, something were—*Cimic.*
Penetrate into female organs, something strove to—*Pip. n.*
Plug, dull, were driven from right ovary to uterus—*Iod.*
Pregnant—*Verat. a.*
Press out, something would—*Eupi.*
　–out, uterus were swollen and would—*Pyrus*
　–left ovary, she must—*Med.*
Pressed out of vagina, uterus would be—*Graph.*
　–out of uterus, something would be—*Ant. c.*
Pressing on cervix uteri, finger were—*Cast.*
　–outward in mamma, bladder were—*Lact.*
　–a piece of wood stretched across back, from within (before menses)—*Nux m.*
Pressure of a sharp stone in abdomen, at menses—*Cocc.*
　–in uterus as if something would come out—*Ant. c.*
　–in vagina or uterus when stooping—*Lyc.*
Pricking in vagina—*Syph.*
Prolapse from weight and bearing down, uterus would—*Pall.*
　–during stool, uterus would—*Dirc.*
　–during hard stool, uterus and vagina would—*Podo.*
Prolapsus would occur and internal organs would pass out—*Calc. c.*
Protrude, uterus would—*Nat. c.*
　–through the vagina, all would—*Lil. t.*
Protruded from the uterus, something—*Aster.*
Pulled inward, left mamma were—*Aster.*
Pulling downward on female sexual organs, something heavy were—*Merc.*
　–ovary down, something were—*Med.*

Pushed up when she sat down, uterus were—*Nat. h.*

   –out, internal genitals were being—*Murx.*

   –out of genitals, everything would be—*Kali c.*

   –against ovary by legs, something were—*Med.*

Pushing out of uterus—*Aster.*

   –in the uterus, something were—*Aster.*

   –up in the vagina when sitting, something were—*Am. c., Ferr. i., Nat. h.*

Raw near nipple, left chest were—*Ars. h.*

Rawness in genitals after washing—*Eupi.*

Rising from uterus to throat, round body were—*Raph.*

Rivet or bullet in region of breasts—*Lil. t.*

Rolling over to right side of ovarian region, something were—*Lach.*

Room for fœtus in uterus, there were not enough—*Plb.*

   –were not sufficient for uterus—*Tarent.*

Rose higher, hard induration in breast—*Carb. an.*

Round body rising from uterus to throat—*Raph.*

Sac were distended and if pressed would burst in ovary—*Med.*

Salt on pudenda—*Caust.*

Short, muscles and tendons were too—*Merc.*

Shut and opened, uterus—*Nat. h.*

Sinking, uterus were—*Pall.*

Slivers or sticks in or about uterus—*Arg. n.*

Somersaults in uterus, fœtus were turning—*Lyc.*

Sore, parts were—*Zinc.*

   –and biting, were—*Thuj.*

   –left ovary were—*Syph.*

   –in vagina—*Kreos.*

Splinter were in labia—*Hep.*

Squeezed by a hand, uterus were—*Gels.*

   –during menses, uterus were—*Kali i.*

   –in a vise, left ovary were—*Coloc.*

Stabbing in uterus, knife were—*Crot. c.*

Steam were pouring into vagina, scalding—*Pulx.*

Sticking in ovaries, needles were—*Coloc.*

   –into left thigh and vulva, a needle were—*Goss.*

   –in left breast, needles were—*Con.*

Sticks or slivers in or about uterus—*Arg. n.*

Stitches with needles in small spot between left nipple and axilla deep in—*Calad.*

Stone, sharp, pressing in abdomen at menses—*Cocc.*
Strained when walking, ovary were—*Apis*
String were pulling in right breast—*Sumb.*
   —were tied to nipple and pulled through to back—*Crot. t.*
   —around them, nipples had a tight—*Pyrog.*
   —were pulling from breast into axilla—*Brom.*
   —between uterus and sacrum—*Nat. m.*
Stung by a bee in ovaries—*Apis*
Substance would come out of genitals—*Inul.*
Support the part, would be forced through vulva and she must
   —*Vib.*
Supported by the hand, vulva must be—*Senic.*
Suppurate, breast would—*Calc. c., Clem.*
   —breast would if touched—*Calc. c.*
Swelling, uterus were—*Ang., Sarr.*
   —in uterus from a tumor—*Sarr.*
   —immense in ovarian region—*Arg. n.*
   —of clitoris, with sticking in—*Bor.*
   —mammæ were—*Benz. ac., Berb.*
Swollen, breasts were—*Berb.*
   —genitals were—*Graph., Zinc.*
   —in uterine region—*Lach.*
   —and burning, uterus were—*Pyrus*
Tearing below left nipple, something were—*Ran. b.*
Tendons and muscles were too short—*Merc.*
Thrust into left nipple, knife were—*Paull.*
   —into breast, knives were—*Hydrs.*
   —suddenly from pudendum into right thigh, knife were—*Croc.*
Tick of watch in left side of vagina—*Alum.*
Tight bandage in uterine region—*Hyper.*
Tongs, left mammary region were torn with red-hot—*Chin. a.*
Torn toward abdomen, breasts were—*Bufo*
   —toward body, breasts were—*Bufo*
   —with red-hot irons in left breast—*Chin. a.*
   —to pieces, heart and breasts were—*Hyos.*
Touch of the uterus, she could not bear the least—*Cham.*
Touched, mammary glands would suppurate if—*Calc. c., Clem.*
Turning somersaults in uterus, fœtus were—*Lyc.*
Ulcer, a deep, had formed in left breast—*Iodof.*
   —an internal, at menses—*Cocc.*

Ulcerate, breasts would—*Merc.*
   —in the whole abdomen from uterine troubles—*Arg. m.*
Urethra lay on clitoris—*Alumn.*
Vise, left ovary were squeezed in a—*Coloc.*
Watch, tick of, in left side of vagina—*Alum.*
Water, boiling, were running from vulva up to mouth—*Sec.*
   —hot, were pouring from breast into abdomen—*Sang.*
   —warm, were flowing down in leucorrhœa—*Bor.*
Wave went from uterus to throat—*Gels.*
Weight hung to uterus bearing down—*Ovi g. p.*
   —were in uterus—*Alet.*
   —and bearing down in pelvis causing uterus to prolapse—*Pall.*
Wet, external organs were—*Eup. pur.*
Wind were in cellular tissues above nipple—*Merc. i. f.*
   —in uterine region—*Hydrs.*
   —uterus were full of—*Phos. ac.*
Wounded by cutting instrument in uterus—*Murx.*
Wood, a piece of, stretched across back pressing from within—
   Nux m.

INTERNAL CHEST

Act, muscles failed to—*Vib.*
Adhered to chest, lungs had—*Cadm. s., Gad., Kali n., Lac c., Mez., Ran. b., Seneg., Thuj.*
 –in left scapular region, on deep inspiration—*Form.*
Air in—*Sulph.*
 –a cavity in, filled with burning air which dilated in puffs—*Med.*
 –chest were filled with cold—*Corn. a.*
 –were retained when coughing—*Dros.*
 –into the chest, did not get enough—*Brom., Gins.*
 –in, there were no—*Kali c.*
 –were forcibly kept out of—*Phos.*
 –out of chest, she could not get—*Naph.*
 –did not penetrate—*Rumx.*
 –escaped into the pleural cavity—*Chlor.*
 –would pass through chest more rapidly than through the larynx—*Chlor.*
Alive in chest, something were—*Colch.*
 –in chest on breathing, something were—*Led.*
 –beneath the ribs, something were—*Croc.*
 –jumping in, something were—*Croc.*
Animal were wriggling in epigastric region—*Chel.*
Anxiety below left breast—*Phos.*
Asleep, chest were—*Merc.*
Ball, hard, in the middle of—*Kali c.*
 –in left chest—*Hura*
 –ascended from epigastrium along thorax to throat where it causes suffocation—*Plb.*
 –a large ball rising from upper end of sternum to upper end of the œsophagus—*Lac d.*
 –going to and fro under ribs—*Cupr.*
 –twisting in epigastrium—*Inul.*
Beaten in—*Apis, Cham., Kreos., Mur. ac., Zinc.*
Bladder hung in left—*Aur.*
Blood, chest were too full of—*Calc. c., Lil. t.*
 –upper part were too full of—*Sang.*
 –left chest were too full of—*Cyc.*

Blood—Continued

 —accumulated in—*Cupr.*

 —rushed to—*Cact., Calc. c., Phos.*

 —rushed from heart into chest and would burst out above—*Spong.*

 —orgasm of blood in chest would take breath away—*Sulph.*

 —surged from chest to throat, hot—*Phos.*

 —warm, were ascending in—*Mill.*

 —into the left lung, it were difficult to force—*Sumb.*

Blow in left chest—*Urt. u.*

 —of hammer in left chest, oft repeated—*Aur.*

 —on chest, constriction from—*Tarent.*

Body, broad, with many points were pressing upward in chest and dorsal muscle of left side—*Spong.*

 —a foreign, were rising up in—*Zinc.*

 —a foreign, were rising from uterus to chest—*Raph.*

 —foreign, sticking in cardiac orifice and behind sternum—*Nat. m.*

 —foreign, behind sternum with prickles in it, with slight motion causes cough and tears—*Rumx.*

 —a hollow, were turning rapidly in—*Sol. t. æ.*

Boiling and bubbling in chest, something were—*Lachn.*

Bound, chest were—*Cact.*

 —with a narrow tape—*Phos.*

 —together, throat and chest were—*Ars., Tril.*

Breaking open with a crash—*Paull.*

Breath, on account of sense of weight in, he could not draw a deep—*Phos.*

 —pain would arrest—*Dios.*

 —did not reach lower—*Lob. s.*

 —could not be expelled—*Dros.*

Brick, an iron, were being forced from stomach to chest—*Ornith.*

Broke inside left chest after feeling as if pressed by fingers in costal cartilages, something—*X-ray*

Broken and sharp points were sticking in flesh, ribs were—*Sep.*

 —bones of chest were—*Kali bi.*

Bruised, chest were—*Carb. v., Kreos., Murx., Staph.*

 —spot in upper chest were—*Zinc.*

 —and corroded, spot as large as hand in left chest were—*Zinc.*

 —on motion, joints in chest were—*Arn.*

Bubbles in—*Mill.*

 —burst in—*Sulph.*

Bubbling in—*Lach., Lachn.*
  –and boiling in—*Lachn.*
  –of liquid in—*Ol. an.*
  –in region of heart—*Lach., Lyc.*
Bundles, lungs were tied in—*Dig.*
Burning in flesh of—*Lach.*
Burst, chest would—*Aur. m., Merc., Seneg., Zinc.*
  –head and chest would—*Bry.*
  –upper part of chest would—*Arg. n.*
  –in, something would—*Rhus t.*
Bursting, chest were—*Carb. an., Merc., Ol. an., Sil., Zinc.*
Cask, chest were a big empty—*Phyt.*
Cavity in chest were filled with burning air which dilated in puffs
      —*Med.*
  –extended from side to side about middle of chest—*Med.*
Chains were tightened around chest, contracting it—*Glon.*
Choked in chest—*Lil. t.*
Clawing in left chest—*Seneg.*
Clogged, left chest were—*Sumb.*
Close and oppressed breathing, sternum were lying too—*Cina*
Closing, lungs and bronchi were—*Oxyt.*
Coal of fire in chest—*Carb. v.*
Cold air or ice, chest were filled with—*Corn. a.*
  –breathing on a cold spot in—*Brom.*
  –and hollow, chest were—*Zinc.*
  –feeling in left chest after drinking—*Sol. o.*
  –wet cloths applied to three different parts of wall of thorax
      —*Ran. b.*
Compressed, chest were—*Cact., Paraf.*
  –by an iron armor—*Crot. c.*
  –contents of thorax were—*Agar.*
  –in a vise, in front of—*Helon., Nux m.*
Congested, both lungs were becoming—*Equis.*
Constricted, chest were—*Bufo, Caps., Coloc., Cupr. ar., Ferr.,*
      Plat., Valer.
  –everything in chest were tightly—*Plat.*
  –by a thin wire around both lungs—*Asar.*
  –walls of chest were being—*Dig.*
Constriction of—*Plat.*
  –great, in middle of sternum—*Cact.*
Contact with back, lungs came in—*Sulph.*

Contents, chest were deprived of its—*Stann.*
    –of stomach were passing into chest—*Cham.*
    –of lower chest and stomach were pressed upon each other—
      Med.

Contracted, chest were—*Cinnb., Med.*

Contraction or drawing together within lower portion of
    sternum, diaphragm—*Pyrog.*

Convex, chest were—*Aml. n.*

Cord pulling from suprasternal fossa downward and sideways
    —*Apis*

Corroded in chest, parts were—*Zinc.*
    –bruised spot as large as hand in left—*Zinc.*

Cough up hard substance lying under sternum, must—*Abies n.*
    –but without ability, he would—*Tanac.*

Cracked by mall of lead, chest would be—*Plat.*

Crawling beneath sternum—*Samb.*

Crowbar were pressed tightly from right to left breast until it
    came and twisted a knot around the heart, which stopped
    it—*Tab.*

Crushed, chest were—*Juncus*
    –when stooping, left chest were—*Anac.*
    –by a mass of lead, chest would be—*Plat.*
    –in, sternum were being—*Kreos.*

Cupping glass had been applied inside of chest—*Pin. s.*

Cut to pieces, chest were—*Kali i., Zinc.*

Dagger were stabbing in chest—*Crot. c.*

Depression bent in toward spine, lower end of sternum made a
    deep—*Aml. n.*

Deprived of its contents, chest were—*Stann.*

Dislocated, right clavicle were, < moving the shoulder—*Lac c.*
    –one rib had been, and snapped back again—*Calad.*

Distended, chest could not be sufficiently—*Con.*
    –which could not be completely, something in chest were being
      —*Bry.*
    –chest were—*Brom., Cadm. s., Caps., Cinch., Cocc., Gua., Olnd.,*
      Stann.

Dragging in sides of chest—*Corn. c., Sep.*

Drawing together, chest were—*Pyrog.*

Drawn together, chest were—*Nux v.*
    –toward dorsal vertebræ, chest were gradually being—*Syph.*
    –toward spine, sternum were gradually—*Syph.*

Drawn—*Continued*
  –back in left side of—*Ind.*
  –inward, ribs would be—*Eug.*
  –upward, contents of chest and abdomen were—*Antip.*
  –right side of chest were repeatedly—*Cham.*
  –back in left breast by means of a thread, something were—*Croc.*

Drops, warm, were running over chest—*Ars. h.*
  –falling in—*Thuj.*

Dropped down in chest, something had—*Bar. c.*
  –rapidly in a vessel in right chest, liquid—*Stann.*

Dropping and gurgling in chest, fluid were—*Puls.*

Dry in chest, everything were—*Merc.*

Dust in trachea, throat and behind the sternum—*Chel.*

Empty, chest were—*Chr. ac., Stann., Vinc.*
  –feeling in—*Olnd.*
  –behind sternum—*Zinc.*

Enlarged ten fold, caliber of chest were—*Phyt.*

Eructations would relieve chest—*Cist., Crot. c.*

Eviscerated, chest were—*Phos., Stann.*

Excoriated and raw, chest were—*Ars.*

Excoriation in chest—*Phos., Rumx.*

Expand in chest, something should but would not—*Bry.*
  –lungs had no room to—*Nat. m.*

Expanded, chest were—*Olnd.*

Fall in, dorsal vertebræ would—*Bar. c.*
  –down in chest, something would—*Nux v.*

Falling in chest, a hard body were—*Corn. c.*
  –together, chest were—*Juni.*

Feather fluttering across clavicle, causing a cough; preceded by a feeling of a bar at the same place—*Hæm.*
  –in center of chest oscillating with every breath—*Rumx.*
  –tickling in chest—*Morph., Phos. ac.*

Fæces ascended to chest—*Lach.*

Feel every muscle and fiber in the right side, she could—*Sep.*

Fell forward in thorax on turning on right side, something—*Sulph.*

Filled with mucus, chest were—*Zinc.*
  –chest could only be half—*Dig.*

Fire from chest to shoulder, coals of—*Lach.*

Fixed in upper chest, something were—*Fl. ac.*

Flatus were rising in chest—*Lach.*
Fluid dropping in left chest—*Puls.*
　　–in lower part of right lung wanted to discharge itself into region of duodenum—*Chen. v.*
　　–ran through narrow opening, on turning in bed—*Ign.*
Fluttering of bird's wing in chest—*Nat. m.*
Fly to pieces, chest would—*Lact., Sulph.*
Food lodged in chest—*Am. m.*
　　–in region of heart—*Acon.*
　　–in upper end of sternum—*Lac. ac.*
　　–were lying under sternum—*All. c., Bry., Chin., Puls.*
Forced from stomach to chest, an iron brick were being—*Ornith.*
Full, chest were too—*Agar., Lyc., Nit. ac., Puls.*
　　–on waking, chest were—*Sep.*
　　–and not enough room in it—*Caps.*
　　–and tight—*Puls.*
　　–in morning, lower part of chest were—*Puls.*
　　–thorax were—*Med.*
Give way, something in chest must—*Arg. n.*
　　–way at touch, walls of chest would—*Pin. s.*
Gnawing in front of chest, something were—*Nat. h.*
Grasp sternum and twist it, lift it up, rub it to pieces or burst it, someone would—*Sulph.*
Grasped, sternum were—*Sil.*
Grating in chest on inspiration, something were—*Eup. pur.*
Grown fast in the chest, something had—*Sulph.*
　　–fast in region of lower ribs, something had—*Thuj.*
　　–to sore spot in chest, something had—*Med.*
　　–together, internal parts of chest were—*Dig.*
Gurgling and dropping in chest, fluid were—*Puls.*
Hammer in left chest, repeated often, a strong blow as with—*Aur.*
Hand grasped her breast bone—*Sil.*
Hanging in chest, bladder were—*Aur.*
　　–down, everything in chest were—*Crot. t.*
Hard body were falling in chest—*Corn. c.*
　　–substance under sternum must be coughed up—*Abies n.*
Hawk mucus from chest, inclination to—*Stann.*
Heavy lay under sternum, something—*Cast.*
　　–oppressed her on all sides from neck to diaphragm, something—*Sin.*

Hollow, chest were—*Ars., Aspar., Chin., Chin. a., Chin. s., Coca, Crot. t., Sep.*

–and cold—*Zinc.*

–and sore—*Sep.*

Hopping in chest, something living and—*Croc.*

Hornets going from pectoral region to head, swarms of—*Cact.*

Hot inside the chest, something were—*Spong.*

–in small spot beneath ensiform cartilage, something were— *Spire.*

Hunger affected the chest—*Rhus t.*

Hung suspended from the chest, all internal organs were—*Lil. t.*

Hypertrophied, all tissues in chest were—*Chlor.*

Ice in right chest, a lump of—*Sulph.*

–or cold air, chest were filled with—*Corn. a.*

Incarcerated flatus in chest—*Phos.*

Inflamed and raw in chest when breathing frosty air—*Apis*

Instrument, dull, behind right false ribs—*Ran. s.*

Iron, hot, had been run into chest and hundred weight put on it—*Naja*

Knife plunged into chest—*Nux m., Sumb.*

–dull, thrust into chest between fifth and sixth ribs—*Dulc.*

–transfixed with, through xiphoid appendix to back—*Cupr. s.*

–were thrust through right—*Con., Corn. f.*

–were plunged into left chest on bending to right side—*Rhod.*

–were thrust into top of left lung and then turned around— *Sep.*

Knives cutting in chest—*Psor.*

–were thrust into—*Hydrs.*

–two, going toward each other in—*Kali c.*

Laced, chest were—*Ferr., Glon.*

–were tightly—*Card. b., Plat.*

Lancinating from stiletto in—*Amph.*

Large, chest were too—*Alum.*

Lead, would be cracked by a mall of—*Plat.*

–would be crushed by a mass of—*Plat.*

Living and hopping in chest, something were—*Croc.*

Load, heavy, were in chest—*Nat. s.*

–heavy, in side of—*Stann.*

Loaded in thoracic viscera—*Atham.*

Lodged in the chest, food had—*Am. m.*

Lodged—*Continued*

    –under mid-sternum, lump of hot lead were—*Nux v.*

    –in chest the size of a fist, something were—*Cic.*

    –in sternum, something indigestible had—*Chin. s.*

    –in upper end of sternum, food were—*Lac. ac.*

    –in chest, mostly on right side of sternum which must be coughed up, something were—*Abies n.*

    –in region of heart, food had—*Acon.*

Loose, everything in chest were—*Bry., Kali n., Mez., Phos., Rhus t.*

    –short, or wabbling about, everything in chest were too—*Spig.*

    –under left rib, something were—*Ambr.*

Lump in chest—*Ambr., Chin.*

    –in left chest—*Both. a.*

    –in lower end of sternum and back—*Ovi g. p.*

    –under sternum—*Chin.*

Morsel of food in chest—*Am. m.*

    –he had swallowed too large a—*Spire.*

Move in chest, so full nothing could—*Con.*

Mucus in chest, he had much—*Cina*

Narrow, chest were too—*Agar., Ars., Graph., Lil. t., Nux m., Ol. an., Seneg., Sulph.*

    –when walking, upper part of chest were too—*Bry.*

Narrowed, cavity of thorax were—*Agar.*

Needle sticking in left chest—*Spig.*

    –red hot, burning in upper part of chest—*Ol. an.*

Needles in middle of chest, pricked by, < on breathing—*Elæis guin.*

Opened on drawing a breath—*Paull.*

Oppressed by nerves, chest were—*Puls.*

Out of chest, she could not get air—*Naph.*

Pain would arrest the breath—*Dios.*

    –were between ribs—*Nat. n.*

Passing into chest, contents of stomach were—*Cham.*

Peppermint rising in chest, effects of eating—*Æsc.*

Pieces, chest would fly to—*Lact., Sulph.*

Pins, pricked by a cushion full of—*Anag.*

    –thousand, pricking on inner surface of sternum—*Sol. t. æ.*

    –struck in the lungs with a cushion of—*Anag.*

    –and needles under the sternum—*Kali bi.*

Plug of mucus moving in chest—*Coc. c.*

  –in chest—*Anac.*

  –in right side of chest—*Sphin.*

Plugged in right side of chest—*Anac.*

Point, sharp, pressed in chest—*Pers.*

  –sharp, pressed under scapula—*Pers.*

  –sharp, were being turned about an old sore at end of sternum
      —*Samars.*

  –dull, were being thrust about an old sore at sternum—*Samars.*

Pounded, muscles of chest had been—*Ran. b.*

Pressed inward from both sides, chest were—*Bell., Cina*

  –inward, sternum were—*Con., Rhus t.*

  –together, ribs were—*Calend.*

  –upon, sternum were—*Rhod.*

  –in, lower sternum were—*Juncus*

  –away from under the sternum, something were being—*Kalm.*

  –upon each other, contents of lower chest and stomach were—
      Med.

  –out of lower chest, something were—*Valer.*

  –against lower front—*Sulph.*

  –with point of finger in xiphoid cartilage—*Asaf.*

  –by fingers in left costal cartilages, followed by a sensation as
      if something broke inside—*X-ray*

  –a sharp point, under scapulæ—*Pers.*

  –tightly from right to left breast until it came and twisted a
      knot around heart which stopped it, a crowbar were—*Tab.*

  –out of lower chest, something were—*Valer.*

Pressing inward, sternum were—*Rhus t., Syph.*

  –upon it with hand, chest were oppressed by someone—*Ferr.*

  –upon chest, under sternum—*Sabin.*

Prevented exhalation when talking or coughing, something in
    chest—*Dros.*

  –free passage of air to chest, something in throat—*Fel t.*

Pricking the flesh, ribs were broken and points were—*Sep.*

  –dull stick in chest were—*Pall.*

Pried out, ribs were being—*Samars.*

Pulled from spleen into chest, something were—*Bor.*

  –off, pleura were—*Elaps*

Raw, chest were—*Gamb., Psor., Rhus t.*

  –and excoriated in—*Ars.*

Raw—*Continued*

–and inflamed in chest when breathing frosty air—*Apis*

–under clavicle—*Rumx*.

Respiration were tremulous—*Mag. p. Aust.*

Resisted the expansion of the chest, something—*Iod.*

Rising in chest, flatus were—*Lach.*

–in chest, worm were—*Merc.*

Rolled up, chest were—*Carb. v.*

Room, chest were too full and not enough—*Caps.*

Rose in œsophagus and remained in chest, something—*Crot. h.*

Rub it to pieces or burst it, someone would grasp the sternum, twist it and lift it up—*Sulph.*

Rumbling in left chest and in intestines—*Cocc.*

Rushed into chest, wind—*Sabin.*

Scraped by a shell, chest were—*Plb.*

Screwed together, chest were—*Glon.*

–together in right lower ribs—*Sulph.*

Screwing together in epigastrium—*Sil.*

Shell, chest were scraped by a—*Plb.*

Short, chest were—*Sars.*

–everything in chest were too—*Spig.*

–on straightening up and walking erect, chest were too—*Sars.*

–everything in chest were too loose, short, or wabbling about—*Spig.*

Sink in, walls would—*Ptel.*

Sleep in clavicle, chest had gone to—*Ferr.*

–under right ribs, chest had gone to—*Apis*

Small, chest were too—*Cupr. ar., Ign.*

–too, for heart—*Cean.*

Something size of fist were in the throat and chest—*Cic.*

Sore and hollow, chest were—*Sep.*

–one great, in chest—*Cinch. b.*

–everything were, on stepping—*Seneg.*

–spot in—*Zinc.*

–low down in—*Spong.*

Spasm of suffocating—*Sep.*

Sprained, chest were—*Agar.*

–sternum were—*Rumx.*

–bones and cartilage were—*Arn.*

Stabbed in chest, squeezed between iron plates and then—*Paull.*

Stabs of a dagger in chest, two—*Crot. c.*

Steam, hot, passing from chest to abdomen—*Sang.*
  –hot wavelike, moving through abdomen, chest and throat—*Lyss.*
Sternum lying too close and oppressed breathing—*Cina*
Stick, dull, pricking in right—*Pall.*
Sticking behind sternum, food remains—*All. c.*
Stitch would appear behind the heart—*Fl. ac.*
Stone in chest—*Puls.*
  –pressing in—*Rat.*
  –heavy, in—*Alum.*
  –under sternum—*Sil.*
  –pressing at lower sternum—*Lil. t.*
  –pressing down in pleura—*Cor. r.*
Stopped up, chest were—*Phos.*
  –up and could not get air—*Bry.*
  –up in lower—*Phos.*
Strained in chest—*Sulph.*
Strangling from mucus in chest—*Ip.*
Stretched fibers returned to their places causing drawing pains between shoulders and chest—*Raph.*
String were stretched from chest to groin—*Plb.*
  –left breast were drawn toward back by a—*Croc.*
Struck with a cushion full of pins in inner chest—*Anag.*
  –with hammer in left chest, repeated often—*Aur.*
Stuffed, chest were—*Ambr., Lach.*
Substance, a hard brittle, rose into—*Sul. ac.*
  –a broad and pointed, were forced up in—*Spong.*
  –lying under the sternum, must cough up hard—*Abies n.*
  –had swallowed a hard, and were sticking behind mid-sternum—*Abies n.*
  –were between lungs and sternum—*Brom.*
Suffocate, he must—*Phos.*
Suppurating behind sternum—*Staph.*
Surged from chest to throat, hot blood—*Phos.*
Suspended from chest, all internal organs were—*Lil. t.*
Swallowed a piece of hard-boiled egg, he had—*Spire.*
  –hot food had been—*Euph.*
  –hot water, in right chest—*Saba.*
  –too large a morsel, he had—*Spire.*
Swelled with painful soreness, sternum had—*Osm.*
Swelling of front of chest—*Aml. n.*

24

Sympathy, mutual, between ovaries and lungs—*Apis*
Talk, she would lose the power to—*Prun.*
Tear asunder, chest would—*Zinc.*
Tearing in chest, something were—*Ran. b., Spig.*
Tension from a cold in chest—*Sep.*
Thin, walls of chest were—*Pin. s.*
Throbbing, undulation, as from wind balls under ribs—*Tell.*
Thrust in the middle of sternum—*Sul. ac.*
   –into top of left lung then turned around, knife were—*Sep.*
   –into left inner chest, blunt knife were—*Dulc.*
Tickling with a feather in chest—*Morph., Phos. ac.*
   –in chest would provoke cough—*Verat. a.*
Tied in bundles, lungs were—*Dig.*
Tight, chest were too—*Mez., Squill., Tab.*
   –lower part of chest were too—*Lact.*
   –chest were too full and—*Puls.*
   –laced too—*Plat.*
Tightened around chest, contracting it, chains were—*Glon.*
Torn, everything in chest were—*Psor.*
   –loose in chest, something were—*Nux v.*
   –open, chest would be—*Nat. m.*
   –out of chest, something were—*Rhus t.*
   –out by cough, something would be—*Rhus t.*
   –and he would spit blood with each coughing spell, chest would
      be—*Pip. n.*
   –loose, something in middle of sternum were—*Phos.*
   –away under sternum, something would be—*Psor.*
   –loose under sternum, something were being—*Phos.*
   –in two, sternum were—*Nat. p.*
   –to pieces, sternum were—*Dig.*
   –out of chest in sternum, a piece were—*Æsc.*
   –away, thoracic walls anterior to heart were—*Cere. b.*
   –ribs were being—*Samars.*
Touch, walls would give way at—*Pin. s.*
Turned around in chest, a button—*Lach.*
   –around in, something—*Stram.*
Twist it, lift it up, rub it to pieces or burst it, someone would
      grasp sternum and—*Sulph.*
Ulcer in middle of thorax—*Puls.*
   –in chest—*Caust.*

Ulcerated, two surfaces in contact in right chest—*Iodof.*
  –in left chest—*Gels.*
Undulation or throbbing from wind balls under ribs—*Tell.*
Vise, chest were in a—*Æth., Bufo, Raph., Tab.*
  –front of chest had been compressed in a—*Helon., Nux m.*
Wabbling about, everything in chest were too loose, short or—
    Spig.
Walled up in chest—*Carb. v.*
Walls were thin—*Pin. s.*
Water in chest—*Crot. c.*
  –were rolling or grumbling about in left—*X-ray*
  –hot, in chest—*Acon., Cic.*
  –hot, were floating in—*Hep.*
  –hot, moved about in—*Hep.*
  –hot, in right chest, he had swallowed—*Saba.*
  –boiling, poured into—*Acon.*
  –boiling in left—*Sul. ac.*
  –drops of, trickling down inside of—*X-ray*
  –drops of, in left chest—*Hep.*
Wave, cold, in chest—*Camph.*
Waves, lungs moved in—*Dulc.*
  –rising in chest—*Verat. v.*
Weight, heavy, in chest—*Am. c., Lact., Nat. s.*
  –in left chest—*Both. a.*
  –he could not draw a deep breath on account of—*Phos.*
  –great, lying in middle of sternum—*Phos.*
  –crushing, under sternum, on walking up hill—*Aur.*
  –seems to fall from pit of chest to pit of stomach—*Nat. h.*
Whirled from chest to head, something—*Cact.*
Wide, chest were—*Alum.*
  –enough, chest were not—*Cham.*
Wind, chest were full of—*Lach.*
  –suffocative feeling in chest from—*Ovi g. p.*
  –rushed into chest—*Sabin.*
Wire around both lungs, constricted by a thin—*Asar.*
Working in hot room, weakness in chest came from—*Glon.*
Worm were rising in chest—*Merc.*

EXTERNAL CHEST

Abscess on left chest—*Med.*
Air, cold, blowing through hole in clothes on chest—*Chin., Culx.*
Ants were running over chest—*Mez.*
Armor of iron compressed chest—*Crot. c.*
Band across chest—*Lob.*
  –around chest—*Acon., Æth., Cact., Lob., Mag. c., Phos., Pic. ac., Sil., Upas*
  –around clavicles—*Chlor., Thuj.*
  –around lower chest—*Chlor.*
  –of iron around chest—*Arg. n., Cact., Nit. ac., Paull.*
  –chest were compressed by an iron—*Paull.*
  –constricting chest transversely—*Zinc.*
  –drawn across chest—*Aml. n.*
  –encircling chest—*Æth., Op.*
  –encircling chest at line of pleura—*Caps.*
  –chest were encircled in a tight—*Phos., Pic. ac.*
Bandage, chest would be squeezed in a tight—*Colch.*
Bar across chest, impeding respiration—*Vichy*
  –across chest on level with clavicles—*Hæm.*
Beaten, bones and cartilages were—*Arn.*
  –in pectoral muscle—*Staph.*
  –on sternum—*Sul. ac.*
  –ribs had been—*Calad.*
Biting between mammæ, fleas were—*Phos. ac.*
Bitten off, nipple were—*Tab.*
Blow, chest were constricted from—*Tarent.*
Blowing through hole in clothes, cold air were—*Chin., Culx.*
Bound, chest were—*Cact.*
  –up, chest were—*Tril.*
  –with a hoop, chest were—*Ars.*
  –with an iron band, chest were—*Nit. ac.*
Broken around chest, in evening—*Zing.*
  –bones of chest were—*Kali bi.*
Bruised about chest—*Cham.*
  –sternum were—*Sars.*
  –in lower end of sternum—*Cic.*
  –all ribs were—*Arn.*

Bruised—*Continued*
 –in dorsal ribs—*Ran. b.*
 –cartilages were—*Arn., Cere. s., Tax.*
Burning from glowing coals, chest were—*Carb. v.*
 –from nettles—*Pæon.*
 –from electric sparks—*Phel.*
Burst open with crack, chest would—*Paull.*
 –it, someone would grasp the sternum, twist it, lift it up, rub it to pieces or—*Sulph.*
Choke from pressure on chest, she would—*Aloe*
Clothing were too tight during respiration—*Ery. a.*
Cloths applied to anterior walls of thorax when walking in open air, she had wet—*Ran. b.*
Coals, glowing, burning chest—*Carb. v.*
Compressed in a vise, chest were—*Helon.*
 –by a weight, chest were—*Nux v.*
 –by an iron band, chest were—*Paull.*
 –by iron armor, chest were—*Crot. c.*
Constricted across chest—*Phos.*
 –by a blow—*Tarent.*
 –by emotion, chest were—*Hura*
 –and stiff, chest were—*Op.*
 –chest, lips were pressed together and—*Cinch.*
 –by vise, chest were—*Bufo, Tab.*
 –by tight waistcoat, chest were—*Lyc.*
Constricting chest transversely, band were—*Zinc.*
Contracting, pectoral muscles were—*Brach.*
Contused, skin on chest were—*Chel.*
Cord about chest causing oppression of breathing—*Stann.*
 –tied tightly about chest—*Cact.*
Cords around chest and waist, ligated with—*Arg. n.*
Crack open, chest would—*Paull.*
Creeping over short ribs, snake were—*Murx.*
Crushed, chest were—*Juncus*
 –by a mass of lead, chest would be—*Plat.*
Drawn across chest, band were—*Aml. n.*
 –tight around right lower chest, something were—*Culx.*
 –together, chest were—*Nux v.*
 –intercostal muscles were—*Nat. p.*
 –up, skin of chest were—*Syph.*
Drops, warm, were running over chest—*Ars. h.*

Electric sparks, fine, on sternal end of right clavicle—*Carb. ac.*
 –sparks burning chest—*Phel.*
Emotion, chest were constricted from—*Hura*
Encircled by band, chest were—*Acon., Æth., Cact., Caps., Lob., Op., Phos., Pic. ac.*
Falling together, chest were—*Juni.*
Flannel caused itching on chest—*Hipp.*
Fleas biting between mammæ—*Phos. ac.*
 –caused itching on chest—*Nat. c.*
Garments were too tight about chest—*Caust., Meli., Nux v., Phos.*
Give way under pressure, chest were thin and would—*Pin. s.*
Grasp sternum, twist it, lift it up, rub it to pieces or burst it, someone would—*Sulph.*
Hand upon chest, someone pressed with—*Ferr.*
Heavy were resting on chest, something—*Iodof.*
 –weight on chest—*Cact., Phos., Prun., Valer., Zinc.*
Hoop about chest—*Lyc.*
 –chest were bound by—*Ars.*
Induration, hard, rose higher in breast—*Carb. an.*
Instrument passed through sternum—*Calc. p.*
Iron armor compressed chest—*Crot. c.*
 –band around chest—*Arg. n., Cact.*
 –band, chest were bound with—*Nit. ac.*
 –band, chest were compressed with—*Paull.*
Lay on sternum, something—*Ran. s.*
Lead, chest would be crushed by a mass of—*Plat.*
Lice on chest—*Led.*
Ligated with cords around chest and waist—*Arg. n.*
Load, heavy, on chest—*Æth., Arg. m., Carb. ac., Elaps, Nux v., Phos., Samb., Stront., Verat. v.*
 –heavy, on chest when waking—*Kali bi.*
 –heavy, lying on chest all night—*Ars. m.*
 –pressing on front of chest—*Carb. ac.*
Lying on chest all night, a heavy load were—*Ars. m.*
 –on chest, a stone were—*Viol. o.*
Needles and pins at sternum—*Kali bi.*
 –were pricking from right side of chest down to scrotum—*Antip.*
Nettles were burning chest—*Pæon.*
Passed through sternum, an instrument were—*Calc. p.*

Peg were stuck in lower false ribs—*Elæis guin.*

Pincers, iron, causing constriction in middle of sternum—*Çact.*

Pressed, see also INTERNAL CHEST

Pressed inward from both sides, chest were—*Bell.*

  –inward, sternum were—*Rhus t.*

  –upon chest, a hand were—*Ferr.*

  –upon, sternum were—*Coloc.*

Pressing on front of chest, load were—*Carb. ac.*

Pricking of needles extending down from right side of chest to scrotum—*Antip.*

Resting on chest, something heavy were—*Iodof.*

Running over chest, ants were—*Mez.*

Scraped by a shell, chest were—*Plb.*

Scratched as far as arm, chest were—*Paull.*

Short, chest were too—*Nux v.*

Slip from their sockets, clavicles would—*Lyss.*

Snake were creeping over region of short ribs—*Murx.*

Sore in left clavicle near sternum, bones were—*Sal. ac.*

Sparks, fine electric, on sternal end of right clavicle—*Carb. ac.*

  –electric, burning chest—*Phel.*

Splinter in pimples on sternum—*Am. c.*

Squeezed in a tight bandage, chest would be—*Colch.*

Stone were lying on chest—*Viol. o.*

Stove on chest, heat from—*Lach.*

Strapped, chest were—*Ail.*

Stuck in lower false ribs, peg were—*Elæis guin.*

Tape, chest were tied with—*Sil.*

Thin and would give way under pressure, chest were—*Pin. s.*

Tied tightly about lower part of chest, cord were—*Cact.*

Tight about chest, clothing were too—*Ery. a.*

  –about chest, garments were too—*Caust., Meli., Mill., Nux v., Phos.*

Vise, chest were compressed in—*Helon.*

  –chest were constricted by—*Bufo, Tab.*

Weight on chest—*Kali bi., Phos., Sanic., Sec., Spong., Stann.*

  –on chest, awakening him at night—*Viol. o.*

  –in region of sternum—*Chlor.*

  –on sternum—*Aml. n.*

  –heavy, on chest—*Cact., Phos., Prun., Zinc. val.*

  –compressed chest—*Nux v.*

Wet cloths were applied to walls of thorax—*Ran. b.*

RESPIRATORY ORGANS

Adhered to walls of chest, lungs were—*Cadm. s., Euph., Gad., Kali n., Lac c., Mez., Ran. b., Seneg., Thuj.*
  —to ribs, lower lobe of left lung were—*Euph.*
Adhering, left lung were—*Euph.*
  —to ribs, lower lobe of lungs were—*Kali c.*
  —tightly to larynx, mucus were—*Alum.*
Adhesions in lungs—*Mez.*
Air, cannot inspire enough—*Bry., Meli.*
  —cells were stuck together—*Ail.*
  —into cells, he could not get enough—*Crot. t.*
  —cold, streaming through air passages—*Cor. r.*
  —could not get deep enough into lungs—*Caps.*
  —could not long survive for want of—*Apis*
  —could not pass through in larynx—*Chel.*
  —in larynx—*Mez.*
  —were withheld on talking or coughing—*Dros.*
  —she inhaled did not reach pit of stomach—*Prun.*
  —were too close—*Sars.*
  —room had been exhausted of—*Nux v., Plan.*
  —in chest, something kept—*Dros.*
  —open cavity in lower right lung were exposed to cold—*Culx.*
  —cavity in upper part of lungs filled with burning—*Med.*
  —inspired, were cold—*Cor. r., Lith.*
  —filled with cold, or ice—*Corn. a.*
  —were too cold in larynx—*Hipp.*
  —breathing hot—*Trif. p.*
  —escaped from lungs into pleural cavity—*Chlor.*
  —breathing difficult as from want of—*Trades.*
  —passed into glands of neck on breathing—*Spong.*
  —passing through passages were icy cold—*Cor. r.*
  —expired were warmer than usual—*Coc. c.*
  —expired smelled putrid—*Chr. ac.*
  —passages were full of smoke—*Brom.*
  —passages were lined with thick stiff mucus—*Sang. n.*
  —breathless from passing rapidly through—*Rumx.*
  —rose through trachea in waves—*Lyc.*

Apple-seed cell lodged in upper larynx or rima glottidis—*Bry.*
Attention, whole, must be centered on act of respiration—*Chlor.*
Ball were rolling loose in trachea—*Chen. a.*
  —were rising from pit of stomach into larynx—*Kali ar.*
Band, rubber, were drawn around right lung—*Culx.*
Beaten, lung were—*Med.*
Blistering sore in lung, her breath were forming—*Med.*
Blood, lungs were full of—*Trif. p.*
  —were forcing its way into finest vessel of lungs—*Zinc.*
  —any minute he might raise—*Rumx.*
Blow in lower lung—*Tarent.*
Body, foreign, in larynx—*Bell., Cop., Cub., Ptel.*
  —foreign, in air passages—*Hyos.*
  —small foreign, in larynx with desire to swallow—*Calc. f.*
  —foreign, lying over larynx—*Ign.*
  —foreign, stopped up larynx—*Arg. m.*
  —foreign, in windpipe—*Brom., Ter.*
Brain would be brought into contact with cold air at every inhalation—*Cimic.*
Break on coughing, skull would—*Nux v.*
Breath, could not get her—*Calc. c., Rumx., Spong.*
  —after warm drinks could not get her—*Phos.*
  —would be his last, each—*Dig.*
  —would cease—*Apis, Olnd., Ter., Trom.*
  —would leave her on lying down—*Lac c.*
  —would be taken away from riding rapidly downhill—*Bor.*
  —not able to draw a long—*Rhus t.*
  —would be impeded in trachea—*Laur.*
  —larynx closed upon—*Mosch.*
  —he were holding—*Dros.*
  —he would sink together and lose his—*Sep.*
  —if she cannot expectorate would lose her—*Sep.*
  —awakes from loss of—*Kali c., Lach., Sep.*
  —were stopped up by a spasm—*Sars.*
  —were stopped at pit of stomach—*Rhus t.*
  —remained stopped between scapulæ—*Calc. c.*
  —must take a deep—*Card. m., Fl. ac.*
  —exhaled a cold—*Rhus t.*
  —were forming a blistering sore in lung—*Med.*
Breathe for two, she had to—*Samb.*
  —again, would not be able to—*Apis*

Breathing, clothes hindered—*Lach.*
　—from a tight girdle, hindrance to—*Chel.*
　—hot air—*Trif. p.*
　—a membrane prevented—*Kali c.*
　—through a sponge—*Phyt., Spong.*
　—would stop—*Apis*

Breathless from passing rapidly through air—*Rumx.*

Bruised, trachea were—*Still.*

Bubbling in middle lobe of right lung, fluid were—*Tell.*

Bundles, lungs were constricted and tied up in—*Dig.*

Buried in right lung, dagger were—*Chin. b.*

Burning air, cavity in upper part of lungs were filled with—*Med.*
　—in lungs with smoke, paper were—*Coff.*
　—of peppermint in larynx—*Elaps*

Burst while coughing, forehead would—*Nat. m.*

Caliber of larynx were diminished—*Euphr.*

Catarrh were coming on—*Stict.*

Cavity, open, in lower right lung, exposed to cold air—*Culx.*

Cease, breath would—*Apis, Olnd., Ter., Trom.*

Chewing peppermint, he had been—*Spire.*

Choke, she would—*Crot. h., Naja, Nux v.*

Clogged, lungs were—*Phos.*

Close, air were too—*Sars.*

Closed, air passages and lungs were—*Gad.*
　—larynx were—*Aur. m., Tarax.*
　—by pressure, when lying on back with head forward, larynx were—*Ol. an.*
　—upon breath, larynx were suddenly—*Mosch.*
　—trachea were—*Mez.*
　—by a film or leaf, trachea were—*Mang.*

Coated, larynx were—*Phos.*

Clothes hindered breathing—*Lach.*

Collapsed, lungs were—*Osm., Phys.*
　—left lung were—*Med.*

Cold air, filled with—*Corn. a.*
　—inspired air were—*Cor. r., Lith.*
　—icy, passing through passages—*Cor. r.*
　—larynx were—*Brom.*
　—heavy, settled on both lungs—*Iodof.*
　—in larynx, air were too—*Hipp.*

Cold—*Continued*

   –air would be brought into contact with brain at every inhalation—*Cimic.*

Come out on coughing, a piece of lung would—*Mag. s.*

Compressed, larynx were—*Tarax.*

Compression of lungs—*Iris fœ., Lipp.*

Congested, lungs were—*Pyrus*

Constricted, air passages were internally—*Puls.*

   –larynx were—*All. c., Bell.*

   –larynx causing suffocation, someone—*Caust.*

   –in lungs—*Nat. m., Phos.*

   –with fine threads, lungs were—*Kali chl.*

   –and tied in bundles, lungs were—*Dig.*

   –from a wire around left lung—*Asar.*

   –upper portions of both lungs were—*Coca*

   –small spot in lungs were—*Thuj.*

Constricting larynx, vapors of sulphur were—*Mosch.*

Constriction, breath could not get through larynx because of—*Spong.*

Contact with back, lungs came in—*Sulph.*

Contracted, air passages to pit of stomach were—*Sep.*

   –in middle of left lung—*Ail.*

   –larynx were—*Alum.*

Cord were drawn around treachea—*Cham.*

Cotton, larynx were stuffed with—*Pyrus*

   –lungs were stuffed with—*Kali bi., Med.*

Cough enough to start mucus, she could not—*Caust.*

   –did not reach low enough to raise mucus—*Rumx.*

   –he would have to—*Chlor.*

   –wanted to but could not—*Alet.*

Coughing, skull would break on—*Nux v.*

   –larynx would be torn when—*All. c.*

Crackling in trachea—*Arn.*

Covered with a glutinous substance, trachea were—*Lipp.*

   –with a dry mucus, larynx were—*Coff.*

Crawling in upper part of—*Nux m.*

   –in larynx—*Con., Sabin.*

Crumb were in larynx—*Tril.*

Crushed, sides of larynx were—*Brom.*

Cutting in larynx, knife were—*Manc.*

Dagger buried in right lung—*Chin. b.*

Deep enough into lungs, he could not get—*Caps.*

Denuded, larynx were—*Acon.*

Depressed by diaphragm, lungs were—*Carb. ac.*

Die from suffocative attacks, she will—*Tub.*

Diminished, caliber of larynx were—*Euphr.*

Discharge in middle lobe of right lung, some fluid wanted to—*Tell.*

—fluid from right lung into duodenum, wanted to—*Chen. v.*

Dislodged, something low down in trachea which must be—*Sin.*

Down were in larynx—*Phos. ac., Sulph.*

—were tickling in trachea—*Calc. c.*

Draw a long breath, not able to—*Rhus t.*

Drawing on a thread in larynx, from front backwards, one were —*Calc. ar.*

Drawn shut, larynx were—*Am. c.*

—together as far as pit of stomach, air passages were—*Sep.*

—through bronchi, rough cord were—*Anan.*

—around trachea, a cord were—*Cham.*

—apart, lung were violently—*Elaps*

—to right side, left lung were—*Med.*

—up in hand and then let loose, left lung were—*Med.*

—tight around right lung, a rubber band were—*Culx.*

—down when standing, lungs were—*Am. c.*

Drop of liquid had entered trachea—*Gels.*

Dry, inspired air were very—*Stann.*

—spot in larynx—*Crot. h.*

—mucous membranes were too—*Laur.*

—in evening, lungs were—*Kali bi.*

Dust, one had inhaled—*Bell., Mar.*

—in throat and lungs—*Calc. c.*

—in lungs—*Calc. c., Hep.*

—inhaling—*Ars., Ign., Ip.*

—he had swallowed—*Ferr. ma.*

—in air—*Ars.*

—in larynx—*Calc. s.*

—in trachea—*Chel., Ferr. ma.*

—or feather-down tickling in trachea—*Calc. c., Mar.*

—in trachea and throat and behind sternum—*Chel.*

Eaten rancid fat, causing cough, he had—*Eupi.*

Effort to relieve himself by expelling air from his lungs, he made a sudden—*Ox. ac.*

Empty, upper part of left lung to axilla were—*Iris fœ.*
Enlarged, bronchial tubes were—*Med.*
Enough air into cells, he could not get—*Crot. t.*
Escaped from lungs into pleural cavity, air—*Chlor.*
Ether, inhaling—*Glon.*
Eviscerated, lungs were—*Phos.*
Excites cough, sulphur vapor—*Ars., Carb. v.*
Exciting cough, something in pit of stomach were—*Bell.*
Exhalation, something in chest prevented—*Dros.*
Exhausted of air, room had been—*Nux v., Plan.*
Expand, lungs had no room to—*Carl., Nat. m.*
   –lungs could not—*Chr. ac., Crot. h., Laur.*
   –root of lung could not—*Chr. ac.*
Expanded, lungs could not be—*Asaf.*
Expiration were prevented by talking or coughing—*Dros.*
Exploded in right lung, awakening him from sleep, something
     were—*Helod.*
Failed her, causing weakness, respiration—*Plat.*
Fallen into trachea with whistling in throat, something had
     —*Aloe*
Falling, with sudden pain in left lung—*Form.*
Fanning a blistering sore in lungs, her breath were—*Med.*
Fast to chest, especially when writing, lungs were—*Lac c.*
Fatigued by respiration, he were greatly—*Senec.*
Fat, causing cough, he had eaten rancid—*Eupi.*
Feather in larynx—*Dros., Lyc.*
   –larynx were tickled with a—*Lyc.*
   –dust or feather-down tickling in trachea—*Calc. c.*
   –swaying to and fro in bronchi—*Rumx.*
   –in upper bronchi, tickled with—*Laur.*
Feathers in throat—*Calc. c.*
   –he were inspiring—*Ign.*
Filled with burning air, cavity in upper part of lungs were—*Med.*
   –with cold air or ice—*Corn. a.*
   –with foreign body, larynx were—*Arg. m.*
   –with mucus, respiratory organs were—*Cop.*
   –with mucus, bronchi were—*Cupr.*
   –with thick tenacious mucus, bronchi—*Chlf.*
   –with a plug, larynx were—*Ant. c.*
Filling up, lungs were—*Lycps.*
Film, trachea were closed by a—*Mang.*

Fire, lungs were on—*Pyrog.*

Foreign substance obstructing larynx—*Lach.*

 —substance in larynx—*Ptel., Tril.*

 —substance, soft, in larynx—*Dros.*

 —body in larynx—*Bell., Cop., Cub., Ptel.*

 —body, small, in larynx with desire to swallow—*Calc. f.*

 —body, larynx were filled or stopped with—*Arg. m.*

 —body were lying over larynx—*Ign.*

 —body in windpipe—*Brom.*

Fluid were bubbling in middle lobe of right lung and wanted to discharge—*Tell.*

Fluttering during cough, something in lungs were loose and—*Phos.*

Formication in lungs—*Sapon.*

Forced asunder, larynx were—*Kali ar.*

Forcing its way into finest vessel of lungs, blood were—*Zinc.*

Full of blood, lungs were—*Trif. p.*

 —of mucus, lungs were—*Med.*

 —of smoke, air passages were—*Brom.*

 —of smoke, lungs were—*Bar. c., Coff.*

 —of smoke of paper burning, lungs were—*Coff.*

Fullness of trachea as if from chest—*Lob.*

Fumes—see also SULPHUR and VAPOR.

 —he had inhaled sulphur—*Lyc., Puls.*

 —he were inspiring sulphur—*Ign.*

 —in larynx, sulphur—*Camph., Ip., Par.*

 —sulphur in trachea—*Bry.*

 —of a burning match causing desire to cough—*Aml. n.*

Fur, larynx were lined with—*Phos.*

Get breath, he could not—*Calc. c., Rumx., Spong.*

 —breath after warm drinks, he could not—*Phos.*

Girdle, tight, hindered breathing—*Chel.*

Granulated, larynx were—*Kali i.*

Grasped firmly, trachea were—*Phyt.*

Grating in chest on deep inspiration—*Eup. pur.*

Grown together in suffocative attacks, parts were—*Dig.*

Hæmorrhage from left lung would follow—*Hydrs.*

Hæmoptysis would follow—*Sep.*

Hair in larynx—*Naja*

 —in trachea—*Naja, Sil.*

Hangs in larynx, a string of mucus—*Osm.*

Hanging loose in larynx, a piece of flesh were—*Phos.*
Hard, right lung and liver were small and—*Abies c.*
Hard mass collected in lungs—*Stict.*
Hindered by clothes, breathing were—*Lach.*
Holding the breath—*Dros.*
Hooks, little, in larynx (sometimes below)—*All. c.*
Ice or cold air, filled with—*Corn. a.*
   —water rising and falling through cylindrical opening in left
      lung after drinking—*Elaps*
Impeded in trachea, breath would be—*Laur.*
Impediment existed deep in chest—*Dig.*
Impurities, trachea were loaded with—*Trif. p.*
Inflamed, larynx were—*Bell.*
Inflated, lungs remained partly—*Euph. amyg.*
Inhaled air did not reach pit of stomach—*Prun.*
   —smoke or pitch—*Bar. c., Nat. a.*
   —hot steam, he had—*Med.*
   —dust, one had—*Bell., Mar.*
   —peppermint, he had—*Sanic.*
   —sulphur fumes, he had—*Lyc., Puls.*
Inhaling dust—*Ars., Ign., Ip.*
   —ether—*Glon.*
Inspire enough air, he cannot—*Bry., Meli.*
Inspired air were cold—*Cor. r., Lith.*
Inspiring fumes, he were—*Ign.*
Interrupted breathing, something suddenly ran from neck to
      larynx and—*Lach.*
Jarred on coughing, whole chest were—*Chlor.*
Kept air in chest, something—*Dros.*
Knife were cutting in larynx—*Manc.*
   —thrust into top of left lung—*Sep.*
Knives were stitching in lungs—*Iris fœ.*
   —two, going toward each other in abdomen when coughing—
      Kali c.
Large, lungs were too—*Mag. s.*
Last, each breath would be the—*Dig.*
Leaf, trachea were closed with—*Mang.*
   —small, obstructed windpipe on hawking—*Ant. t.*
Leave her on lying down, breath would—*Lac c.*
Lid in larynx—*Phyt.*
Liquid had entered trachea, a drop of—*Gels.*

Lined with fur, larynx were—*Phos.*
Load on upper part of lungs, she had a—*Ars.*
  –on upper part of both lungs, she had a—*Cupr. ac.*
Loaded with impurities, trachea were—*Trif. p.*
Lodged in upper larynx, apple-seed cell were—*Bry.*
Loose and fluttering in lungs during cough, something were—
     Phos.
  –on riding, lungs were—*Caj.*
  –in brain when coughing, something tore—*Sep.*
  –in trachea, ball were rolling—*Chen. a.*
  –in larynx, a piece of flesh were hanging—*Phos.*
  –left lung were drawn up in hand and then let—*Med.*
Loosened from pleura when lying, lungs were—*Caust.*
  –during respiration, something would be—*Raph.*
Lose her breath if she cannot expectorate, she would—*Sep.*
  –his breath, he would sink together and—*Sep.*
Loss of breath, awakens from—*Kali c., Lach., Sep.*
Lump in upper part of larynx—*Kali bi.*
  –in larynx—*Lob., Med.*
  –behind larynx—*Ust.*
  –the size of walnut were sticking behind larynx—*Coc. c.*
  –of phlegm moving up and down in windpipe on coughing—
    Calc. c.
  –rose up to meet food and obstructed it—*Lob.*
Lying over larynx, foreign body were—*Ign.*
Mass, hard, collected in lungs—*Stict.*
Membrane, tough, were moved about by cough—*Kali c.*
  –prevented breathing—*Kali c.*
Moved painfully up and down, right lung—*Æsc.*
  –in a wave, left lung—*Dulc.*
Moving in bronchi, plug of mucus were—*Coc. c.*
  –up and down in larynx, a plug were—*Lach.*
  –up and down in windpipe on coughing, lump of phlegm were
    —*Calc. c.*
Mucus would cause suffocation—*Calad.*
  –respiratory passages were filled with—*Cop.*
  –larynx were covered with dry—*Coff.*
  –hangs in larynx, a string of—*Osm.*
  –were adhering tightly to larynx—*Alum.*
  –in trachea which he cannot get up—*Rhod.*
  –bronchi were filled with—*Cupr.*

Mucus—*Continued*
  –bronchi were filled with thick tenacious—*Chlor.*
  –lungs were full of—*Lyc.*
  –tenacious, in lungs—*Crot. t.*
  –obstructed lungs—*Nux m.*
  –passages were lined with thick stiff—*Sang. n.*
Nail pressing in larynx—*Spong.*
Narrowed, larynx were—*Eug.*
Narrower, larynx and trachea were—*Spong.*
Obstructed by a small leaf, trachea were—*Ant. t.*
  –larynx were partly—*Arum d.*
  –larynx, foreign substance—*Lach.*
  –by mucus, lungs were—*Nux m.*
  –lungs were—*Kali i., Nat. ar., Phos.*
Overworked, lungs had been—*Lyc.*
Oppressed by a heavy weight, lungs were—*Nat. ar.*
Paper burning in lungs, smoke of—*Coff.*
Paralysis of diaphragm oppressed respiration—*Stach.*
Paralyzed, lungs were—*Phos.*
Pass through in larynx, air could not—*Chel.*
Passed into glands of neck on breathing, air—*Spong.*
Passing through passages were icy cold, air—*Cor. r.*
Pepper, red, were throughout nostrils and air passages—*Seneg.*
Peppermint, he had inhaled—*Sanic.*
  –he had been chewing—*Spire.*
  –were burning in larynx—*Elaps*
Phlegm were rattling in lungs, a large quantity of—*Phos.*
  –viscid, in larynx—*Par.*
Piano notes vibrated in larynx—*Calc. c.*
Piece of lung would come out—*Mag. s.*
Pieces when coughing, head would fly to—*Bry., Caps.*
Plug were moving up and down in larynx—*Lach.*
  –in trachea—*Lach.*
  –of mucus were moving in chest—*Coc. c.*
  –sticking in larynx—*Spong.*
  –throat were filled with—*Ant. c.*
  –in region of cricoid cartilage from current of air; feels bruised
      when pressed upon—*Arg. m.*
Pneumonia, he were in first stages of—*Trif. p.*
Pressed up into throat, lungs were—*Lach.*
  –against spine, lungs were—*Laur.*

25

Pressed—*Continued*

  –back against lungs, ribs were—*Iris*

  –back against œsophagus, larynx were—*Chel.*

Pressing windpipe between thumb and finger, someone were—*Lach.*

  –in larynx, a nail were—*Spong.*

Pressure when lying on back with head forward, larynx were closed by—*Ol. an.*

Prevented exhalation when talking or coughing, something in chest—*Dros.*

Pushed back to spine, lungs were—*Seneg.*

Putrid, expired air smelled—*Chr. ac.*

Raise a great deal, she wants to—*Bapt.*

  –blood any minute, he might—*Rumx.*

  –almost anything when coughing, she would—*Senec.*

  –phlegm, did not reach low enough to—*Rumx.*

Ran suddenly from neck to larynx and interrupted breathing, something—*Lach.*

Rancid fat, he had eaten, causing cough—*Eupi.*

Rattling in lungs, a large quantity of phlegm were—*Phos.*

Raw, whole larynx were—*Chlor.*

  –lungs were—*Aral., Carb. v., Chl... s., Kali bi., Phos.*

Removed, larynx and trachea were—*Spong.*

Respiration were impeded in trachea—*Laur.*

  –whole attention must be centered on act of—*Chlor.*

Rested against back when coughing, lungs—*Sulph.*

Rising from pit of stomach into larynx, ball were—*Kali ar.*

  –and falling through cylindrical opening in left lung, ice water were—*Elaps*

Rivet from upper part of left lung to scapula, there were a—*Sulph.*

Rolling loose in trachea, ball were—*Chen. a.*

Rose in larynx threatening respiration, something—*Con.*

  –to meet food and obstructed it, a lump—*Lob.*

  –through trachea in waves, air—*Lyc.*

Rubber band were drawn tight around right lung—*Culx.*

Ruffling, painful, of lungs—*Gad.*

Ruptured, inner and lower third of right lung were—*Chlor.*

Scraping in epiglottis—*Bell., Lach., Osm., Puls.*

  –in glottis after heartburn—*Nux v.*

Seized by talons, windpipe were—*Ind.*

Shut, larynx were drawn—*Am. c.*

Sink together and lose his breath, he would—*Sep.*

Sinking down, lower lobe of left lung were—*Bad.*

Skin in larynx—*Lach., Phos., Thuj.*

Small and hard, right lung and liver were—*Abies c.*

Smoke, air passages were full of—*Brom.*

  —lungs were full of—*Bar. c., Coff.*

  —of paper burning, lungs were full of—*Coff.*

  —or pitch, inspiring—*Bar. c., Nat. ar.*

  —in larynx, inspired oily—*Bar. c.*

Smother, he would—*Ars., Arum t., Coloc.*

Smothering—*Iodof., Meli.*

  —on falling asleep—*Am. c., Ant. t., Aur., Bad., Carb. an., Carb. v., Dig., Graph., Grin., Lach., Op., Ran. b.*

  —before cough—*Cor. r.*

  —before expectoration—*Ail.*

  —him when lying down, something behind trachea were—***Ter.***

Soft substance were in trachea—*Dros.*

Softened, entire parenchyma of lungs were—*Lyc.*

Solidified, lungs were—*Ery. a.*

Something were in larynx—*Ferr., Sulph.*

  —came from larynx when coughing—*Raph.*

  —were in pit of stomach exciting cough—*Bell.*

  —low down in trachea which must be dislodged—*Sin.*

  —in trachea that might be raised but cannot—*Lach.*

Space enough, windpipe had not—*Cist.*

Spasm, breath were stopped by a—*Sars.*

Splinter in larynx—*Arg. n.*

Split, when coughing, head would—*Calc. c.*

Sponge, breathing through—*Spong.*

  —in throat, breathing through—*Brom.*

Stagnated in upper part of lungs—*Seneg.*

Steam, he had inhaled hot—*Med.*

Sticking in larynx, something were—*Raph.*

  —behind larynx, lump size of walnut were—*Coc. c.*

  —below larynx, something were—*Eupi.*

  —in larynx, plug were—*Spong.*

  —in larynx, talons were—*Lach.*

Stitching of knives in lungs—*Iris fœ.*

Stone in trachea—*Sanic.*

Stop, breathing would—*Apis*

Stoppage in trachea—*Sol. t. æ.*
Stopped, larynx were—*Cur., Verb.*
  –up larynx, foreign body—*Arg. m.*
  –right half of larynx were—*Prim.*
  –by a spasm, breath were—*Sars.*
  –at pit of stomach, breath were—*Rhus t.*
  –between scapulæ, breath remained—*Calc. c.*
Stopper in larynx——*Spong.*
Strained after coughing, lungs were—*Calc. s.*
Streaming through air passages, cold air were—*Cor. r.*
Stretched across larynx, something were—*Meny.*
Stuck together, air cells were—*Ail.*
Stuffed with cotton, lungs were—*Kali bi., Med.*
  –larynx were—*Naja, Nat. ar.*
Substance, soft, were in trachea—*Dros.*
Suffocate, one would—*Calc. ar., Cham., Cupr., Ferr., Hep.,*
    Lach., Lact., Lyss., Rhus t., Verat. a.
  –when going to sleep, he were about to—*Graph.*
  –after coughing, he would—*Tab.*
  –he were about to—*Vesp.*
Suffocated from sulphur vapors—*Brom.*
  –with cough, she would be—*Syph.*
Suffocating—*Ars., Der., Dig., Dirc., Guai., Hydr. ac., Tarent.,*
    Tub.
  –at night, runs to window to breathe—*Arg. n.*
Suffocation, someone constricted larynx causing—*Caust.*
  –mucus would cause—*Calad.*
Sulphur vapors in air passages—*Ars.*
  –vapors in larynx—*Camph., Ip., Par.*
  –vapors suddenly caused constriction of larynx—*Mosch.*
  –vapors in larynx excites cough—*Ars., Carb. v.*
  –fumes in trachea—*Bry.*
  –fumes, he had inhaled—*Lyc., Puls.*
Support abdomen when coughing, he must—*Con.*
Survive for want of air, he could not long—*Apis*
Swallowed dust, he had—*Ferr. ma.*
Swaying to and fro in bronchia, feather were—*Rumx.*
Swelling, larynx were—*Lyc.*
Swollen in larynx—*Hydr. ac., Iod.*
  –mucous membrane of throat were—*Samb.*
  –trachea were—*Chel.*

Take a deep breath, he must—*Card. m., Fl. ac.*

Taken away from riding rapidly downhill, breath would be—*Bor.*

Talons were sticking in larynx—*Lach.*

–windpipe were seized by—*Ind.*

Tear bronchi, cough would—*Cub.*

Tearing away from lung, something were—*Nit. ac.*

Thickened, mucous membrane of bronchi were—*Kali bi.*

Thread, lungs were tied with—*Kali m.*

–in larynx from front backwards, one were drawing on a—*Calc. ar.*

Threads, lungs were constricted with fine—*Kali chl.*

Thrust into top of left lung, knife were—*Sep.*

Tickled with a feather, larynx were—*Lyc.*

–with a feather in upper bronchi—*Laur.*

Tickling in air passages would provoke cough—*Rhus t.*

–in larynx were caused by down—*Sulph.*

–soreness in trachea—*Stann.*

–in trachea from dust or feather-down—*Calc. c.*

Tied with a thread, lungs were—*Kali m.*

–up in bundles, lungs were constricted and—*Dig.*

Tight, lungs were too—*Nat. m.*

–around right lung, rubber band were drawn—*Culx.*

Tore loose in brain when coughing, something—*Sep.*

Torn to pieces, larynx were—*Med.*

–by a broken rib on walking fast, lungs were—*Naja*

–when coughing, larynx would be—*All. c.*

–off larynx, mucous membranes were—*Med.*

–off larynx with every cough, mucous membranes were—*Osm.*

–loose during inspiration, something were—*Berb.*

–out on coughing, lungs were—*Elaps*

–loose in larynx on coughing, something were being—*Calc. c.*

Turned over, lungs—*Ang.*

Ulcer were in larynx—*Bell., Kali bi., Nat. m.*

Ulcers, small, were in larynx—*Nit. ac.*

Ulcerated, larynx were—*Med.*

–surfaces in lungs in contact when breathing—*Iod.*

Ulceration in larynx—*Kali bi.*

Valve or stopper in larynx—*Spong.*

Vapor in trachea causing cough—*Bry.*

Vapors, dry, irritating, caused choking—*Crot. h.*
  –breathing sulphur—*Ip., Kali m., Meph.*
  –of sulphur constricting larynx—*Mosch.*
  –of sulphur in trachea—*Par.*
  –of sulphur, suffocated from—*Brom.*
  –of sulphur, suffocative fits from—*Mosch.*
  –in trachea caused cough—*Bry.*
  –hot, rising from trachea—*Ferr.*
Vibrated in larynx, notes of piano—*Calc. c.*
Want of air, he could not long survive for—*Apis*
  –of air, breathing difficult as from—*Trades.*
Warmer than usual, expired air were—*Coc. c.*
Water flowing into windpipe, quantity of—*Spig.*
  –ice, rising and falling through cylindrical opening in left lung
      after drinking—*Elaps*
Waves, left lung moved in—*Dulc.*
  –air rose through trachea in—*Lyc.*
Wedge in larynx in morning—*Caust.*
Weight in lungs—*Merc.*
  –oppression on lungs from a heavy—*Nat. ar.*
Wet, trachea were (sensation passes downward)—*Pen.*
Whizzing in larynx from movement of blood—*Arg. n.*
Wide enough, chest were not—*Euph.*
  –on breathing, air passages were too—*Acon.*
Wire, left lung were constricted by—*Asar.*
Withheld on talking or coughing, air were—*Dros.*

HEART AND CIRCULATION

Aching from sorrow, heart were—*Pyrus*

Action, no action in—*Asaf.*

–of heart were being interfered with—*Mit.*

Aglow in veins, blood were—*Agar.*

Air, lack of—*Vib.*

Alive in heart, something were—*Cyc.*

–running in heart, something were—*Cyc.*

–struggling about the heart, something were—*Cast. eq.*

Artery were pulsating on upper surface of heart while walking —*Coc. c.*

Ascending to throat, heart were—*Podo.*

Band, heart were restricted by an iron—*Cact.*

–narrow, encircling body and lying upon heart—*Phos.*

Bands tightly drawn around it, heart were hanging by—*Kali c.*

–about the heart—*Lyss.*

Bar were pressing in region of heart—*Bell.*

–were lying transversely across region of heart, extending to right side—*Hæm.*

Beat violently, pulse—*Coc. c.*

–heart could not—*Asaf.*

–heart had not room enough to—*Cact.*

–felt all over head—*Parth.*

–heart were bound together and could not—*Asaf., Ether., Lach.*

–would tear it off, heart were hanging by a thread and—*Lach.*

–intermitted a single—*Lach.*

Beating from above downward, heart were—*Crot. c.*

–on dorsal spine, heart were—*Carb. s.*

–conscious of—*Sin.*

–all arteries were—*Saba.*

–hard, yet it could hardly be discovered, heart were—*Phys.*

–if she moved, heart would stop—*Dig.*

–of heart were louder—*Cupr. s.*

–heart were overloaded with—*Lil. t.*

–in the heart, all pulses were—*Paraf.*

–on retching > eructations < lying—*Luna*

–would stop—*Onos.*

–heart had stopped—*Aster., Cic., Lach., Pyrus*

Beating—*Continued*

—stopped, then started suddenly—*Conv.*

—stopped for a while, then a hard thump—*Aur.*

—after waking at midnight, heart had almost stopped—*Sac. lac.*

—in water, heart were—*Sumb.*

Beats of heart were felt through whole thorax—*Olnd.*

Belching, something in heart prevented—*Calc. ar.*

Bird, wounded, fluttered in heart—*Stry.*

Bird's wings fluttering in heart—*Cact.*

Blood would go to heart, all—*Puls.*

—went to heart, all blood—*Lil. t.*

—in heart, too much—*Pyrog.*

—all parts contained large amounts of—*Æsc.*

—were boiling in body—*Aur., Chim. mac., Kali c.*

—boiling hot in arteries—*Ars.*

—were boiling hot in veins—*Med.*

—ceased to flow into head—*Seneg.*

—had ceased to circulate—*Gels.*

—in head could not circulate—*Bar. c.*

—circulated hot through vessels—*Rhus t.*

—circulated rapidly and violently—*Tab.*

—all parts contained large amounts of—*Æsc.*

—were cold water—*Verat. a.*

—difficult for blood to get in or out of heart—*Helod.*

—distended arteries—*Daph. o.*

—were dissolved—*Crot. h.*

—were flowing backward—*Elaps*

—merely gurgling through heart—*Spig.*

—would be jerked out of veins—*Nux v.*

—heart were overloaded with—*Lil. t.*

—in region of heart, there were too much—*Cyc.*

—had suddenly been retained in one of the large veins of the neck—*Tell.*

—were running cold through veins—*Pyrog., Rhus t.*

—rush of blood, especially on ascending—*Sulph.*

—rushed from heart to chest and would burst out above—*Spong.*

—were rushing to heart and then head—*Nux m.*

—were shut up in heart—*Lil. t.*

—stagnated in arteries—*Carl.*

—could scarcely struggle through veins—*Zinc. s.*

—heart were swimming in blood or water—*Bufo*

Blood—*Continued*

  —were too thick to circulate—*Pyrus*

  —were as thin as paper—*Bell.*

  —were transparent—*Bell.*

  —turned into ice water—*Abies c.*

Blow in heart—*Agar., Carl.*

  —heavy, or thump in the heart—*Ovi g. p.*

Boiling, blood were—*Aur., Chim. mac., Kali c.*

  —and bubbling around heart—*Lachn.*

  —hot in arteries, blood were—*Ars.*

  —hot in veins, blood were—*Med.*

  —in body, blood were—*Kali c.*

Bolts were holding heart—*Cact.*

Bound down or hadn't room enough to beat, heart were—*Cact.*

  —together and could not beat, heart were—*Asaf., Ether., Lach.*

Breaking away about heart, something were—*Apis*

  —through back < leaning back in chair, heart were—*Chin. a.*

Broken, heart were—*Nat. m., Ol. an.*

  —out or torn away, walls of chest anterior to heart were—*Cere. b.*

Bruised, region of heart were—*Arn.*

  —at base of heart—*Arn.*

Bubble or lump started from heart and forced through arteries—*Nat. p.*

Bubbling in region of the—*Lach., Lyc.*

  —and boiling around the—*Lachn.*

Bubbles were forcing through arteries—*Nat. p.*

Burst, heart would—*Asaf., Ether., Kalm., Lyss., Sac. lac.*

  —heart and veins would—*Am. c.*

  —at night, heart and veins would—*Am. c.*

  —out above, blood rushed from heart to chest and would—*Spong.*

Bursting about heart, sudden spasmodic—*Zinc.*

  —feeling, heart with a—*Med.*

Cap over heart—*Zinc.*

Cavities of the body, heart filled all the—*Sep.*

Cavity where the heart ought to be—*Med.*

Ceased beating, heart had—*Aster., Cic., Lach., Pyrus*

  —to circulate, blood had—*Gels.*

  —in limbs, circulation had—*Lyc.*

  —on the outer side of thigh, circulation had—*Thea*

Ceased—*Continued*
  –to flow into head, blood—*Seneg.*
  –then gave one hard thump, heart—*Aur.*
Circulate in head, blood could not—*Bar. c.*
  –blood had ceased to—*Gels.*
  –blood were too thick to—*Pyrus*
Circulated hot through vessels, blood—*Rhus t.*
  –rapidly and violently, blood—*Tab.*
Circulating more quickly than usual, blood were—*Ment. pu.*
Circulation after constriction of leg were removed, starting of
  —*Vib.*
Claw, iron, grasping the heart—*Lach.*
Cloud, a heavy, weighed down on her heart—*Cimic.*
Clutched, heart were—*Cact.*
Cold in heart—*Graph., Helod., Kali bi., Kali chl., Kali n., Nat. m.,
  Petr.*
  –about the heart from mental exertion—*Nat. m.*
  –through veins, blood were running—*Pyrog., Rhus t.*
  –water, blood were—*Verat. a.*
Coldness in blood vessels—*Acon., Ant. t.*
Compression about heart—*Agar., Bufo, Tarent.*
Confusion about heart—*Dig.*
Congested, capillary circulation were—*Pop.*
Constricted, heart were being—*Bufo, Glon.*
Constriction in and about heart—*Arn., Bufo, Iod., Lil. t., Nux m.*
  –starting of circulation after constriction of leg were removed
  —*Vib.*
  –violent in heart—*Nat. m.*
Contracted, heart were being—*Glon.*
Corroded, heart were—*Eup. per.*
Crawling about the heart—*Canth., Nux v.*
  –below the heart—*Abrot.*
  –in veins like tightening up of parts—*Tril.*
Crowbar were pressed tightly from right to left breast and
  twisted a knot around heart which stopped it—*Tab.*
Crushed, heart were being—*Spig.*
Crushing about heart—*Ol. an.*
Cutting up and down in heart, knife were—*Lac d.*
  –about heart, knives were—*Sulph.*
Dagger-stroke in heart region—*Gins.*

Difficult for blood to get in or out of heart—*Helod.*
Dilated, heart were—*Stann.*
  –heart vessels were—*Kali i.*
Dipped into a liquid, heart were—*Crot. c.*
Dissolved, blood were—*Crot. h.*
Distended or swelled to fill chest, heart were—*Cench.*
  –with blood, arteries were—*Daph. o.*
Drawing in heart region—*Cact., Calc. ac., Canth., Chr. ox., Croc., Ferr., Meny., Olnd., Phel.*
Drawn up together, heart and ovary were—*Naja*
Driven to part touched with magnet, blood were—*Mag. p. Arct.*
Drowned in water, heart were—*Bufo*
Dying with weakness of heart—*Merc.*
Electric shock in heart—*Sep.*
  –shocks from heart to front of neck—*Graph.*
  –wires, pains traveled on, starting from left side and returning
      to left side—*Samars.*
Encircling body and lying upon heart, narrow band were—*Phos.*
Enlarged, heart were—*Cench., Med., Pyrog., Sulph.*
Faint, he would—*Sulph.*
Fall down, heart would—*Hyper.*
Falling suddenly from above toward middle, heart were—*Arg. n.*
Fell into abdomen, heart—*Cench.*
Filled the chest, heart—*Cench.*
  –with lead, blood vessels were—*Nabalus*
  –blood vessels were over—*Guaj.*
Fire were in heart region—*Sac. lac.*
Flopped over, heart fluttered and—*Tub.*
Floundered, heart—*Gins.*
Flow into head, blood ceased to—*Seneg.*
Flowing backward, blood were—*Elaps*
Fluid, hot, were running through vessels—*Vib.*
Fluttered and flopped over, heart—*Tub.*
  –in heart, wounded bird—*Stry.*
Fluttering of heart—*Tub.*
  –in region of heart—*Laur.*
  –below cardiac region—*Calad.*
  –in pit of stomach—*Nux v.*
  –of bird's wing in—*Cact.*
Food remained in region of heart—*Acon.*

Force out upward from surging into chest, heart would—*Spong.*
Forced out upward, heart would be—*Spong.*
 –itself out, heart would—*Apoc.*
 –toward the heart, something were—*Coc. c.*
 –through arteries, a bubble or lump started from heart and—
    Nat. p.
Forcing through arteries, bubble were—*Nat. p.*
Fright, palpitations came from—*Nat. p.*
Frogs, a dozen, leaped about the heart, then heart missed every
    fourth beat—*Tab.*
Full, heart were too—*Asaf.*
 –of blood, heart were too—*Pyrog.*
 –and swollen, heart were too—*Asaf.*
 –and wants to get away from it, heart were too—*Iod.*
 –of quicksilver, veins were—*Raph.*
Glowing in veins, blood were—*Agar.*
Grasped, heart were—*Cact., Lil. t.*
 –by a hand, heart were—*Cact., Dig., Lil. t., Nux m.*
 –with an iron hand, heart were—*Cact., Iod.*
 –the heart, something—*Nux m.*
 –violently and relaxed alternately, heart were—*Lil. t.*
Grasping the heart, iron claw were—*Lach.*
 –at base of heart, hand were—*Iod.*
Grown too fast, heart had—*Rhus t.*
 –fast, heart had—*Phos.*
Gurgling through heart, blood were merely—*Spig.*
Hand grasping at the base of the heart—*Iod.*
 –heart were grasped by an iron—*Cact., Iod.*
Hanging by a thread and every beat would tear it off—*Lach.*
 –by tightly drawn bands, heart were—*Kali c.*
Hard substance extending from heart region to stomach—*Nat. c.*
Heat in heart—*Sul. i.*
Heated, blood were—*Chim. mac.*
Heavy, heart were—*Ovi g. p.*
 –weighted heart down, something—*Cham., Ovi g. p., Sac. lac.*
Hollow in region of heart—*Croc., Graph., Sulph.*
Hornets, swarms of, going from pectoral region to head—*Cact.*
Hot in veins, blood were boiling—*Med.*
 –in arteries, blood were boiling—*Ars.*
 –through vessels, blood circulated—*Rhus t.*
 –water in blood vessels—*Sin., Syph.*

Hung by a thread, heart were—*Lyc.*

Hurt, heart were—*Cham.*

Ice water, blood had turned into—*Abies c.*

Impeded, heart action were—*Grat.*

Impediment in region of heart—*Mez.*

Iron, hot, had been run into the chest and heavy weight were put on it—*Naja*

Jerked out of veins, blood would be—*Nux v.*

  —suddenly shut, valves of heart were—*Alumn.*

Jumped out of its place, heart suddenly—*Merc. i. f.*

Jumping, heart were—*Thyroid.*

Knife were cutting up and down in apex of heart—*Lac d.*

  —were piercing heart > pressure—*Lepi.*

  —a dull-pointed knife were drawn slowly through heart—*Spig.*

  —were stabbing in arteries with burning—*Card. b.*

Knives were cutting about the heart—*Sulph.*

Knocked together, heart and knees were—*Nat. m.*

Knot, crowbar twisted a knot around the heart which stopped it—*Tab.*

Laced, heart were tightly—*Merl.*

Large, heart were—*Med.*

  —heart were too—*Bov., Bufo, Lach., Med., Pyrog., Sulph.*

  —heart were too large for containing cavity—*Lach., Sulph.*

  —heart were enormously, with oppression of chest—*Bov.*

Lay on heart region causing tension, something—*Gins.*

Lead, blood vessels were filled with—*Nabalus*

Leaped about heart, a dozen frogs—*Tab.*

Lesion, there must be fatal organic heart—*Pop.*

Lightness at heart—*Chr. ac.*

Liquid, heart were dipped into a—*Crot. c.*

Lump or bubble started from heart and forced through the arteries —*Nat. p.*

  —throbbing inside the heart—*Cupr. s.*

Lying transversely across region of heart, extending to right side, bar were—*Hæm.*

Marble were pressing from epigastrium to heart—*Kalm.*

Misfortune had happened causing oppression about the heart—*Tarent.*

Moved, heart would stop beating if she—*Dig.*

  —heart were swung by a thin thread and moved back and forth —*Tub.*

Moving in cardiac region, reptile were—*Cact.*

Narrow on left and smaller than right, heart were too—*Ovi g. p.*

Needle were crosswise in ventricles and pricked at each contraction—*Iber.*

Needles were pricking in heart—*Lyss., Manc.*

 —were pricking in region of heart—*Asc. t.*

 —were running into heart—*Lyss.*

Nerve were tense in precordial region—*Sep.*

Noise from escaping steam in carotid artery on turning head—*Sulph.*

Numb, heart feels—*Ovi g. p.*

Occupied body, heart had—*Sep.*

Ovary and heart were drawn together—*Naja*

Overloaded with blood, heart were—*Lil. t.*

Pains traveled on fine electric wires starting left side of heart and returning to left side—*Samars.*

Palpitations in pit of stomach—*Med.*

Paper, blood were as thin as—*Bell.*

Piercing the heart, knife were, > pressure—*Lepi.*

Place, heart were in too small a—*Eup. per.*

Poked with a finger, heart were—*Jac.*

Pressed against side of chest and had not room enough—*Lach.*

 —down, heart were—*Ars., Cham.*

 —down, heart would be—*Carb. v.*

 —down with suppressed menses, heart would be—*Cham.*

Pressing against heart, something were—*Eup. per.*

 —from epigastrium to heart, marble were—*Kalm.*

 —in region of heart, bar were—*Bell.*

Pressure came from abdomen and compressed heart—*Nat. m.*

 —upon a nerve in heart—*Nat. m.*

Prevented belching, something in heart—*Calc. ar.*

Pricked at each contraction, needle were crosswise in ventricle and—*Iber.*

Pulled up suddenly and let go again, heart were—*Mag. c.*

Pulling backward or to the right by a string, heart were—*Arg. n.*

Pulsating on upper surface of heart while walking, artery were—*Coc. c.*

Pumping cold water, heart were—*Pyrog.*

Purring or thrilling over cardiac region—*Spig.*

 —noise in region of heart—*Glon.*

Quicksilver, veins were full of—*Raph.*

Quivering in heart—*Med.*

Relaxed, heart were grasped violently and relaxed alternately—*Lil. t.*

Reptile from before backward in left cardiac region, annoying movement of—*Cact.*

Restricted by a band of iron, heart were—*Cact.*

Retain blood, vessels had no power to—*Crot. h.*

Retained in one large vein, blood had suddenly been—*Tell.*

Rise to throat, heart would—*Glon.*

Rising into throat, heart were—*Caust., Podo.*

Rolling through arteries, shot were—*Nat. p.*

Room enough, heart had not—*Helod., Sulph.*
   –enough to beat, heart bound down or had not—*Cact.*
   –enough, heart were pressed against side of chest and had not—*Lach.*

Rubbed against ribs on breathing, heart were—*Cann. i.*

Running in heart, something alive were—*Cyc.*
   –cold through veins, blood were—*Pyrog., Rhus t.*
   –through veins, cold water were—*Rhus t.*
   –through veins, hot water were—*Ars., Rhus t.*
   –through veins all night long, hot water or oil were—*Syph.*
   –palpitation came from—*Cot.*

Rupture in precordial region—*Guare.*

Ruptured in heart region—*Guare.*
   –cardia were—*Calend.*

Rush of blood on ascending—*Sulph.*

Rushed from heart to chest and would burst out above, blood—*Spong.*

Rushing to heart then head, blood were—*Nux m.*

Scraping in the heart—*Rhus t.*

Screwed up in heart—*Atrop.*
   –together, heart were—*Naja*

Shock, heart had a—*Arn.*
   –electric, from heart to neck—*Graph.*

Shocks in heart region—*Arn., Glon., Phyt., Tab.*

Shot, heart were—*Lil. sup.*
   –were rolling through arteries—*Nat. p.*

Shut up in heart, blood were—*Lil. t.*
   –suddenly, valves of heart were jerked—*Alumn.*

Sickness in heart—*Cann. i., Lycps.*

Side, heart were on the right—*Bor., Sin.*

Sinking in heart region—*Jatr., Tarax.*
Small a place, heart were in too—*Eup. per.*
Sore in pericardium—*Crot. h.*
Sorrow, heart were aching from—*Pyrus*
Sparks, electric, from heart to front of neck—*Graph.*
Spasm, muscle fibers of heart participated in general—*Mag. p.*
Squeezed, heart were—*Arn., Bor., Iod., Lil. t., Tarent.*
  –heart were suddenly—*Arn.*
  –together, heart were—*Iod.*
  –together in region of heart—*Arn.*
  –by a hand, heart were—*Lil. t., Spig.*
  –by a vise, heart were—*Lil. t., Tab.*
  –off, heart would be—*Cham., Nux m.*
Stabbing in arteries with burning—*Card. b.*
Stagnated in arteries, blood—*Carl.*
Start out of vessels, blood would—*Nux v.*
Sticking through heart—*Pæon.*
Stiff with blood, arteries were—*Daph. o.*
Still, heart stood—*Aur., Dig., Sep.*
  –heart would stand—*Lob.*
  –heart were suddenly—*Arg. m.*
  –circulation stood—*Gels., Lyc.*
Stone, cold, in heart—*Petr.*
  –great, laid upon heart—*Cere. b.*
Stop, heart would—*Onos.*
  –beating if she moved, heart would—*Dig.*
  –if she stood still, heart would—*Gels.*
Stopped, heart had—*Arg. n., Aster., Aur., Cact., Chin. a., Cic.,*
    Cimx., Dig., Dign., Lil. t., Luna, Lyc., Pyrus, Rumx., Serp.,
    Tab.
  –frequently—*Lil. t.*
  –after waking at midnight, heart had almost—*Sac. lac.*
  –beating for a while then a hard thump—*Aur.*
  –then started suddenly, heart had—*Conv.*
  –suddenly, heart had—*Rumx.*
  –by a crowbar which pressed tightly from right to left breast
    and twisted a knot around heart—*Tab.*
  –blood had, then began to flow again—*Stry.*
  –in arms, circulation had—*Glon.*
Stopping, heart were—*Nux m.*
Strained, heart had been—*Ant. t.*

Stream, a hot wave-like, were moving from heart—*Lyss.*
String, heart were pulling backward or to the right by a—*Arg. n.*
Strings breaking at apex of heart—*Caust.*
Struggle through veins, blood could scarcely—*Zinc. s.*
Struggling about the heart, something alive were—*Cast. eq.*
Substance, hard, extending from heart region to stomach—*Nat. c.*
Suppuration in spot in heart region, on pressure—*Coc. c.*
Suffocating, heart were—*Lact.*
Surrounded with water, heart were—*Pip. n.*
Suspended, circulation were—*Saba.*
  –from left rib, heart were—*Kali c.*
  –in legs, circulation were—*Lact.*
Swaying to and fro by a thin thread, heart had torn itself loose
    and were—*Dig.*
Swelled or distended to fill chest, heart were—*Cench.*
  –preventing inspiration, heart were—*Ether., Lach.*
Swimming in blood or water, heart were—*Bufo*
Swollen, heart were—*Ars., Asaf., Bapt., Bell., Cent., Kali i.,*
    Med., Plb., Sulph., Thea
  –heart were too full or—*Asaf.*
  –when lying on left side, heart were—*Ang.*
Swung by a thin thread and moved back and forth, heart were
    —*Tub.*
Tear it off, heart were hanging by a thread and every beat would
    —*Lach.*
Tense in precordial region, blood were too—*Pyrus*
Thin as paper, blood were—*Bell.*
Thread, heart were hung by a—*Lach., Lyc.*
  –heart had torn itself loose and were swaying to and fro by a
    thin—*Dig.*
  –and every beat would tear it off, heart were hanging by a—*Lach.*
  –and moved back and forth, heart were swung by a thin—*Tub.*
Thrilling or purring over cardiac region—*Spig.*
Throat, heart came into—*Lyss., Podo., Stry.*
Throbbing about heart—*Scut.*
  –of a lump in heart—*Cupr. s.*
  –heart suddenly stopped beating, followed by a heavy—*Rumx.*
Thud in the heart, something went—*Ovi g. p.*
Thump in heart, heavy blow or—*Ovi g. p.*
  –heart had stopped beating for a while and then a hard—*Aur.*
Tick of watch, pulse in body were—*Ambr.*

Tightening up of parts from crawling in veins—*Tril.*
Tired, heart were—*Nux v., Pyrog.*
  –after a long run, heart were—*Pyrog.*
Torn, heart were—*Tarent.*
  –out, heart were being—*Elaps*
  –to pieces, heart were—*Pyrog.*
  –to pieces, heart and breast were—*Hyos.*
  –to pieces on moving arm, heart would be—*Carb. an.*
  –away or broken, walls of chest anterior to heart were—
      Cere. b.
  –out when walking, heart would be—*Hipp.*
  –itself loose, heart had, and were swaying to and fro by a thin
      thread—*Dig.*
Transfixed by a blunt instrument, heart were—*Cere. b.*
Transparent, blood were—*Bell.*
Trembled, heart—*Crot. h.*
Tumbled about or over—*Crot. h.*
Turn over, heart would—*Camph., Sol. t. æ.*
Turned over, heart—*Aur., Cact., Lach., Op., Tarent.*
  –over and forward, heart—*Camph.*
  –over and ceased beating for a while—*Lach.*
  –and twisted around—*Tarent.*
  –into ice water, blood—*Abies c.*
Turning around, heart were—*Aur.*
  –around rapidly, heart were—*Sol. t. æ.*
Twisted and turned around, heart—*Tarent.*
  –heart feels—*Tarent.*
  –a knot around heart which stopped it, crowbar—*Tab.*
  –pulse were—*Ars. h.*
Vacuum in heart—*Chr. ac.*
Vibrating, all blood vessels in body were—*Phel.*
Vise, heart were squeezed in a—*Tab.*
  –heart were squeezed or grasped in a—*Lil. t.*
Warmth about heart—*Cann. s.*
Watch, pulse felt like a tick of a—*Ambr.*
Water, heart were beating in—*Der., Sumb.*
  –blood were cold—*Verat. a.*
  –cold, dropped from heart—*Cann. i.*
  –blood turned to ice—*Abies c.*
  –cold, running through veins—*Rhus t.*
  –drowned in water, heart were—*Bufo*

Water—*Continued*

   –hot, in blood vessels—*Sin., Syph.*

   –hot, were running through veins—*Ars., Rhus t.*

   –hot, or oil running through veins all night long—*Syph.*

   –heart were pumping cold—*Pyrog.*

   –heart were surrounded with—*Kali i., Pip. n.*

   –swimming in blood or water, heart were—*Bufo*

   –heart were working in—*Bov.*

Weight, a heavy, were lying on heart—*Sac. lac.*

   –over heart—*Naja*

Weighted heart down, something heavy—*Cham., Ovi g. p., Sac. lac.*

   –down by a heavy black cloud that settles over her, heart were —*Cimic.*

Whirled around first one way and then the other, heart were— *Cact.*

Whirling, heart were—*Ant. t.*

   –in heart region—*Merl.*

Wind about the heart—*X-ray*

Wires, pains traveled on electric, starting from left side and returning to left side—*Samars.*

Wood were in region of heart, a blunt piece of—*Ran. s.*

Working in water, heart were—*Bov.*

NECK AND BACK

Abraded, skin on back were—*Petr.*
Adhesive plaster near inner margin of right scapula—*Zinc.*
Air, cold, blowing on back—*Camph.*
  –cold, spreading from spine over the body—*Agar.*
  –cold, over lumbar region—*Sumb.*
  –cold, blowing on left lumbar region—*Castor.*
  –soft, blowing through the back—*Sec.*
  –warm, streamed up the spine to the head—*Ars.*
Alive in back, something were—*Mag. p. Ambo*
  –in gluteal muscles, something were—*Juncus*
  –in sacrum, mouse were—*Mag. p. Arct.*
Ants crawling in back—*Graph.*
  –crawling in back and legs—*Alum.*
  –creeping along back, spine and neck—*Agar.*
Asleep in nape of the neck—*Agar.*
  –cervical muscles were—*Rhus t.*
  –back were—*Sep.*
  –after midday nap, back were—*Phos.*
  –on sitting down, back were—*Merc.*
  –in shoulder—*Sep.*
  –lumbar region were—*Berb.*
Aura about neck in damp situations—*Chin. s.*
Ball, elastic, pressed in head and spine—*Benz. ac.*
Balls, hot, dropped from each breast through to back, rolling down back, along each limb and dropping off at heels; followed by balls of ice—*Lyc.*
Band, tense, reaching from nape of neck to ears—*Anac.*
  –around neck—*Bell.*
  –were too tight, neck—*Bry.*
  –from shoulder to and around neck—*Lepi.*
  –pressed through small of back and everything were constricted—*Puls.*
Bandaged, small of back were tightly—*Puls.*
Bar of iron pressing on small of back—*Elaps*
Bathed in hot water, right scapula were—*Na:. s.*
Battery, galvanic, applied to spine—*Agar.*

396

Bearing down extending to back with weakness—*Kali fer.*

Beaten in back—*Ars. i., Berb., Calc. ar., Maland., Nat. m., Ruta, Stram., Syph., Zinc.*

  –muscles of back had been—*Agar.*

  –shoulder had been—*Lepi., Lyss.*

  –between shoulder blades—*Ang.*

  –in upper part of back—*Anac.*

  –to pieces, back were—*Mag. c.*

  –and sore in back—*Sul. ac.*

  –violently along back—*Ang.*

  –whole back had been—*Arn.*

  –and sore, back were—*Sul. ac.*

  –or lame, spine were—*Ruta*

  –in small of back—*Ang., Eup. per., Sil., Sulph.*

  –in flesh of small of back—*Rhus t.*

  –in sacral region—*Agar., Nat. m., Staph.*

  –in lower back—*Zing.*

Beating in left shoulder, someone were—*Pip. n.*

  –in dorsal spine, heart were—*Carb. s.*

Bed were hard—*Acon., Arn., Bapt., Bry., Caust., Con., Dros., Graph., Kali c., Mag. c., Mag. m., Nux m., Nux v., Phos., Plat., Pyrog., Rhus t., Ruta, Saba., Sil., Stann., Sulph., Tarax., Thuj., Verat. a.*

Beetles were crawling in spine—*Acon.*

Bending backward would > pain in small of back—*Æth.*

Bent back, spine were—*Mag. c.*

  –backward, dorsal vertebræ would be—*Juncus*

  –too long, back had been—*Rhod.*

  –inward, back were—*Podo.*

Biting in back—*Lyc., Merc., Mur. ac., Sulph.*

  –on back from minute insects—*Chlor.*

Blood dripping through a valve in left scapulæ—*Spig.*

  –had suddenly been retained in one of the large veins of the neck—*Tell.*

Blow, severe, in left brachial plexus—*Chr. ac.*

  –on neck, he had a—*Lach.*

  –on neck as if eyes would spring out of head, when pressing on throat—*Lach.*

  –of fist in back—*Nux m.*

  –in back on stooping—*Sep.*

  –in coccyx, numbness from—*Plat.*

Blowing on back, cold air were—*Camph.*
  –on back, wind were—*Hep.*
  –on back, cool wind were—*Asar., Chin.*
  –on parts between scapulæ—*Caust.*
  –on spine, someone were—*Tab.*
  –on back through hole in clothes, wind were—*Chin., Culx.*
  –through back, soft air were—*Sec.*
  –on left lumbar region, cold air were—*Cast.*
Body, foreign, passed through spine from top to bottom and
      stopped at pointed obstacle—*Raph.*
  –heavy, were moving down back—*Bar. c.*
Boil were hanging on left flank—*Rhus t.*
Boils were on back—*Cimic.*
Bound too tight, neck were—*Con.*
  –tight with a napkin, neck were—*Chel.*
  –tightly, nape of neck were—*Plat.*
  –in hips and small of back, wants to be, with hæmorrhage—
      Tril.
Break, nape of neck would—*Bell.*
  –left side of neck would—*Form.*
  –with pain, neck and left shoulder would—*Thlaspi*
  –back would—*Alum., Bell., Form., Kalm., Lil. t., Sanic., Vib.*
  –in bed, back would—*Ferr. i.*
  –in back, something were going to—*Sep.*
  –just above the waist, back would—*Alet.*
  –small of back would—*Ham., Lyc.*
  –in two, back and hips would—*Æsc.*
  –at top of sacrum, back would—*Cupr. ac.*
  –with hæmorrhoids, back would—*Ham.*
Breaking, cords of neck were—*Lyc.*
  –back were—*Bell.*
  –off, shoulder were—*Chel.*
  –in back with piles—*Bell.*
Breath, cool, passed over small of back—*Sulph.*
  –stopped between scapulæ—*Calc. c.*
Broken, nape of neck were—*Chel.*
  –in nape, on looking up—*Graph.*
  –scapulæ were—*Anan.*
  –back were—*Clem., Ferr. i., Kali c., Lyc., Mag. c., Mag. p.
      Arct., Nat. m., Nux v., Ox. ac., Plat., Rhus t., Vacc., Vario.,
      Verat. a., Xanth.*

Broken—*Continued*

  –joints of spine would be—*Hyos.*

  –and tied together with a piece of string, back were—*Ovi g. p.*

  –< sitting or lying, back were—*Carb. an.*

  –or bruised in back—*Conv.*

  –small of back were—*Ars., Bell., Carb. an., Cham., Clem., Cor. r., Graph., Kali c., Lyc., Nat. m., Nux v., Phos., Plat., Sep., Staph.*

  –small of back were, only at night—*Ferr. i.*

  –to pieces, small of back were—*Staph.*

  –in left loin—*Coc. c.*

  –in across loins with loss of sexual power—*Coc. c.*

  –cracking in sacrum as if bones were—*Mag. p. Arct.*

  –in lumbar and sacral region—*Meli.*

Bruised, neck were—*Arg. m., Caust., Ferr., Naja, Nat. m., Zinc.*

  –upper part of neck were—*Elaps*

  –nape of neck were—*Agar., Ars., Asar., Bell., Cann. i., Dig., Iod., Merc. i. r., Nat. m., Nat. s., Nux v., Phos. ac., Ruta, Sulph., Tep., Thuj.*

  –back of neck were—*Iodof.*

  –and stiff, neck were—*Sol. n.*

  –glands of neck were—*Psor.*

  –and swollen, submaxillary glands were—*Staph.*

  –in cervical muscles—*Asar.*

  –scapulæ were—*Kreos., Merc. i. f., Nux v.*

  –right shoulder had been—*Coloc.*

  –and swollen in right scapula to shoulder—*Berb.*

  –in left shoulder—*Ind.*

  –back were—*Dros., Eup. per., Gamb., Nat. m., Ox. ac., Psor., Vib.*

  –or broken in back—*Conv.*

  –in muscles of back—*Cinnb.*

  –in loins—*Sulph. i.*

  –and weary in loins, belly and thighs—*Bov.*

  –in small of back—*Graph., Mag. m., Nat. s.*

  –in right side of small of back—*Rhus t.*

  –or crushed in small of back—*Am. m.*

  –in right side of lumbar vertebræ—*Rhus t.*

  –in back and sacrum—*Stront.*

Bubbling in muscles of back and arms, something were—*Petr.*
　—beneath scapulæ—*Squill.*
　—in lumbar region, < lying—*Berb.*
Bumped the coccyx, he had—*Samars.*
Burning from nettles, in neck—*Pæon.*
　—under skin of back—*Mur. ac.*
　—in upper spine, a fire were—*Tub.*
　—sore, in loins—*Murx.*
　—in left lumbar region, from a hot needle, sudden—*Æth.*
Burnt when turning head, neck were—*Calc. c.*
Carried something heavy on right shoulder, he had—*Cast.*
Chafed, neck were—*Ox. ac.*
Charred after sensation of red hot iron rod passing up spine to atlas—*Cann. i.*
Choking from a cold wet string tied about neck—*Sanic.*
Circulation would aggravate pain in left shoulder—*Cist.*
　—in neck would be hindered by clothes—*Lach.*
Clammy cold on back of neck—*Sanic.*
Close together, abdomen and back were too—*Plb.*
Cloth, lying on a roll of—*Euon. atrop.*
　—cold, on lumbar region—*Sanic.*
　—on back, cold wet—*Cast.*
Clothes on spine were damp—*Tub.*
　—were on fire in lumbar region—*Ars. i.*
Coal, red hot, on shoulder—*Phos. ac.*
Coals, hot, between scapulæ—*Lyc.*
Cold wet string were tied about neck choking her—*Sanic.*
　—feeling on back of neck—*Sanic., Sil.*
　—clammy feeling on back of neck—*Sanic.*
　—air down back—*Coff. t.*
　—air were blowing on back—*Camph.*
　—air spreading from spine over body—*Agar.*
　—hand between shoulders—*Sep.*
　—perspiration between shoulder blades—*Lachn.*
　—wind were blowing on parts between scapulæ—*Caust.*
　—ice against back—*Cocc.*
　—iron pressed upon back—*Phyt.*
　—water between shoulders—*Abies c.*
　—water were dropping down back—*Caps.*
　—water were dashed on back—*Lil. t., Puls., Saba.*

Cold—*Continued*

    –water were poured down back—*Alumn., Puls., Stram., Zinc.*

    –water on back when leaning against chair—*Agar.*

    –were trickling down back—*Ars.*

    –wet cloth on back—*Cast.*

    –cloth in lumbar and sacral region—*Sanic.*

    –air were blowing over lumbar region—*Sumb.*

    –air were blowing in left lumbar region—*Cast.*

Coldness between shoulders—*Am. m.*

    –running over back—*Quass.*

Collar were too tight—*Aml. n., Ant. t., Lach., Sep.*

Compressed, neck were—*Crot. h., Pip. m.*

    –between fingers, skin of neck were—*Spong.*

Constricted, neck were—*Lyc.*

    –with a napkin, neck were—*Chel.*

    –nape of neck were—*Puls.*

    –and swollen, muscles of neck were—*Chin. s.*

    –a band passed through small of back and everything were—*Puls.*

Contract backward, back would—*Brach.*

Contracted in muscles of back—*Cinnb.*

Cool wind were blowing on back—*Asar., Chin.*

    –drops of sweat were going down left side of spine—*X-ray*

    –breath passed over small of back—*Sulph.*

Cord tied tightly around neck—*Lach.*

    –in back were pulling down, during pregnancy—*Plb.*

    –around loins—*Gent. l.*

    –were drawn tightly across lower part of loins—*Arn.*

Cords of neck were breaking—*Lyc.*

    –of nape of neck were loose—*Verat. v.*

    –of neck were pulled—*Sil.*

Cracked across sacrum when stooping, something were—*Kali bi.*

Cracking in sacrum as if bones were broken—*Mag. p. Arct.*

Cramped position, back were lying in a—*Ferr. i., Zinc.*

Cravat, tight, in muscles of neck—*Arn., Asar.*

Crawling over shoulders and neck, insects were—*Kali n., Lac c., Nat. c., Phos. ac., Sec., Tab.*

    –on neck, worms were—*Arund.*

    –on back and shoulders when going to bed, insects were—*Osm.*

    –as from beetles in spine—*Acon.*

Crawling—*Continued*

–in back, ants were—*Graph.*

–on back, vermin were—*Agn., Bell., Mag. s., Nat. c., Osm., Zinc.*

–beneath skin on right knee and back—*Rat.*

–under skin, insects were—*Con.*

–over back and scrotum, worms or insects were—*Staph.*

Creeping along spine, ants were—*Agar.*

–through back, soft air were—*Sec.*

–or running in right shoulder blade when urinating, something were—*Hep.*

–through back from below upward, hot water were—*Nit. s. d.*

Crept up back from extremities, an icy feeling—*Saponin.*

Cricked, back were—*Calc. c.*

Crooked, middle of back were—*Raph.*

Crushed, back were—*Phos.*

–bones of dorsal vertebræ were—*Med.*

–or bruised in small of back—*Am. m.*

–lumbar region were—*Berb.*

Crust, sharp, sticking in middle of spine on swallowing food—*Caust.*

Cut in two, back were—*Hep.*

Cutting head off from body—*Phys.*

Damp, clothes on spine were—*Tub.*

Darting through back, something were—*Aspar.*

Dashed on back, cold water were—*Lil. t., Puls., Saba.*

Denuded on left side of back—*Plat.*

Detached from sacrum, something became—*Sol. t. æ.*

Disjointed, neck were—*Calc. c.*

–nape were—*Lachn.*

–cervical vertebræ were—*Ang.*

–neck would be—*Pic. ac.*

–in middle of spine—*Thuj.*

–in right loin—*Carb. s.*

–in last lumbar vertebræ—*Sanic.*

Dislocated, neck were—*Asar.*

–when turning head, neck were—*Lachn.*

–neck would be—*Pic. ac.*

–back were—*Bell.*

–right lumbar region were—*Carb. s.*

–in cervical vertebræ—*Cinnb.*

Distended between shoulders—*Bell.*
Draw head to right side, cervical vertebræ would—*Juncus*
Drawing in from abdomen to back—*Plb.*
  –in spinal cord—*Schinus*
  –through scapulæ, thread were—*Elect.*
Drawn up, tendons of neck were—*Stront.*
  –toward neck, shoulder would be—*Carb. v.*
  –backward, back were—*Lil. t.*
  –along skin of back on waking, a hot sponge were—*Wild.*
  –in region of spine as if convexity were interior and back were
      drawn far forward—*X-ray*
  –tightly across lower part of loins, cord were—*Arn.*
Dripping down spine from nape of neck, water were—*Tub.*
Dropped out of lumbar region, vertebræ had, and spine were
      tied together with a string—*Ovi g. p.*
Dropping down back, cold water were—*Caps.*
  –on flesh of back, liquid were—*Kali bi.*
  –in left loin, fluid were—*Zing.*
  –out of bottle in lumbar region, water were—*Med.*
Drops of cool sweat going down left side of spine—*X-ray*
Dryness of os coccygis—*Agar.*
Effort to support spinal column, it were an—*Phos.*
Elastic ball pressed in head and spine—*Benz. ac.*
Electric shocks on neck above larynx—*Manc.*
  –shocks from heart to neck—*Graph.*
  –shocks on back—*Nux v.*
Emaciated, left shoulder were—*Sumb.*
Enlarged on right side of neck, gland were—*Med.*
  –neck and back were—*Sanic.*
Envelope, neck were in some unyielding—*Lyc.*
Fall apart, bones of sacrum would—*Calc. p., Tril.*
  –apart after splitting, back would—*Lyss.*
  –in while sitting, dorsal spine would—*Bar. c.*
Falling to pieces, hips and small of back were—*Tril.*
  –in lumbar region, sparks of fire were—*Sec.*
Filled upper part of sacrum, something size of hand—*Ars. h.*
Finger were pressing on right side of neck when talking—*Zinc.*
  –pressed over spinous process of scapulæ—*Chen. v.*
Fire burning in upper spine—*Tub.*
  –in lumbar region, clothes were on—*Ars. i.*
  –were falling in lumbar region, spark of—*Sec.*

Firmness in lumbar region and limbs, there were no—*Carl.*
Flannel shirt, he wore a stout—*Ferr. s.*
  —on back causing itching, > scratching—*Hipp.*
Flesh were pinched up and shaken back and forth by a hand—
  Sol. m.
Flowing from sore in lumbar region, warm liquid were—*Hura*
Fluid were dropping in left loin—*Zing.*
Fluttering in sacrum rising gradually to occiput—*Ol. j.*
Fly to pieces, shoulder would—*Rhus t.*
Forced inward below left scapula, plug were—*Prun.*
Fracture in back—*Sul. ac.*
Fractured, left shoulder were—*Chel.*
  —on inclining backward, a vertebra between shoulders were—
    Crot. c.
Galvanic battery attached to spine—*Agar.*
Gimlet running into spine—*Lyc.*
Give way, muscle in right side of neck would—*Pic. ac.*
  —way, back would—*Æsc.*
  —out soon, back would—*Phos.*
Gliding over each other, vertebræ in lumbar region were—*Sanic.,*
  Sulph.
  —past each other, vertebræ of lower back were—*Sanic.*
Glued to spine, pain as if parts were—*Cinnb.*
Goiter and she could not see over it, she had a large—*Zinc.*
Gnawing in coccyx—*Kali c.*
Grasped by a hand on lying down, neck were—*Glon.*
  —with a hand, neck were—*Grat.*
  —and twisted around, flesh between shoulders were—*Sars.*
Gurgling and rolling in scapula—*Tarax.*
Hammer were striking upon back—*Lyss.*
  —in small of back, struck by a—*Sep.*
Hand grasped neck on lying down—*Glon.*
  —neck were seized by a—*Grat.*
  —were laid between scapulæ, an icy cold—*Sep.*
Hanging between scapulæ, heavy load were—*Carb. s., Lyss.*
  —from back, clothes were—*Saponin.*
  —on left flank, boil were—*Rhus t.*
Hard, back were—*Sep.*
  —several places on back were—*Coc. c., Guare.*
  —mass pressed against sacrum—*Chin. s.*

Hard—*Continued*

   –bed were—*Acon., Arn., Bapt., Bry., Caust., Con., Dros., Graph., Kali c., Mag. c., Mag. m., Nux m., Nux v., Phos., Plat., Pyrog., Rhus t., Ruta, Saba., Sil., Stann., Sulph., Tarax., Thuj., Verat. a.*

Heartburn down back—*Acon., Alumn.*

Heat rushed up spine to head—*Phos.*

   –from nettles on back—*Pæon.*

Heavy load on nape of neck—*Par.*

   –on shoulder, he had carried something—*Cast.*

   –load were hanging between scapulæ—*Carb. s.*

   –weight on back—*Saponin.*

   –body were moving down back—*Bar. c.*

Held in some unyielding envelope, neck were—*Lyc.*

Hole in clothes on back and wind were blowing on—*Chin., Culx.*

   –in back above sacrum, a large—*Sac. lac.*

Hot—see also RED HOT

Hot sponge were drawn along skin of back on waking—*Wild.*

   –stove, sitting with back to—*Dulc.*

   –water were running upward from nape of neck—*Glon.*

   –water, right scapula were bathed in—*Nat. s.*

   –coals between scapulæ—*Lyc.*

   –water were creeping through back from below upward—*Nit. s. d.*

Humpbacked, she would become—*Raph.*

Hung between shoulders, heavy weight were—*Lyss.*

Hungry along spine—*Lil. t.*

Ice lay on vertex then forehead, then to nape of neck and then to small of back—*Laur.*

   –lying on—*Lyc.*

   –below shoulder blade, touched by a piece of—*Agar.*

   –were between scapulæ, a piece of—*Lachn.*

   –were in lumbar region, a lump of—*Agar., Laur.*

   –water were running down back in streams—*Vacc., Vario.*

Icy cold hand were laid between scapulæ—*Sep.*

   –feeling crept up back from extremities—*Saponin.*

Injured, spine had been—*Paraf.*

   –small of back had been—*Prun.*

   –coccyx were—*Ruta*

Insects, minute, were biting back—*Chlor.*

Insects were crawling over shoulders and neck—*Kali n., Lac c., Mag. c., Nat. c., Phos. ac., Sec., Tab.*
—were crawling on back and shoulders—*Osm.*
—were crawling over back and scrotum—*Staph.*
—on back, stings of—*Chlor.*
Instrument, pointed, thrust into scapula—*Spong.*
Iron, red hot, passed up spine to atlas, around head leaving a charred feeling—*Cann. i.*
—red hot, were moving along close to left side of neck below jaw—*Phel.*
—pressed upon back, piece of cold—*Phyt.*
—bar were pressing on small of back—*Elaps*
—were thrust through lower vertebræ—*Alum.*
Jerk in nape of neck—*Corn.*
Knife lancinating back—*Mim.*
—stabbing from within outward in vertebræ—*Bell.*
—were thrust through back—*Cupr., Pyrog.*
—were thrust through side and back—*Ran. b.*
—were through loins—*Ign., Kali bi.*
Knives pierced between scapulæ—*Nat. s.*
—pierced in sacrum—*Nat. s.*
Knocked away, small of back had been—*Arg. m.*
Laced in about neck—*Glon.*
Laid between scapulæ, icy cold hand were—*Sep.*
Lain on back too long while sitting, he had—*Rhod.*
Lame, shoulder were—*Kali i.*
—back were—*Nux v.*
—and beaten, spine were—*Ruta*
—in small of back in morning—*Sel.*
—sacrum were—*Ang.*
Lancinating back, knife were—*Mim.*
Large, neck were too—*Kali c.*
—for parts, bones of spine were—*Cinnb.*
Larger, neck were—*Acon. l.*
Lay on head, then nape of neck and small of back, ice—*Laur.*
Lead, shoulders contained—*Nux m.*
Ligature around neck prevented return of blood from head—*Glon.*
Liquid were dropping on back—*Kali bi.*
—were flowing from sore in lumbar region, warm—*Hura*

Load, heavy, on nape of neck—*Par.*
　–heavy, were hanging between scapulæ—*Carb.* .
Loose, cords of nape of neck were—*Verat. v.*
　–in shoulder, flesh were—*Staph.*
　–on lower back, flesh were—*Lyc.*
Lump between shoulders—*Arn., Mag. s.*
　–of ice in lumbar region—*Agar., Laur.*
　–size of hen's egg rising and falling in right iliac and lumbar region—*Hydrs.*
　–in right lumbar region—*Equis.*
Lying in an uncomfortable position, head and neck had been—*Dulc., Ferr., Puls.*
　–in an uncomfortable position, one had been—*Zinc.*
　–in a cramped position—*Ferr. i.*
　–on a roll of cloth—*Euon. atrop.*
　–improperly, back had been—*Ferr. ma.*
　–unsupported, back had been—*Ind.*
　–on cervical muscles and back, weight were—*Vinc.*
Missing, a section of vertebræ were—*Ovi g. p.*
Moist on back, clothes were—*Tub.*
Mouse were alive in sacrum—*Mag. p. Arct.*
　–were running up back—*Sulph.*
Moving down in small of back, heavy body were—*Bar. c.*
　–along close to left side of neck below jaw, a red hot iron were—*Phel.*
Mumps were coming on—*Lyss., Trif.*
Nail were sticking in lumbar region—*Berb.*
　–were in back—*Lepi.*
　–were driven in on each side of vertebræ—*Cinnb.*
Needle pricks in back—*Tub.*
　–in left side of nape of neck, sticking with a somewhat blunt—*Tarax.*
　–in left lumbar region, sudden burning from hot—*Æth.*
Needles, muscles of left side of face from forehead to neck and axilla were pierced with red hot—*Spig.*
　–and pins pricking on skin of forehead, neck and arms—*All. c.*
　–sticking into mole on neck when touched—*Tarent.*
　–blunt, sticking in left side of neck—*Tarax.*
　–stinging middle of spine when walking in open air—*Calc. c.*
Nettles were burning on neck—*Pæon.*
　–on back, heat from—*Pæon.*

Off shoulders, head were—*Puls.*

   –the body, head were being cut—*Phys.*

Overlifting in loins—*Valer.*

Oyster shell in right side of neck, piece of—*Sil.*

Pain extending through coccyx in spinal marrow—*Lact.*

Pains would twist her body when they run up her back—*Corn.*

Paralyzed, anterior cervical muscles were—*Dig.*

   –nape of neck were—*Cina*

   –in back and neck—*Cocc.*

   –back were—*Euph.*

   –shoulder were—*Lyss.*

   –by stroke of lightning, right shoulder had been—*Ign.*

Passed up spine to atlas, and around head, leaving a charred feeling, a red hot iron—*Cann. i.*

   –through spine from top to bottom, a foreign body, and stopped at pointed obstacle—*Raph.*

   –over small of back, cool breath—*Sulph.*

Perspiration between shoulders, wet with—*Lachn.*

Piece of flesh were being forcibly twisted out under left scapula —*Corn.*

   –were gone in lower spine, lameness—*Pic ac.*

Pieces, shoulder would fly to—*Rhus t.*

   –hips and back were falling to—*Tril.*

   –back were in two—*Sanic.*

Pierced by knives between scapulæ and sacrum—*Nat. s.*

   –with red hot needles in axilla—*Spig.*

Pincers in muscles of left side, pulled by—*Inul.*

   –in muscles of left side of neck extending to right chest, abdomen and side of scrotum—*Antip.*

   –back were pressed with—*Carl.*

Pinched by pinchers in back—*Cann. s.*

   –up and shaken back and forth by a hand, flesh were—*Sol. m.*

Pins were pricking back—*Guan.*

Plaster, adhesive, near inner margin of right scapula—*Zinc.*

   –on lumbar region—*Hura*

Plug in back—*Carb. v.*

   –in back when lying or sitting—*Carb. v.*

   –were stuck in spine < by motion—*Anac.*

   –forced inward two inches below left scapula—*Prun.*

Pointed instrument were thrust into scapula—*Spong.*

Points, sharp, in coccyx—*Cann. s.*

Position, he had been lying in a cramped—*Ferr. i.*

  –one had lain in an uncomfortable—*Zinc.*

  –head and neck had lain in an uncomfortable—*Dulc., Ferr., Puls.*

Pounded, back had been—*Conv.*

Poured down back, cold water were—*Alumn., Anac., Puls., Stram., Zinc.*

  –over small of back and through pelvis, boiling water were—*Verat. v.*

Power going, back were turning to pulp and—*Colch.*

Pressed like an elastic ball in head and spine—*Benz. ac.*

  –by a dull wedge or tight cravat, muscles of neck were—*Asar.*

  –asunder, bones in back and shoulders were—*Berb.*

  –by a weight on right shoulder—*Am. br.*

  –by two or three fingers over spinous process of scapulæ—*Chen. v.*

  –against chest, back were—*Tarent.*

  –upon back, a small piece of cold iron were—*Phyt.*

  –with pincers, back were—*Carl.*

  –outward in back, something were—*Ruta*

  –upon the back, thumb were—*Meny.*

  –inward from both sides, small of back or sacrum were—*Kali c.*

  –through small of back, band were; and everything were constricted—*Puls.*

  –against sacrum, hard mass were—*Chin. s.*

Pressing on right side of neck when talking, a finger were—*Zinc.*

  –between scapulæ, a stone were—*Chin., Nux v.*

  –on left shoulder, someone were—*Rhus t.*

  –from within, a piece of wood stretched across back (before menses)—*Nux m.*

  –on small of back, an iron bar were—*Elaps*

Pressure around loins—*Gent. l.*

Prevented return of blood from head, ligature around neck—*Glon.*

  –circulation of blood in shoulder, tape—*Saba.*

Prick of needles in back—*Tub.*

Pricking of pins and needles on skin of forehead, neck and arms—*All. c.*

  –back, pins were—*Guan.*

Pricking—*Continued*

–of pins down each side of neck, right chest, abdomen and scrotum—*Antip.*

Protrude on turning head, a tumor in neck would—*Calc. c.*

Pulled from shoulder to ear, a string were—*Lepi.*

–on cords of neck, someone—*Sil.*

–by pincers in muscles of left side—*Inul.*

Pulling upward from tip of coccyx, something were—*Lil. t.*

–down, during pregnancy, cord in back were—*Plb.*

Pulp and all power going, back were turning to—*Colch.*

Pushed into back, large splinters were—*Agar.*

Quicksilver moved up and down in spinal cord—*Phos.*

Raise or turn herself, she could not—*Sep.*

Red hot iron were moving along close to left side of neck below jaw—*Phel.*

–hot iron rod passed up spine to atlas, around head, leaving a charred feeling—*Cann. i.*

–hot needles pierced axilla—*Spig.*

–hot coal on shoulder—*Phos. ac.*

Retained in one of the large veins of left side of neck, blood had been—*Tell.*

Rising and falling in right iliac and lumbar region, lump size of hen's egg, were—*Hydrs.*

Rod passed up spine to atlas and around neck, leaving a charred feeling, red hot iron—*Cann. i.*

–of iron were thrust in lower vertebræ—*Alum.*

Roll of cloth, lying on a—*Euon. atrop.*

Rolling and gurgling in scapulæ—*Tarax.*

Running or creeping in right shoulder blade when urinating, something were—*Hep.*

–up arms and back, a mouse were—*Sulph.*

–down the back, large spider were—*Dulc.*

–internally in right loin, something were—*Hep.*

–up to brain, a stream of warm water were—*Cann. i.*

–down back, cold water were—*Agar., Alum., Alumn., Ars., Puls., Stram., Zinc.*

–down back if he leans against chair, cold water were—*Agar.*

–down back in streams, ice water were—*Vacc., Vario.*

–upward from nape of neck, hot water were—*Glon.*

–down back, warm water were—*Tep.*

–into spine, a gimlet were—*Lyc.*

Rushed up spine to head, heat—*Phos.*
Scraped out with an instrument, spine were—*Cinnb.*
Screwed together, spine were—*Colch.*
  –back were—*Æth.*
  –in on rising from a seat, small of back were—*Zinc.*
  –in in lumbar region—*Kali i.*
Seized by a hand, neck were—*Grat.*
Separate, lower vertebræ would—*Chel.*
  –everything inside of back would—*Cinnb.*
Shaken back and forth by a hand, flesh were—*Sol. m.*
Sharp crust sticking in middle of spine on swallowing food—*Caust.*
  –sitting on something—*Lach.*
Shell were in right side of neck, a piece of oyster—*Sil.*
Shirt on skin of back, he wore a stout flannel—*Ferr. s.*
Shocks, electric, on neck above larynx—*Manc.*
  –electric, from heart to neck—*Graph.*
  –electric, on back—*Nux v.*
Short, neck were too—*Lac. ac.*
  –muscles of neck were too—*Aur., Cic., Macrot.*
  –on bending head forward, neck muscles were—*Hyos.*
  –tendons in sides of neck were too—*Nux v.*
  –back and neck muscles were too—*Sulph.*
  –cervical muscles were too—*Hyos.*
  –muscles of back were too—*Caust., Thuj.*
  –sinews of back were too—*Lach.*
  –to allow stooping, back were too—*Phys.*
  –in back, ligaments were too—*Prun.*
  –right side of psoas magnus were too—*Coloc.*
  –lumbar muscles were too—*Sulph.*
  –gluteal muscles were too—*Dios.*
Singing sensation were coming from nape of neck—*Chlol.*
Sitting on something sharp—*Lach.*
  –with back to the stove—*Dulc.*
Small, neck were too—*Chim. mac., Chin.*
Sore burning in loins—*Murx.*
  –and beaten in back—*Sul. ac.*
Soreness, internal, from leaning back upon cushions and back—*Am. be.*
Space were vacant in region of sacrum—*Culx.*
Sparks of fire falling in lumbar region—*Sec.*

Spider running down back, a large—*Dul.*
Splinters, large, pushed into back—*Agar.*
  –thousand, in deltoid muscle—*Agar.*
  –in dorsal vertebræ—*Agar.*
Split and fall apart, back would—*Lyss.*
Sponge, hot, drawn along skin of back on waking—*Wild.*
Sprain in neck—*Nicc.*
Sprained, nape of neck were—*Ars., Coloc., Lyc., Nicc., Ruta, Sulph.*
  –on turning, neck were—*Agar.*
  –transversely through nape—*Wild.*
  –back were—*Gamb., Mur. ac., Rhus t.*
  –in forenoon, back were—*Cocc., Petr.*
  –in muscles of back—*Chin. a.*
  –in whole vertebral column—*Sol. t. æ.*
  –in shoulder—*Ambr., Ign., Rhus t.*
  –between shoulders—*Ant. c., Bell., Petr., Stann.*
  –in left shoulder—*Chel., Nicc.*
  –in small of back—*Puls., Sep.*
  –in lumbar region—*Æsc., Agar., Arg. n., Ars., Caust., Gamb., Gran., Hall, Hep., Kali bi., Lach., Narz., Ol. an., Petr., Puls., Rhod., Sep.*
  –deep in lumbar and sacral region—*Arg. m.*
  –in sacrum and coccyx—*Lach.*
Spurted on back, water were—*Lyc.*
Squeezed, neck were being—*Ferr.*
  –in loins—*Dulc.*
  –in lumbar region—*Caust.*
Stabbing with a knife from within outward in vertebræ—*Bell.*
Sticking with a somewhat blunt needle in left side of nape of neck—*Tarax.*
  –into mole on neck when touched, needles were—*Tarent.*
  –fast to back on deep inspiration, something were—*Sars.*
  –below right shoulder blade, something were—*Ars. h.*
  –in spine, something were—*Eug.*
  –in middle of spine on swallowing food, sharp crust were—*Caust.*
  –like a blow on back—*Cina*
  –into lumbar region, nail were—*Berb.*
Stiff, neck were—*Pall., Zinc.*
  –cervical vertebræ were—*Calc. c.*

Stiff—*Continued*

  —and bruised, neck were—*Sol. n.*

  —nape of neck were—*Rhod.*

Stinging of needles in spine—*Calc. c.*

Stings of insects on back—*Chlor.*

Stone pressing between shoulders—*Chin., Nux v.*

Stooped too long, he had—*Mur. ac.*

Stooping a long time. pain in back after—*Dulc.*

Straighten back, she could not—*Cob.*

Strained, neck were—*Ant. c., Sil.*

  —from lifting, neck were—*Ambr.*

  —muscles of back were—*Form., Thuj.*

Streams of ice water were running down back—*Vacc., Vario.*

Strength had left back, all—*Zinc.*

Stretch, back were put on the—*Arg. n.*

Stretched from back of neck to eyes, thread were—*Lach.*

  —neck were—*Carl.*

  —muscles above right spine of ilium were—*Stann.*

  —across back from within, and pressing, a piece of wood were (before menses)—*Nux m.*

Striking upon back, a hammer were—*Lyss.*

String were pulled from shoulder to ear—*Lepi.*

  —about neck were tight—*Elæis guin.*

  —a cold wet, were tied around neck causing a choking sensation—*Sanic.*

  —between uterus and sacrum, there were a—*Nat. m.*

  —lumbar vertebræ had dropped out and spine were tied together with a—*Ovi g. p.*

Struck by a blow of fist in back—*Nux m.*

  —with a hammer in back—*Sep.*

Stuck in spine, a plug were—*Anac.*

Support spinal column, it were an effort to—*Phos.*

Suppurating in shoulder blade, everything were—*Calend.*

  —in back, at night before menses—*Berb.*

Sweat, cool drops of, going down left side of spine—*X-ray*

Swelling, neck were—*Carl., Mang., Par., Ptel., Rhod.*

  —muscle of neck were—*Ail.*

  —back were—*Berb.*

Swollen and bruised, submaxillary glands were—*Staph.*

  —and constricted, muscles of neck were—*Chin. s.*

Swollen—*Continued*

–vessels in left side of neck were—*Sil.*

–though it is not, coccyx were—*Syph.*

Tape prevented circulation of blood in shoulder—*Saba.*

Tear off, shoulder would—*Sep.*

Tense band reaching from nape of neck to ear—*Anac.*

–tendon from right shoulder along neck—*Crot. h.*

–and swollen, sides of neck were—*Sep.*

–in back, nerves and vessels were—*Coloc.*

Tension, external, over thyroid gland—*Agar.*

Thickened, neck were—*Canth., Con., Iod., Kali c., Pip. m.*

Thread, tight, around neck just below ears—*Rumx.*

–were drawing through scapulæ—*Elect.*

Threads stretched from back of neck to eyes—*Lach.*

Throbbing would arise in neck—*Fl. ac.*

Thrust through back, a knife were—*Cupr., Pyrog.*

–through side and back, knife were—*Ran. b.*

–into scapula, a pointed instrument were—*Spong.*

–into lower vertebræ, an iron rod were—*Alum.*

Thumb pressed upon back—*Meny.*

Tied tightly around neck, a cord were—*Lach.*

–too tight, cravat were—*Arn., Asar.*

–or constricted with a napkin, neck were—*Chel.*

–about neck, a ligature were—*Glon.*

–together with a string, lumbar vertebræ had dropped out and spine were—*Ovi g. p.*

Tight, collar were too—*Aml. n., Ant. t., Lach.*

–cravat, in muscle of neck—*Arn., Asar.*

–necktie were too—*Sep.*

–about neck, something were—*Dios.*

–string about neck—*Elæis guin.*

Tired, neck were—*Chim. mac.*

–and unable to support head, neck were—*Fago.*

Tongs twisting lumbar region—*Graph.*

Torn on moving and touch, left side of neck were—*Puls.*

–asunder, shoulder would be—*Mez.*

–apart on stooping, vertebræ were being—*Chel.*

–in lumbar region, parts were—*Sabin.*

Touched by a piece of ice below shoulder blade—*Agar.*

Trickling down back, cold water were—*Ars.*

Tugging at os coccygis, weight were—*Ant. t.*

Tumor in neck would protrude on turning head—*Calc. c.*

Turn or raise herself, she could not—*Sep.*

Twanging in left side of face and neck, wires were—*Kali bi.*

Twist her body when they run up her back, pains would—*Corn.*

Twisted about, neck would be—*Dulc.*

—out under left scapulæ, a piece of flesh would be forcibly—*Corn.*

—flesh were grasped between shoulders and—*Sars.*

Twisting lumbar region, tongs were—*Graph.*

Twitching from liquid dropping on flesh, back were—*Kali bi.*

—in back from electric shocks—*Nux v.*

Ulcerated, coccyx were—*Phos.*

Uncomfortable position, head and neck were lying in an—*Dulc., Ferr., Puls.*

—position, back had been—*Ferr. ma., Zinc.*

Uncovered all night, shoulder had been—*Kreos.*

Uneasiness, painful, in coccyx—*Tarent.*

Vermin were crawling on back—*Agn., Bell., Con., Mag. s., Nat. c., Osm., Zinc.*

Vise, back were in a—*Kali i., Nux m.*

—small of back were in a—*Æth., Kali i.*

Water, cold, were dashed against back—*Lil. t., Puls., Saba.*

—were dripping down spine from nape of neck—*Tub.*

—cold, dropping down back—*Caps.*

—cold, between shoulders—*Abies c.*

—cold, were poured down back—*Alum., Anac., Puls., Stram., Zinc.*

—cold, were poured down back, with headache—*Alumn.*

—cold, poured over back—*Anac.*

—ice cold, were poured down back—*Alumn.*

—cold, were running down back—*Agar., Alum., Alumn., Ars., Puls., Stram., Zinc.*

—cold, were running down back, if he leans against chair—*Agar.*

—cold, were trickling down back—*Ars.*

—streams of ice, were running down back—*Vacc., Vario.*

—spurted on back—*Lyc.*

—hot, were running upward from nape of neck—*Glon.*

—hot, in back—*Phos.*

—hot, were creeping through back from below upward—*Nit. s. d.*

Water—*Continued*

    —boiling, poured over small of back and through pelvis—*Verat. v.*

    —right scapula were bathed in hot—*Nat. s.*

    —dropping out of a bottle in lumbar region—*Med.*

    —warm, running up to brain, a stream of—*Cann. i.*

    —warm, were running down back—*Tep.*

Weak, neck were too—*Cocc., Plat., Stann., Staph., Verat. a., Zinc.*

Weary in back—*Puls.*

    —and bruised in loins, belly and thighs—*Bov.*

Wedge, muscles of neck were pressed by a dull—*Asar.*

Weight, hundred, on nape of neck—*Rhus t.*

    —great, on nape of neck and shoulders—*Par.*

    —heavy, on back—*Saponin.*

    —were lying upon cervical muscles—*Vinc.*

    —in back and shoulders—*Nat. m.*

    —on shoulder—*Sulph.*

    —on right shoulder, pressed by a—*Am. br.*

    —heavy, hung between shoulders—*Lyss.*

    —between scapulæ were compelling her to bend forward—*Carb. s.*

    —were lying on muscles of back—*Vinc.*

    —in small of back—*Kali c.*

    —around loins—*Gent. l.*

    —heavy, in lumbar region—*Coloc.*

    —tugging at os coccygis—*Ant. t.*

Weighted down by a heavy weight on shoulder—*Carb. s.*

Wet, collar or neck band were—*Tub.*

    —cold string were tied around neck causing choking—*Sanic.*

    —with cold perspiration between shoulder blades—*Lachn.*

    —cloth on back—*Cast.*

    —and moist, clothes on back were—*Tub.*

Wind, cold, were blowing on parts between scapulæ—*Caust.*

    —were blowing on back—*Hep.*

    —were blowing on back through a hole in clothes—*Chin., Culx.*

    —cool, were blowing on back—*Asar., Chin.*

Wires were twanging in left side of face and neck—*Kali bi.*

Withered in lumbar region—*Podo.*

Wood across back, pressing outward, a piece of—*Nux m.*

Worms crawling on neck—*Arund.*

  –crawling over back and scrotum—*Staph.*

Wound were in lower dorsal vertebræ and ribs—*Chel.*

Wrenched, sacral region had been—*Calc. c.*

  –in joints of sacrum—*Mag. p. Aust.*

Wrenching between shoulders—*Am. m.*

UPPER EXTREMITIES

(Aching in arms) weather were going to change—*Lyss.*

Act, limbs would refuse to—*Sep.*

Air blew on arms—*Tep.*

–were passing from shoulder joints to fingers—*Fl. ac.*

Affected, marrow of bones were—*Pip. m.*

Alive running in arm, something were—*Ign.*

–were jumping in arms, something—*Croc.*

–gurgling in shoulder joint, especially about midnight, something were—*Berb.*

–crawling under skin on tips of fingers, something were—*Sec.*

Ants were creeping in limbs—*Phos.*

–were running in fingers and left foot, with stiffness—*Mag. p. Arct.*

Armor encased joints of arms—*Psor.*

Asleep in arms—*Ail., Apis, Aran., Cast. eq., Caust., Cocc., Dub., Eucal., Graph., Kreos., Manc., Nux v., Puls.*

–arms would fall—*Carb. s., Mill., Puls.*

–in shoulder joint—*Zinc.*

–shoulder were—*Merc., Sep.*

–right arm were—*Am. m.*

–elbow were—*Coll., Dig., Graph., Nat. s., Tetrad.*

–hands were—*Agar., Aloe, Alum., Am. c., Aran., Bar. c., Bor., Bry., Calc. c., Calc. p., Cann. s., Carb. an., Carb. v., Caust., Croc., Dios., Euphr., Eupi., Fl. ac., Form., Gas., Graph., Hyos., Kali c., Kali n., Lyc., Merc., Mez., Naja, Nat. c., Nat. m., Nit. ac., Nux v., Petr., Phos., Pic. ac., Plb., Rhod., Sep., Sil., Squill., Sulph., Tep., Verat. a., Zinc.*

–hands had been—*Colch., Lyc., Verat. a.*

–hands and fingers were going to fall—*Dub., Dulc., Puls.*

–back of hand were—*Agar., Laur.*

–wrist were—*Carb. v., Ign.*

–fingers were—*Ail., Alum., Aran., Bar. c., Chlf., Dios., Lipp., Lyc., Nat. c., Nat. m., Par., Rat., Rhod., Saba., Sec., Sulph., Thuj.*

–finger joints were—*Euphr.*

–little finger were, with crawling—*Sul. ac.*

Asleep—*Continued*

   –left little finger were—*Calad., Dios., Med.*

   –finger tips were—*Rhus t.*

   –left thumb were—*Calad.*

   –phalanges were—*Euphr., Kreos.*

Balls, small, coursing along through hands and feet—*Zinc.*

Band—see also CORD and HOOP

Band just beneath axilla—*Magnol.*

   –or ligature around arms, causing blood to rush into hands in evening—*Nux m.*

   –on ring joint, encircled by—*Lyc.*

Bands tied around different parts of arms and legs—*Chin.*

   –bones of upper and lower extremities surrounded by tight—*Con.*

Bandage stopped circulation in arms—*Saba.*

Bandaged tightly in limbs—*Arund.*

   –to body, left arm were tightly—*Cimic.*

Battery, galvanic, were attached to arms—*Dor.*

   –hands were holding poles of galvanic—*Acon.*

Beaten in all limbs after exertion, he had been—*Agar.*

   –limbs were—*Aster., Bov., Dulc., Guaj., Lac c., Stann.*

   –in morning, limbs were—*Sel.*

   –in limbs with trembling—*Alumn.*

   –and sore, limbs were—*Dros.*

   –loose from bones, flesh were—*Thuj.*

   –off the bones, muscles were—*Eupi.*

   –arms were—*Merc., Nit. ac., Sulph.*

   –in middle of humerus—*Puls.*

   –in bones of upper arms—*Ang.*

   –in bones of wrists—*Asaf.*

   –in right wrist—*Calc. p.*

Belong to her, limbs did not—*Agar., Ign.*

Bent transversely, nails were—*Med.*

Biting in arms, electric sparks were—*Phel.*

   –in arms, insect were—*Chlor.*

   –in arms, salt water were—*Hell.*

Black, tips of fingers were dyed—*Sol. n.*

Blew on upper arm, wind—*Tep.*

Blistered, tips of fingers were—*Tarent.*

Blood ceased to circulate in arms—*Phos.*

   –about elbow, skin were infiltrated with—*Chin.*

Blood—*Continued*

  —were trickling down left arm from shoulder to finger joints—*Cot.*

  —streamed from finger tips into body—*Elaps*

  —would burst through veins of arms and hands—*Lil. t.*

  —all rushed to hands—*Nux m.*

  —had been drawn off in hands and fingers, leaving them empty—*Vario.*

  —engorged finger tips—*Rhus t.*

Blow on arm—*Stann.*

  —or thrust on arm—*Sars.*

  —on nerve of arm, tingling—*Scroph.*

Blowing on left shoulder, wind were—*Lyc.*

  —on left arm, cold wind were—*Aster.*

Body, blunt, were pressing in arm—*Ang.*

Boil were forming on hand (but did not)—*Med.*

Boils were in arm pits—*Chim. mac.*

Bound, limbs were—*Tarax.*

  —tightly to body, arms were—*Cimic.*

  —to side, left arm were—*Acon.*

  —stopping circulation, hand were—*Croc.*

Break, arms were brittle as though they would—*Rad.*

  —middle of upper arm would—*Cinnb.*

  —os humerus were about to—*Merc. i. r.*

  —in two, wrist would—*Corn. c.*

  —when touched, wrist would—*Sil.*

  —on flexion, finger joints would—*Iod., Thuj.*

Breaking, hand were—*Bor., Kali n.*

Breath, warm, on arms—*Hyos.*

Brier in middle of left, then right finger—*Dios.*

  —sticking in end of finger—*Sulph.*

Brittle as though they would break, arms were—*Rad.*

Broader, hand were—*Coll.*

Broken, limbs were—*Eup. per., Raph.*

  —shoulder were—*Chel., Cocc., Nat. m.*

  —arms were—*Bry., Cupr., Merc., Ruta, Verat. a., Zinc. ox.*

  —on motion, arms were—*Chel., Puls.*

  —right arm were—*Sphin.*

  —bones of arms were—*Gymn.*

  —elbow were—*Bry., Coc. c., Cur., Phos.*

Broken—*Continued*
  –humerus were—*Bov., Cocc., Cupr., Puls., Samb.*
  –wrist were—*Eup. per.*
  –hands and feet were—*Psor.*
  –in thumb—*Cham.*
  –finger tips were—*Cham.*
  –last phalanx were—*Crot. c.*
Bruise would form on left metacarpal bone—*Rhod.*
Bruised, limbs were—*Ammc., Calend., Cann. s., Led., Staph.*
  –arms were—*Arn., Croc., Verat. a.*
  –in upper arm—*Kreos.*
  –in spots when touching limbs—*Card. b.*
  –in elbow joint and left wrist—*Ammc.*
  –elbow were—*Agar., All. c., Am. c., Ang., Asar., Aur. m. n.,
    Bar. c., Brom., Calc. p., Camph., Carb. v., Caust., Cedr.,
    Con., Cyc., Dulc., Lach., Led., Linum, Nat. s., Phos., Puls.,
    Tell., Thuj., Verat. a., Zinc.*
  –on outside of elbow—*Sul. ac.*
  –severely around left humerus muscle—*Iodof.*
  –wrist were—*Ammc., Aur. m. n., Camph., Cham., Cot., Led.,
    Nat. m., Nit. ac., Nit. s. d., Thuj.*
  –radial artery were—*Bov.*
  –hand were—*Calc. p., Hep., Kali bi., Lil. t., Mag. c., Nicc.,
    Phos. ac., Sil.*
  –back of hand were—*Carb. v., Graph., Hura, Ruta*
  –palm were—*Am. m.*
  –bones of hands were—*Kali bi.*
  –arteries in hands were—*Ill.*
  –fingers were—*Bufo, Camph., Iris fl., Iris fœ., Led., Mez., Nit.
    ac., Peti., Ruta, Vichy*
  –thumb were—*Plat.*
  –nails were—*Jac., Plect.*
Bubbling in muscles of back and arms, something were—*Petros.*
  –in muscles of upper arm, something were—*Cupr.*
  –in left upper arm, something were—*Colch., Squill.*
  –in elbow joint, something were—*Kreos., Mang., Rheum*
  –ends of fingers were—*Ign.*
Burned, left wrist were—*Agar.*
Burning would cut through arms—*Sul. ac.*
  –in spots on shoulder and arms, red-hot coals were—*Phos. ac.*

Burning—*Continued*
   –in biceps muscle—*Raph.*
   –and itching as if frozen, both hands were—*Agar.*
   –and sore in small spots in right middle finger—*Tetrad.*
Burnt along arms—*Cur.*
   –on outer side of right arm—*Prun.*
   –with a hot iron, elbows and fingers were—*Alum.*
   –near wrist, forearm were—*Agar., Cur.*
   –on outer side of little finger—*Prun.*
Bursa would form in wrist—*Prun.*
Burst through veins of arms, blood would—*Lil. t.*
   –hands would—*Vib.*
   –on hanging down, hands would—*Vip.*
Bursting, arms were—*Vip.*
   –in left elbow—*Sil.*
   –finger tips were—*Caust.*
Buzzing in hands—*Vib.*
Chopped with an ax, joints were being—*Phyt.*
Circulation ceased in limbs—*Lyc.*
   –had stopped in arms—*Glon.*
Clawing from hand around elbow—*Caust.*
Closed, hands could not be—*Ars. m.*
Clucking in arm—*Ambr.*
Coal, a red-hot, on shoulder and arms—*Phos. ac.*
Coals glowing in small spots on face and hands—*Caust.*
Cobweb on skin of hands—*Bor.*
Cold as ice, extremities were—*Croc.*
   –limbs were—*Sulph.*
   –in all the limbs, he were getting—*Hep.*
   –hands and arms had been exposed to a temperature of 30° F.
     below zero—*Sanic.*
   –as if he had been handling ice, hands were—*Sanic., Sulph.*
   –from a cold wind, wrist were—*Rhus t.*
   –as ice, fingers were—*Phos. ac.*
Coldness, icy, of joints of middle finger—*Agar.*
Come off, nails would—*Nat. c.*
Compressed by an iron hoop, arm were—*Gas.*
   –nerve of arm had been, causing numbness—*Cimic.*
   –bones of arms were—*Spong.*
   –elbow were—*Chlor., Nat. s.*
   –nerve in forearm from elbow to little finger were—*Æsc.*

Consciousness from pain as of splinters in right forearm, she
would lose—*Agar.*

Constricted, elbow were—*Agar., Petr.*

   –palms would be spasmodically—*Sabin.*

Constriction of elbow as if one had carried a heavy weight—
Elaps

Contracted, skin of hands and fingers were—*Tell.*

   –muscles in palms of hands were—*Coloc.*

Control of will, right arm were not under—*Cupr.*

Contused, wrist joint had been—*Calc. c.*

Cord around shoulder—*Lepi., Plb.*

   –were tied around upper arm—*Alumn.*

   –were drawn tight two inches above and below elbow—*Rat.*

   –were pulling down in arm or hand during pregnancy—*Plb.*

Covered with a glove, hand were—*Carb. s.*

   –with suggillations, hands were—*Rhus t.*

Cracking, wrists were—*Cic.*

Cramp, fingers were about to—*Dios.*

Crawling on neck, shoulders and hands, insects were—*Lac c.*

   –in arms—*Cocc., Ign.*

   –up arms in a straight line, fly were—*Euphr.*

   –up arms during menses—*Graph.*

   –under skin of forearm, mouse were—*Ign.*

   –in hands—*Hyper.*

   –over dorsum of left hand, spider were—*Visc.*

   –and itching in right palm—*Tetrad.*

   –in fingers—*Staph.*

   –in all fingers, worms were—*Goss.*

   –in tips of fingers, something were—*Rhus t.*

   –in tips of three left middle fingers—*Thuj.*

   –and asleep in little finger—*Sul. ac.*

Creeping in limbs, ants were—*Phos.*

   –on limbs, millions of insects were—*Mez.*

Crowded with arms and legs, he were—*Pyrog.*

Crowding through boots, heels were—*Eup. pur.*

Crushed, limbs would be—*Cocc.*

   –bones of arms were—*Gymn.*

   –elbow were—*Thuj.*

   –left humerus were—*Stann.*

   –bones in left forearm were—*Gymn.*

Crushed—*Continued*
  –finger were—*Caust.*
  –bones in fingers were—*Olnd.*
Current, electric, tingling in both arms—*X-ray*
  –galvanic, passed through extremities—*Polyg.*
  –of electricity passed from head to limbs—*Ail.*
  –in hands and fingers, active—*Lil. t.*
Cut, arms were—*Nux v.*
  –through arms, burning would—*Sul. ac.*
Cutting instruments were piercing all joints—*Vesp.*
  –in elbow—*Bell., Cedr., Hydrs., Phos. ac.*
Dangling and turning on a pivot, arms were—*Plb.*
Dashed with cold water, arms were—*Mez.*
Dead, arms were—*Lyc.*
  –right arm were—*Ol. j.*
  –wrist were—*Cann. s.*
  –hands were—*Apis, Ars. h., Bry., Cedr., Cimx., Con., Graph., Guare., Lach., Lyc., Mez., Ox. ac., Phos., Puls., Sep., Sil.*
  –fingers were—*Angel., Calc. c., Hep., Lyc., Par.*
  –little finger were—*Ang.*
  –middle finger were, but remaining very sensitive—*Agar.*
  –phalanges were—*Chel.*
  –tips of fingers were—*Tell.*
Decay, parts in and between wrists were weakened by—*Spong.*
Decayed, nails were—*Sil.*
Detached from body, arms were—*Daph. i., Daph. o.*
Dislocated, shoulder were—*Agar., Anac., Ant. t., Caust., Cop., Ign., Mag. c., Sep., Sulph., Tep.*
  –shoulder joint were—*Caps., Cor. r., Croc., Fl. ac., Ign., Mag. c., Mag. m., Nicc., Olnd.*
  –upper arm were—*Alum.*
  –arm were—*Lac c., Rhod., Thuj.*
  –by a blow, whole right arm were, < axilla—*Paraf.*
  –joints were—*Agn.*
  –head of left humerus were—*Rhus t.*
  –wrists were—*Ang., Arn., Caust., Eup. per., Eupi., Get., Nux v., Ox. ac., Sulph., Thuj.*
  –joints of left hand were—*Get.*
  –first joint of right thumb were—*Laur.*
  –fingers were—*Kiss.*
Dislocation in right carpal joint, severe pain and—*Tub.*

Distended, limbs were—*Chim. mac.*
Dragging in elbow, something were—*Fago.*
Drawing in arms, muscles were tense and—*Zinc.*
   –in bones—*Aloe*
   –in joints of left middle finger—*Bell.*
   –down the arm, left arm in walking presses on elbow—*Ang.*
Drawn together, shoulders would be—*Carb. v.*
   –together on pressure, shoulders would be—*Ferr.*
   –forward (when hanging down), arm were—*Phos.*
   –inward, arms were—*Laur.*
   –asunder, arms were—*Nat. c.*
   –up, arms were being—*Carb. s.*
   –tight two inches above and below elbow, cord were—*Rat.*
   –tightly around upper part of arm causing pain in lines of con-
     striction, ligature were—*Alumn.*
   –skin on finger tips were—*Staph.*
Dripped off right elbow and shoulder, water—*Stry.*
Drop out at shoulder, left arm would—*Lach.*
   –from limbs, flesh would—*Rhus t.*
   –what she had in her hand, she would—*Cyc.*
Dropping from right elbow, cold water were—*Stry.*
Drops of fluid passed from right hand to shoulder during stool
     —*Chin. s.*
   –of blood rolled over each other, gurgling—*Thuj.*
   –of cold water spurted on back of hands on going into open air
     —*Berb.*
Drummed on with a finger, arm were—*Elæis guin.*
Dry, joints were—*Thuj.*
   –as if finger tips were made of paper—*Ant. t., Sil.*
Electric—see also SHOCKS
Electric current passed from head to limbs—*Ail.*
   –current tingling in both arms—*X-ray*
   –shock in shoulder and arm—*Phyt.*
   –shocks in all joints—*Paraf.*
   –sparks, fine, in spots on upper extremities—*Carb. ac.*
   –sparks were biting in arms—*Phel.*
   –shock passed through humerus—*Valer., Verat. a.*
   –shock tingling in left lower arm—*Pip. m.*
   –shock in wrist—*Agar.*
   –sparks on middle finger—*Carb. ac.*
   –current in finger tips—*Lil. t.*

Electricity pricking in fingers and hands—*Glon., Lil. t., Ptel.*

Empty feeling in hands and fingers as if blood had been drawn off—*Vario.*

Encased in armor about joints of arms—*Psor.*

Encircled by band on ring joint—*Lyc.*

Engorged with blood, finger tips were—*Rhus t.*

Enlarged, hands were—*Aran., Lyc.*

 –and thick, fingers were—*Sil.*

 –on waking, finger were—*Coca*

Exercise, had taken violent—*Æsc.*

Exhausted by fatigue, limbs were—*Verat. a.*

Expanded, arm were—*Sep.*

Extension of arms were prevented by string—*Sphin.*

Fall from him, all limbs would—*Merc.*

 –when raised, arm would—*Caj.*

Fallen on her hand, she had—*Lyss.*

Falling from arms, cold water were—*Cann. s.*

Feathers were tickling arms—*Morph.*

Feverish, hands were—*Ham., Phos., Pip. m.*

Fibers or fine wires pulling in continual motion down both arms from elbows to hands—*Cocc.*

Finger, arm were drummed on with—*Elæis guin.*

Fire, arms were on—*Iris, X-ray*

 –were flickering through arm—*Vip.*

 –always burning but <in bed, right forearm and elbow were on—*Lyc.*

 –hands had been exposed to cold, then to heat of—*Phys.*

Fleas were running over arms—*Lyss.*

Flexed on palm, fingers would be—*Com.*

Flickering through arm, flame were—*Vip.*

Fluid passed from right hand to shoulder during stool, drops of —*Chin. s:*

Fly to pieces on coughing, left shoulder would—*Rhus t.*

 –were crawling up limbs in a straight line—*Euphr.*

Forced asunder in middle left finger—*Laur.*

Form in index finger, panaritium would—*Sep., Sil.*

Formication in arms—*Tub.*

Forming, panaritium were—*Gymn.*

Fractured, left shoulder were—*Chel.*

Frostbitten, fingers were—*Bor.*

Frozen, hand were—*Cocc., Dig., Nux m.*
  –with burning and itching, hands had been—*Agar.*
  –palms and finger tips had been—*Spig.*
Full, limbs were—*Spire.*
  –and swollen, arms were too—*Verat. a.*
Fullness in left palm when grasping anything—*Caust.*
Fuzziness in hand—*Hell., Hyper., Merc.*
Fuzzy in limbs—*Sec.*
  –fingers were—*Ars., Colch.*
  –finger tips were—*Kiss., Tab.*
Galvanic current passed through extremities—*Polyg.*
  –passed through forearm—*Gels.*
  –battery, hands were holding poles of—*Acon.*
Glass in finger, a piece of—*Nit. ac.*
  –were in elbow—*Lach.*
Glove, hand were covered with—*Carb. s.*
Glowing in small spot on face and hands, coals were—*Caust.*
Glued together in arms, muscles were—*Rumx.*
Grasped arm tightly, a hand—*Nux m.*
Gurgling in shoulder joint, something alive were—*Berb.*
  –single drops of blood rolled over each other—*Thuj.*
Hairs were rising on back of hands and fingers—*Aloe*
  –on back of little finger—*Fl. ac.*
Hand were clawing around elbow—*Caust.*
Hands all over the bed, one had—*Pyrog.*
  –did not know she had any ; could feel no—*Sec.*
Hanging on upper arm, something heavy were—*Sulph.*
Heat were streaming through arm—*Cic.*
  –gentle, passed from stomach through arms to fingers then
      hands appeared as if dead—*Con.*
Heaviness, leaden, in arms preventing playing piano—*Cur.*
Heavy as lead, limbs were—*Nux v.*
  –load in arms—*Stram.*
  –on right shoulder, he had carried something—*Cast.*
  –arms were too—*Merc.*
  –hanging on upper arms, something were—*Sulph.*
Held in hot water, hands were—*Rhus t.*
Hold a pen, he could not—*Bism.*
Holding her fast in right elbow, something were—*Canth.*
  –poles of galvanic battery, hands were—*Acon.*
  –a book in fingers, he were—*Atro.*

Hoop, iron, compressed arm—*Gas.*
   –were tight about arms—*Gins.*
Ice a long time, penetrating to marrow of bones; he had been holding—*Sulph.*
   –in olecranon process—*Agar.*
   –bones were made of—*Aran.*
   –hands so tingling and cold, he had been handling—*Sanic.*
Infiltrated with blood about elbow, skin were—*Chin.*
Insect were biting in arm—*Chlor.*
Insects were crawling on neck, shoulders and hands—*Lac c.*
   –were creeping on limbs, millions of—*Mez.*
Iron hoop compressed arm—*Gas.*
   –hot, on arms, elbows and fingers—*Alum.*
Itch, ball of thumb would—*Lith.*
Itching and burning in both hands as if frozen—*Agar.*
   –and crawling in right palm—*Tetrad.*
   –in all finger bones—*Lith.*
Joint, left arm were out of—*Caj.*
   –elbow were out of—*Dios.*
Jump, arms would—*Morph.*
Jumping in arms, something alive were—*Croc.*
Knife below head of humerus from within out, stabbing with a blunt—*Bell.*
   –sticking in ball of hand—*Sep.*
   –dull, sticking in flesh between fingers—*Chin. s., Verb.*
Knock on right elbow—*Thuj.*
Knocked against something, upper extremities were—*Arn.*
Knot, nerves of arm had been tied in—*Crot. c.*
Lame, hand were—*Rhus t.*
Lameness were in bones—*Cocc.*
Large and swollen, upper extremities were—*Sec.*
   –hands were—*Ant. t., Bapt., Cann. i., Cupr., Kali n., Mang., Ptel.*
   –hands were too—*Bov., Clem., Hyos.*
   –as sausages, fingers were—*Calad.*
   –finger joints were too—*Eupi.*
Larger than whole body, right arm or hand were—*Cupr.*
   –when grasping anything, thumb and index finger were—*Caust.*
Lashed with a whip, wrist were—*Raph.*
Lead, limbs were heavy as—*Nux v.*

Lead—*Continued*
  –in limbs—*Valer.*
  –arms were filled with—*Sil.*
Lift forearms and hands, he could not—*Aran.*
Light, all limbs were—*Asar., Stict.*
Lightning, right shoulder had been paralyzed by stroke of—*Ign.*
Living were running in arms, something—*Ign.*
Load, heavy, in arms—*Stann.*
Long, arms and legs were two miles—*Cann. s.*
Longer, fingers were—*Tab.*
Loose on thighs and arms, flesh were—*Nat. m.*
  –from humerus, flesh were—*Thuj.*
  –head of humerus were—*Croc.*
  –joints of hand were—*Stram.*
  –finger were—*Spong.*
  –and could be shaken off, finger nails were—*Apis*
Loosely articulated, limbs were—*Laur.*
Loosened from bone, flesh were—*Thuj.*
  –in joints, hands and feet were—*Stram.*
Lose use of limbs on attempting to walk, he would—*Colch.*
Luxated, left shoulder were—*Sulph.*
  –arms were—*Rhus t.*
  –or sprained, right thumb were—*Calc. p.*
Marrow, pain were in—*Ruta*
  –of bones were affected—*Pip. m.*
Mouse were running up arms and back—*Calc. c., Sulph.*
  –were running up and down limbs—*Sep.*
  –were crawling under skin of forearm—*Ign.*
Move limbs but he cannot, he must—*Valer.*
Mummified, hands were—*Ars.*
Needle pricking on skin of elbow, irritated by—*Staph.*
  –raised skin on elbow—*Laur.*
  –raised skin on forearms—*Sulph.*
  –in middle finger, pricked with—*Cupr.*
Needles, red-hot, pierced in muscles of left side of face from
      forehead to neck and axilla—*Spig.*
  –red-hot, in limbs—*Lith.*
  –were pricking in limbs—*Lach.*
  –and pins pricking on skin of forehead, face and arms—*All. c.*
  –shooting into wrist joints—*Acon.*

Nettles, hands had been plunged among—*Arum d.*
  —on last joint of ring finger, stinging from—*Pimp.*
No limbs, he had—*Stram.*
  —hands, she could feel—*Sec.*
Numb, arms were—*Cham.*
  —and paralyzed, left arm were—*Æsc.*
  —hands were—*Hyper.*
  —in left thumb near tip—*Zinc.*
Numbness of fingers as if asleep—*Ail.*
  —in ring and little fingers—*Eupi.*
  —of finger tips—*Apis*
Overheated, limbs were—*Vacc., Vario.*
Panaritium would form in index finger—*Sil., Sep.*
  —were forming—*Gymn.*
Paper, tips of fingers were made of (at night)—*Ant. t., Sil.*
Paralyzed, limbs were—*Azad., Card. b., Kali i., Nat. p., Phos.,*
    Sars., Stann.
  —shoulder were—*Euph., Lact., Puls.*
  —by a stroke of lightning, right shoulder were—*Ign.*
  —arms were—*Crot. h., Hipp., Iod., Lith., Psor., Zinc.*
  —right arm were—*Chim. mac., Ferr. i., Til.*
  —left arm were—*Pall.*
  —and numb, left arm were—*Æsc.*
  —arms and hands were—*Plat.*
  —arms and knees were—*Tab.*
  —elbow were—*Arg. m., Cann. i., Mez., Sulph., Zinc.*
  —if he holds a light weight a short time, arms would be—*Stann.*
  —wrist were—*Acet. ac., Euphr., Lipp., Mez., Plect., Thuj.*
  —hands were—*Carb. an., Elaps, Phos. ac.*
  —fingers were—*Am. m., Ars., Both. l., Bry., Calc. p., Carb. v.,*
    Hell., Lact., Lil. t., Mez., Nat. m., Par., Phos . Plb., Ptel.
  —fingers would be—*Calad.*
Parched, hands and arms were—*Lil. t.*
Passing down right arm from shoulder to fingers, air were—
  Fl. ac.
Pierced with red-hot needles in muscles of left side of face from
    forehead to neck and axilla—*Spig.*
Piercing all joints, cutting instruments were—*Vesp.*
Pin were pricking wrist—*Hura*
  —were thrust through palm of right hand or forefinger—*Anag.*

Pins were pricking skin of forehead, neck and arms—*All. c.*
 –were pricking on palmar surface of phalanges and points of
      fingers—*Rhus t.*
Pithy, palm were—*Bry.*
 –fingers were—*Angel.*
Plunged among nettles, hand had been—*Arum d.*
 –into ice water, hand had been—*Tub.*
 –into boiling water, hand had been—*Arund.*
Position, limbs were kept long in an unusual—*Staph.*
Pounded, hands were—*Lil. t.*
Poured over one side from shoulder to thigh, cold water were—
      Verb.
 –on arms, ice water were—*Lyss.*
Powerless; all power had left arm—*Stront.*
Pressed out first in one arm then the other, head of humerus
      would be—*Cor. r.*
 –bones of forearms were—*Verat. a.*
Presses on bend of elbow in walking as if drawing down arm,
      left arm—*Ang.*
Pressing on left shoulder by clavicle, someone were—*Rhus t.*
 –in arm, blunt body were—*Ang.*
Pressure of fingers would sprain them, least—*Plan.*
Pricked with needle in middle finger—*Cupr.*
Pricking—see PINS and NEEDLES
Pricking on skin of forehead, face and arms, needles and pins
      were—*All. c.*
 –in limbs, needles were—*Lach.*
 –on skin of elbow, needle were—*Staph.*
 –of electricity in fingers and hands—*Lil. t., Ptel.*
Pulled from right shoulder to neck, tendon were—*Crot. h.*
 –out of joint, shoulders and hips were—*Fl. ac.*
 –left arm were—*Lach.*
 –out of socket, joints of right finger were being—*Fl. ac., Sil.*
 –tip of right index finger were—*Arum d.*
 –out, nail of left forefinger were being—*Phos.*
 –through artery, pulse like a thread were—*Spig.*
Pulling down in arm during pregnancy, cord were—*Plb.*
Pulsating under left thumb nail—*Am. m.*
Rain on back of hand when in open air, sprinkles of—*Berb.*
Raise limbs but he could, could not—*Sulph.*
Raised by a needle on arms, skin were—*Laur., Sulph.*

Refuse to act, limbs would—*Sep*.

Relaxed, muscles in hands were—*Gels*.

Restrained in limbs, motor power were (but actually motion is easy)—*Tarax*.

Rolling down arm from shoulder to hand, something were—*Rhus t*.

Room in capsule, head of humerus had not—*Laur*.

Running up arms and back, mouse were—*Calc. c., Sulph*.

  –in arm, something living were—*Ign*.

  –over arms, fleas were—*Lyss*.

  –through bones at elbow, water were—*Graph*.

  –through wrists, water were—*Tub*.

  –through wrists, hot water were—*Rhus t*.

Rushed to hands, all blood—*Nux m*.

Salt water were biting in arms—*Hell*.

Sausages, fingers were—*Calad*.

Sawed at wrists with a dull saw, someone—*Syph*.

Scalded, fingers were—*Nat. c., Rhus v*.

Scraped, elbow were—*Plat*.

  –bones near joints were—*Spig*.

Scratched off arms, skin were—*All. c*.

Seized, arm had been—*Cupr*.

Separate, bones of arms would—*Still*.

  –joints were—*Stram*.

Separated from body, arms were—*Daph., Stram*.

  –from each other, all parts of limbs were—*Stram*.

Separating from attachments, shoulder were—*Kali bi*.

Shaken off, finger nails were loose and could be—*Apis*

Shattered, hand were—*Pall*.

Shock—see also ELECTRIC

Shock, electric, in arms—*Cic*.

  –galvanic, in limbs—*Polyg., Verat. v*.

  –in all joints—*Paraf*.

  –electric, through humerus—*Valer., Verat. a*.

  –electric, tingling in left lower arm—*Pip. m*.

  –electric, in wrists—*Agar*.

  –electric, in hand—*Aloe*

  –of electricity pricking fingers and hands—*Lil. t., Ptel*.

Shooting into wrist joints, needles were—*Acon*.

Short, tendons of limbs were too—*Cimx., Rhus t., Spig*.

  –tendons in arms were too—*Cimx., Kreos., Laur*.

Short—*Continued*

   –elbow joint were too—*Mang.*

   –forearm were too—*Cham.*

   –wrist were too—*Carb. v.*

   –in right wrist, muscles were too—*Zinc.*

   –tendons in hands were too—*Phos. ac.*

   –nerves in hand were too—*Aloe*

   –tendons in fingers were too—*Nux v., Phos. ac.*

   –tendons in left thumb were too—*Sulph.*

Shortened, limbs were—*Mez.*

   –arms were—*Æth., Alum., Bell.*

   –tendon of wrist and hand were—*Carb. v.*

Skin, hard, were over tips of fingers on left hand—*Staph.*

Sleep, limbs were going to—*Gels., Mill., Rheum*

   –arms had gone to—*Croc., Lach., Stram.*

   –right arm had gone to—*Kali bi.*

   –left arm had gone to—*Apis*

   –arms would go to—*Cham., Euphr.*

   –left arm would go to—*Pall.*

   –fingers had gone to—*Cimx.*

Slept on left arm all night, he had—*Iber.*

Snapped from place in elbow, tendon—*Sars.*

Snatched back on taking hold of anything, arm were—*Stry.*

Something were in hand—*Dros.*

Sore and beaten, limbs were—*Dros.*

   –and burning in small spots on right middle finger—*Tetrad.*

Sparkling in elbow—*Verat. a.*

Sparks, electric, in limbs—*Phyt.*

   –fine electric, on middle finger—*Carb. ac.*

Spider, big, crawling on back of hand—*Visc.*

Splinter in pimple near wrist—*Arg. n.*

   –in hand when touching a hair on it—*Ign.*

   –in finger—*Nit. ac., Sil.*

   –in bone of index finger—*Fl. ac.*

   –between thumb and index finger—*Arn.*

   –under thumb nail—*Fl. ac., Hura*

   –under finger nail—*Calc. p.*

   –under right index nail had caused suppuration—*Ran. b.*

Splinters in left elbow, a thousand—*Agar.*

   –in right forearm; would lose consciousness from pain of—*Agar.*

Splinters—*Continued*

   —of fine glass under finger nails—*Coc. c.*

Sprain them, least pressure of fingers would—*Plan.*

Sprained—see also LUXATED

Sprained, limbs were—*Rhus v.*

   —shoulders were—*Agar., Alum., Alumn., Ambr., Arg. m., Asar., Berb., Cere. s., Cyc., Hep., Ign., Lyc., Mang., Mur. ac., Nat. m., Nicc., Petr., Phos., Plect., Ruta, Saba., Sep., Spig., Vesp.*

   —arms were—*Aur. m., Bell., Bor., Jug. c., Merc., Nit. ac., Petr., Phos.*

   —arms had been—*Jug. c., Kalm., Wild.*

   —left shoulder joint were—*Vesp.*

   —right shoulder joint were—*Sabin.*

   —in upper arm—*Sol. t. æ.*

   —muscles of upper arm were—*Ter.*

   —joint of arm were—*Arn.*

   —elbow were—*Alum., Cur., Juncus, Lach., Mang., Tell.*

   —right elbow were—*Gels., Tab.*

   —wrists were—*Berb., Bry., Carb. an., Caust., Hipp., Jug. c., Lach., Ox. ac., Rhod., Rhus t., Ruta, Seneg., Zinc.*

   —right wrist were—*Gels., Zinc.*

   —hand were—*Acon., Carb. v., Dios., Caust., Jug. c., Kalm., Sil.*

   —back of hand were—*Rhus t.*

   —fingers were—*Jug. r., Aloe, Kali n., Phos.*

   —index finger and thumb were—*Lachn.*

   —left little finger were—*Nux m.*

   —thumb were—*Camph., Cham.*

   —right thumb were—*Calc. p., Prun.*

   —left thumb were—*Ang., Kreos.*

   —finger tips were—*Cham., Stann.*

Sprinkled with drops of cold water when going into open air, backs of hands were—*Berb.*

Squeezed together, bones of limbs were—*Alum.*

   —wrists had been—*Euphr.*

   —and gradually let go, wrist were—*Phys.*

   —hands were being—*Spig.*

   —left hand were—*Tarent.*

Squeezing something for a long time, he had been—*Myris.*

Stabbing below head of humerus from within out, blunt knife were—*Bell.*

Sticking between fingers, dull knife were—*Chin. s., Verb.*

   –in ball of hand, knife were—*Sep.*

   –under nail of right index finger—*Sep.*

Stiff, limbs were without joints and—*Petr.*

Stiffen, right hand would—*Asaf.*

Stiffened, palm would be—*Stry.*

Sting of wasp at elbow—*Arg. m.*

   –of bee in palm of left hand—*Crot. h.*

Stinging from nettles on last joint of right ring finger—*Pimp.*

Stitched too tight, skin on fingers were—*Mag. p.*

Strained, limbs were—*Dub.*

   –unduly in left upper arm—*Rhus t.*

   –muscles were—*Form.*

   –right elbow were—*Hyper.*

   –wrists were—*Lyss.*

Streaming into body from finger tips, blood were—*Elaps*

Strength in limbs, there were no—*Staph.*

Stretch limbs, she wanted to constantly—*Rhus t.*

Stretched, limbs were forcibly—*Rhus t.*

   –shoulder were—*Carl.*

Stretching apart when walking or sitting, fingers of right hand were—*Aur. m. n.*

String prevented extension of arms—*Sphin.*

   –tied about arms—*Nux m., Sec.*

   –tight about wrist—*Manc.*

Strong in forearms and hands—*Aran.*

Struck, joint of elbow had been—*Calc. p.*

   –crazy-bone had been—*Cinnb.*

   –violently on fingers leaving warts, she had been—*Phos.*

Supported himself upon it, upper arm would break if he—*Samb.*

Suppurate at roots of nails, it were about to—*Mag. p. Aust.*

Suppurating, finger tips were—*Sil., Sep.*

Swelled, limbs were—*Guaj.*

   –arms and legs suddenly—*Tanac.*

Swollen, arm were—*Hep., Kali br.*

   –and too full, arm were—*Verat. a.*

   –head of humerus were—*Laur.*

   –bend of elbow were—*Lept., Verat. a.*

   –head, hands and face were, < washing—*Æth.*

   –hands and forearms were greatly—*Aran.*

   –hands were—*Cocc.*

Swollen—*Continued*

    —on closing, hands were—*Gins.*

    —left hand were—*Med.*

    —finger joints were—*Calc. c.*

    —when writing, finger joints were—*Bry.*

Tape prevented circulation in arms—*Saba.*

Tearing pain were in bones of wrist—*Benz. ac.*

Tense from shoulder to neck, tendon were—*Crot. h.*

Thick, hand were—*Clem.*

    —and clumsy, hands were too—*Manc.*

    —fingers were too—*Hyos.*

    —and enlarged, bones of fingers were—*Sil.*

Thicker than left, right hand were—*Bry.*

Thread pulled through artery, pulse were—*Spig.*

Threads stretched along arms—*Lach.*

Through elbow, bone would come—*Phos.*

Thumbs, fingers were all—*Phos.*

Thrust or blow on arms—*Sars.*

    —through arms, something were—*Cupr.*

    —through palm of right hand or forefinger, pin were—*Anag.*

Tickled arms and legs, someone suddenly—*Staph.*

Tickling arm, feathers were—*Morph.*

Tied, arm were—*Abrot., Alumn., Caj., Nux m.*

    —with a cord, arm were—*Aml. n.*

    —around arms, string were—*Nux m.*

    —to body, arms were—*Caj.*

    —in knot, nerves of arm were—*Crot. c.*

    —up, right wrist were—*Glon.*

Tight around arms, clothing were too—*Paraf.*

    —two inches above and below elbow, cord were drawn—*Rat.*

    —around arms, garters were too—*Raph.*

    —about wrist, string were—*Manc.*

    —on hand, skin were too—*Gins.*

Tingling, limbs were—*Trios.*

    —from blow, nerve of arm were—*Scroph.*

    —in both arms from electric current—*X-ray*

    —of electric shock in left lower arm—*Pip. m.*

Torn out, limbs were—*Cham.*

    —out, shoulder joint would be—*Sep.*

    —asunder, shoulder joint would be—*Mez.*

    —from bone, flesh were—*Ant. t., Plat.*

Torn—*Continued*
  –from bone, muscles would be—*Dros.*
  –under right index finger nail—*Con.*
  –off, part of nail had been—*Hura*
  –out, nails were being—*Phos.*
Turned outward, arms and feet were—*Graph.*
Turning on a pivot, arms were dangling and—*Plb.*
Twisted, hands were—*Stry.*
Ulcer would form on left arm—*Tab.*
  –would develop at margin of nails—*Tetrad.*
Ulcerate in right thumb, it would—*Olnd.*
Ulcerated, muscles of left arm were—*Iodof.*
  –forearm were—*Lyc.*
  –fingers were—*Ruta*
  –tips of fingers were—*Alum., Graph., Sars.*
Use of limbs would go—*Fil.*
  –his arms, he could not—*Arn.*
Vesicles on left hand—*Tell.*
Vise, forearm were in—*Brom., Kalm.*
  –first phalanx of left thumb were—*Phos.*
Wart were growing on thumb—*Ferr. pic.*
Washed in acid water, hand were dry—*Sumb.*
Wasp sting at knee and elbow—*Arg. m.*
Water, salt, were biting arms—*Hell.*
  –hot, limbs had been a long time in—*Sec.*
  –cold, were dashed on arms—*Mez.*
  –dropped off right shoulder and elbow—*Stry.*
  –cold, were falling from arms—*Cann. s.*
  –cold, were poured over one side from shoulder to thigh—
    Verb.
  –ice, were poured on arms—*Lyss.*
  –hot, were running through arm—*Rhus t.*
  –cold, were dropping from right elbow—*Stry.*
  –were running through bones at elbows—*Graph.*
  –were running through wrist—*Tub.*
  –hands had been long in—*Verat. v.*
  –hands had been held in hot—*Rhus t.*
  –hands were plunged into boiling—*Arund.*
  –hands had been plunged into ice—*Tub.*
  –were sprinkled on backs of hands on going into open air, drops
    of cold—*Berb.*

Weakened by decay, parts in and between wrists were—*Spong.*
Weather were going to change (aching in upper arms)—*Lyss.*
Wedge were in left shoulder > moving—*Mag. m.*
Weight in all limbs—*Hep.*
 —were resting on shoulders—*Hep.*
 —on left shoulder—*Stann.*
 —heavy, were hung to arms—*Chel., Cur.*
 —in arms, he had carried—*Plat., Thuj.*
Whip, wrist were lashed by—*Raph.*
Wind were blowing on left shoulder—*Lyc.*
 —extended up arms—*Croc.*
 —blew on upper arm—*Tep.*
 —cold, blowing on left arm—*Aster.*
 —wrists were cold from a cold—*Rhus t.*
 —cold, passed through hands—*Kreos.*
Wires or fibers were pulling in continual motion down both arms
  from elbows to hands, very fine—*Cocc.*
Withered, hand were—*Rhus t.*
Wood, arms were made of—*Dulc.*
 —hanging to him, arms were of soaked—*Caj.*
 —hands were made of—*Kali n.*
Worked hard with her fingers, she had—*Nux v.*
Worms were crawling in all fingers—*Goss.*
Wound were smarting in wrist—*Puls.*
Wrenched, right arm below elbow were—*Ars. m.*
Writing, she had been doing much rapid (in wrist)—*Cor. r.*

LOWER EXTREMITIES

Abraded on right buttock, skin were—*X-ray*

Abscess were forming on foot—*Tarent.*

Aching in calves from long walking or standing—*Rumx.*

Act, limbs would refuse to—*Sep.*

Air blowing on feet at night, draft of, must get up and tuck bed-clothes in, which >—*Maland.*
  –cool, blowing on lower extremities—*Lil. t.*
  –hot, blowing over lower abdomen and thighs—*Trom.*
  –hot, going through knee joints—*Lach.*
  –legs floating in—*Stict., Verat. a.*
  –walking on—*Lac c.*
  –were moving through sole, a current of—*Valer.*

Alcohol had been spilled over left thigh—*Lob. s.*

Alive in legs causing twitching, something were—*Berb.*
  –in legs, on touch, twitching from something—*Ars.*
  –in calves, something were—*Sil.*
  –in soles, something were—*Caust.*

All over sidewalk, legs were—*Kali br.*

Anthill, lower extremities were in—*Sal. ac.*

Ants were crawling in the back and legs—*Alum.*
  –were biting above right kneee—*Peti.*
  –were crawling on lower limbs—*Alum., Aster.*
  –were crawling on feet—*Dulc.*

Articulated, limbs were loosely—*Laur.*

Asleep, limbs would fall—*Dulc., Puls.*
  –limbs were—*Ail., Dub., Eucal., Graph., Puls.*
  –in buttocks—*Raph.*
  –in thighs—*Asar., Canth., Chin., Cic., Euph., Glon., Guaj., Ign., Merc., Sil., Thuj.*
  –in legs—*Ail., Aran., Chlor., Lob. s., Phos., Syph.*
  –and tingling, legs were—*Merc. i. f.*
  –legs would go to—*Psor., Sep.*
  –left leg were—*Dios.*
  –left leg would go to—*Euph.*
  –left arm and leg would go to—*Nicc.*
  –lower leg were—*Acon., Asaf., Caust., Chin., Cupr., Ign., Iod., Laur., Merc. c.*
  –in calves—*Coloc.*

439

Asleep—*Continued*

  −feet and ankles were—*Rhus t.*

  −feet were—*Acon., Alum., Am. m., Ant. t., Ars., Bry., Calc. c., Calc. p., Cann. i., Caust., Cham., Cob., Coloc., Croc., Euph., Fago., Graph., Ham., Kali c., Lyc., Mag. m., Mez., Nat. c., Nat. m., Nit. ac., Phos., Plb., Plect., Sec., Sep., Sul. ac.*

  −feet would fall—*Stann.*

  −when pressing it to the ground, foot were—*Gamb.*

  −foot had been—*Saponin.*

  −left foot had been—*Cahin.*

  −when walking, right foot were—*Phos. ac.*

  −toes were—*Chlf., Saba.*

  −right great toe were—*Colch.*

  −in soles of feet—*Olnd., Phos.*

  −heel were—*Rhod.*

Away in space, feet were; < eyes closed—*Cann. s.*

Balls, hot, dropped from each breast through to back and rolling down back, along each limb and off at heels, followed by balls of ice—*Lyc.*

  −small, coursing through arms and legs—*Zinc.*

Band tied around different parts of arms and legs—*Chin.*

  −bones of upper and lower extremities surrounded by tight—*Con.*

  −were drawn from crest of one ilium to the other—*Eug.*

  −or ring encircled joints—*Lyc.*

  −around the hip—*Cench.*

  −around thigh—*Sulph.*

  −of iron about thigh—*Tep.*

  −about knees—*Nux v.*

  −around calves—*Card. m.*

  −around calf of leg or pantaloons too tight there—*Card. m.*

  −or ligature around ankles—*Acon.*

  −tight around left ankle—*Helod.*

  −a rubber, about toes—*Syph.*

Bandaged, legs were—*Anac., Arund., Aur., Benz. ac., Nat. m.*

  ··thigh feels as if tightly—*Acon.*

  −knees were—*Anac., Ars.*

  firmly about the knees when sitting—*Aur.*

  −too tightly, calves of legs were—*Nat. p.*

  −tightly, lower part of leg were—*Acon., Cham., Lyc.*

  −tightly, great toe were—*Plat.*

Bands about bones of extremities—*Con.*
Bar of iron pressing on hip joint—*Sol. t. æ.*
   –of iron around foot—*Ferr.*
Beaten in all the limbs after exertion—*Agar.*
   –in limbs in morning—*Sel.*
   –in limbs with trembling—*Alum.*
   –in limbs—*Aster., Bov., Dulc., Gua., Lac c., Stann.*
   –in legs—*Bell., Lyc., Lyss., Sep., Thuj.*
   –loose from bones, flesh were—*Thuj.*
   –in leg muscles—*Helio.*
   –feeling going down right leg and coming up left—*Chim. mac.*
   –in nates—*Calc. p.*
   –in hip joint—*Agar.*
   –in thigh—*Ars., Calc. p., Cocc., Ruta*
   –in inner thighs—*Laur.*
   –in thighs and knees—*Plat.*
   –in knees—*Puls.*
   –in knee joint—*Ars.*
   –in bend of left knee—*Ars. h.*
   –in sore knee—*Led.*
   –in tibia—*Mez.*
   –in calf—*Chim. umb., Eup. per.*
   –feet had been—*Ant. t.*
   –from body, feet were—*Zinc.*
   –soles of feet were—*Puls.*
   –and sore, limbs were—*Dros.*
Belong to her, limbs did not—*Agar., Op.*
   –to him when smoking tobacco, legs did not—*Tab.*
Bent outward when rising, legs were—*Raph.*
   –transversely, nails were—*Med.*
Bite of flea on inner side of right knee—*Zinc.*
Biting above right knee, ants were—*Peti.*
   –above the knee, flea were—*Pall.*
Bitten by dogs, thigh were—*Hura*
Blistered, feet would become—*Merc. sul.*
   –on toe—*Zinc.*
Bloated, feet were—*Ars. m.*
Blood stagnated in thigh after walking—*Nit. ac.*
   –stagnated in left leg—*Zinc.*
   –were dropping through a valve and bubbling in calf—*Spig.*
   –were going into legs when crossing legs—*Nux m.*

Blood—*Continued*
  –settled in legs—*Rhus t.*
  –trickled down calf of leg—*Nat. c.*
Blow in left buttock—*Cist.*
  –in left knee—*Plat.*
  –obliquely above left knee in wave-like intervals—*Sul. ac.*
  –in calf—*Nux m.*
  –on outer side of left calf, struck by—*Euph.*
  –on metatarsal bones—*Tus. f.*
  –on tendo Achillis—*Mill.*
Blowing on lower extremities, cool air were—*Lil. t.*
  –over lower abdomen and thighs, hot air were—*Trom.*
  –on the knees, wind were—*Cimx.*
  –on him from bend of knees, freezing cold wind were—*Helod.*
  –up limbs from heel to popliteal space, cold wind were—*Helod.*
  –on feet at night, draft of air were—*Maland.*
Blown upon by wintry wind, legs were—*Chin.*
Boil were likely to form on left ankle—*Merc. sul.*
  –on left great toe—*Rhus t.*
Boiling in hip joint—*Led.*
  –water or molten metal under skin in hollow of knee and down
      back of leg—*Bar. c.*
Boring deep in bones of lower limbs—*Coloc.*
Bound tight, legs were—*Lyc., Stann., Til.*
  –limbs were—*Tarax.*
  –in evening, legs were—*Ant. c.*
  –with cords around calves—*Lol. tem.*
  –lower leg were—*Cham., Lyc., Petr., Stann.*
  –tightly when walking, legs were—*Til.*
  –too tightly, knees were—*Sil.*
  –right gastrocnemius muscle were swollen, flattened and broad-
      ened and something bound upon it—*Luna*
  –tightly in right calf—*Luna*
  –with garter, legs were—*Raph.*
  –with garter, left leg were—*Cocc.*
  –foot were—*Stann.*
Break, legs would—*Ars., Thuj.*
  –while walking, legs would—*Mag. p. Arct.*
  –while walking, bone would—*Zinc.*
  –bones of legs would—*Puls.*
  –thigh would—*Valer.*
  –tibia would—*Agar.*

Break—*Continued*
  –on walking, foot would—*Kali c.*
  –bone on outer side of foot would—*Zinc.*
Bristling in muscles of nates—*Puls.*
Brittle and would break—*Rad.*
  –hip were—*Calc. c.*
  –as well as short and small, right hip and thigh were—*Calc. c.*
  –while walking, lower leg were—*Guai.*
Broken, legs were—*Dros., Hep.*
  –limbs had—*Eup. per., Raph.*
  –at night on turning in bed, legs were—*Carb. an.*
  –bones of legs were—*Vacc., Vario.*
  –bones above knee were—*Sulph.*
  –in sciatica, bones were—*Ruta*
  –about to fall asunder, bones were—*Ther.*
  –thighs were—*Sulph.*
  –in upper part of thigh—*Nux v.*
  –left thigh were, ceasing on riding—*Ill.*
  –in middle, thigh were—*Sulph.*
  –on sitting down, middle of thigh bone were—*Ill.*
  –femur were—*Pyrog.*
  –in knee—*Cupr., Dros.*
  –tibia were—*Merc. c.*
  –foot were—*Kali bi.*
  –hands and feet were—*Psor.*
  –across instep, bones of feet were—*Lac d.*
  –in ankle joints—*Carb. s.*
  –and too long, toe nails were—*Lyss.*
Bruised, lower extremities were—*Ammc., Calend., Cann. s., Cic.,
      Led., Menis., Sol. n., Staph., Thuj.*
  –in right leg—*Ornith.*
  –loins and legs were—*Nux m.*
  –on crest of ilium from carrying a heavy load—*Kreos.*
  –right hip joint were—*Sep.*
  –when touched, legs were—*Arn., Ferr.*
  –in spots when touching limbs—*Card. b.*
  –in thighs—*Acon., Am. c., Ang., Arn., Ars., Bar. c., Bell., Bry.,
      Caps., Carb. an., Caust., Cham., Clem., Cocc., Dig., Ferr. i.,
      Fl. ac., Grat., Ham., Hyper., Lact., Led., Lyc., Lyss., Merc.,
      Merc. i. f., Merc. sul., Mos., Nit. ac., Nux v., Ol. an., Phos.
      ac., Plat., Plb., Puls., Rhus t., Ruta, Seneg., Squill., Staph.,
      Sulph., Thuj., Viol. t., Zinc.*

Bruised—*Continued*

--all over thighs from exertion—*Stel.*

--in inner thighs—*Laur.*

--and weary in belly, loins and thighs—*Bov.*

--muscles of thigh were—*Calc. ac., Der., Kali n., Lach., Nux v., Phos., Phos. ac., Puls., Seneg., Staph.*

--right rectus cruris muscle were—*Rhus t.*

--above knees—*Ruta*

--in knees—*Sarr.*

--under left patella—*Samars.*

--lower leg were—*Calc. ac., Canth., Chin., Guai., Led., Nat. s.*

--in calves—*Staph.*

--in left calf—*Helod.*

--periosteum were, when standing—*Chin.*

--in feet—*Carb. ac., Cina, Clem., Com., Hyos., Kali bi., Laur., Lyc., Mag. c., Mez., Narz., Phos., Phos. ac., Polyp. p., Zinc.*

--in outer malleolus of right foot—*Valer.*

--in tarsal bones—*Nat. m.*

--in instep—*Kali i.*

--in left toes—*Daph. o.*

--in tendo Achillis—*Bry.*

--in heel—*Bell.*

--in sole—*Cham., Nux m., Plb., Polyp. p., Psor., Puls., Sul. ac., Thuj.*

--veins in right leg were—*Nat. c.*

Bubbles bursting in hollow of right knee—*Sil.*

Bubbling in thigh—*Berb., Olnd., Sil.*

--in leg—*Berb.*

--extending in a streak from toes through leg—*Squill.*

--extending outward in leg—*Rheum*

--from knee to heel, something were—*Rheum*

--in calf—*Crot. h.*

--in calf, blood were dropping through a valve and—*Spig.*

--in left foot—*Berb., Chel.*

Bugs were crawling from feet to knees—*Zinc.*

Bungling when undressing, foot were—*Apis*

Burning ulcer were forming on leg—*Agar.*

--toes were—*Ferr. p.*

Burnt in tibia—*Lach.*

--toes were—*Pip. n.*

Burst, joints of legs would—*Ham.*
  —with fidgety feet, legs would—*Vip.*
  —in hip, something would—*Rhus t.*
  —thigh were about to—*Staph.*
  —below the knee, ready to—*Kali m.*
  —in knee, something would—*Rhus t.*
  —in ankle joint, something would—*Rhus t.*
Bursting, legs were—*Merc., Staph.*
  —bubbles in hollow of right knee—*Sil.*
  —foot were—*Graph.*
  —toes were—*Ferr. p.*
Buzzing in thigh as after a long journey—*Mosch.*
  —in legs—*Olnd.*
  —in all toes like a frost bite—*Nux m.*
Carious in legs—*Bell.*
Chafed on balls of toes—*Ars.*
Chilblains on ball of foot—*Rhod.*
  —on sole of foot—*Morph.*
Chilled, tibia were—*Colch.*
Chilliness were about to creep up legs—*Malar.*
Chopped with an ax, joints were being—*Phyt.*
Circulation, he felt the—*Euph.*
  —in legs were suspended—*Lact., Lyc.*
  —were starting after constriction of leg was removed—*Vib.*
Circulating in parts, cold water were—*Verat. a.*
Claw of bird were clasping the knee—*Cann. i.*
Clawing in legs in morning—*Stront.*
Claws, femur were fastened to os innominatum with iron—
      Coloc.
Coal, hot, were held at center of tibia—*Raph.*
  —of fire burning on or above ulcer on foot—*Puls.*
Cold felt in lower extremities—*Valer.*
  —as ice, extremities were—*Croc.*
  —from being fanned, legs were—*Agar.*
  —from snow-water, at night, legs were—*Verat. a.*
  —from a wind on legs while standing—*Samb.*
  —in all limbs, he were getting—*Hep.*
  —limbs were—*Sep.*
  —in knees—*Carb. v., Daph. o.*
  —feet were—*Verat. a.*

Cold—*Continued*
  –soles were—*Card. m.*
  –toes were—*Card. m.*
  –clammy, feet and soles were sticky like molasses—*Sanic.*
Cold—see also WATER
Compressed, thigh had been—*Saba.*
Congestion of blood in left leg—*Zinc.*
  –of sole on stepping—*Led., Puls.*
Constricted, muscles in sole of foot had been—*Berb.*
Contracted, gluteal muscle were—*Lepi.*
  –in popliteal space—*Sars.*
  –sinews of sole were—*Berb.*
  –lengthwise in sole of left foot—*Ars. h.*
Contraction in right thigh—*Ambr.*
Contused, great toe were—*Nat. c.*
Convulsions in right thigh—*Podo.*
Cord tied around hips—*Cench.*
  –or ligature, limbs were bound with tight—*Alumn.*
  –around leg midway between hip and knee—*Am. br.*
  –tied around leg under knee—*Alumn.*
  –pulling in foot during pregnancy—*Plb.*
  –around left foot in evening—*Am. br.*
Cords of knee were shortened—*Nat. p.*
  –calves were bound with—*Lol. tem.*
  –around calves, when exhausted—*Ruta*
  –pulled left big toe and adjoining parts upward when walking
      —*Psor.*
Corns on every toe, were getting—*Lyss.*
Cotton-wool, the floor were—*Xanth.*
Cracking in foot—*Rhus v.*
Cramp would set in, in right calf—*Sep.*
  –right foot would—*Com.*
  –toes were about to—*Dios.*
Cramped, calf of leg had been—*Lyss.*
Crawled from knees to toes, something had—*Ars.*
Crawling over thigh causing sudden twitching, a worm were—
      Nat. c.
  –in limbs—*Ign.*
  –in one or the other limbs, a fly were—*Euph.*

Crawling—*Continued*
--up limbs in a straight line, fly were—*Euph.*
--in back and legs, ants—*Alum.*
--in legs—*Arg. n.*
--in tendons of legs—*Rhus t.*
--and formication on legs—*Nux v.*
--up legs and under the skin from feet to uterus, something
  were—*Tarent.*
--beneath skin on right knee and back—*Rat.*
--from feet to knees, bugs were—*Zinc.*
--like ants on lower legs—*Alum., Aster.*
--on feet, ants were—*Dulc.*
--in feet—*Hyper.*
--in whole left foot—*Tax.*
--on ball of great toe—*Caust.*
--in left sole—*Coloc.*
--in soles of both feet as if asleep—*Staph.*
--and warmth in sole of foot—*Berb.*
--in left heel, worm were—*Lach.*
Creak on motion, knee joint would—*Croc.*
Creeping on limbs, millions of insects were—*Mez.*
--above right knee—*Cinnb.*
--of insects on legs—*Helod.*
--sudden, every morning in feet—*Spig.*
--in limbs, ants were—*Phos.*
--in the limbs like a mouse—*Arn., Aur., Bell., Calc. c., Nit. ac.,*
  Rhod., Sep., Sil., Sulph.
Crookedness of left leg and left side—*Ovi g. p.*
Crowded with arms and legs, he were—*Pyrog.*
Crowding through her boots, heel were—*Eup. pur.*
Crush the toes, weight of sheet on feet would—*Thea*
Crushed, hip were—*Euph.*
--ball and socket of hip joint were—*Ferr.*
--limbs would be—*Cocc.*
--legs were—*Agar., Dig., Goss.*
--marrow of bones were being—*Coloc.*
--inwardly, in left knee—*Ars. h.*
--in knees and ankles, bones had been—*Nux m.*
Current, galvanic, passed through extremities—*Polyg.*
--galvanic, passed through right leg—*Dor.*

Cushion when sitting, foot were—*Fl. ac.*
Cushioned when walking, soles of feet were—*Apis*
Cut off, back of leg would be—*Ign.*
Cutting instrument piercing all joints—*Vesp.*
  –in flesh of legs—*Alco.*
Dead, legs were—*Hyper.*
  –feet were—*Cimx., Lyc., Ox. ac., Phos., Phos. ac., Sil.*
  –up to knees, feet were—*Ars. h.*
  –toes were—*Chel.*
  –soles of feet were—*Plb.*
Decayed, nails were—*Sil.*
Decaying, bones of legs were—*Sep.*
Detached from body, legs were—*Stram., Tarent.*
  –from the thigh bone, flesh had become—*Elect.*
Disjointed in right foot—*Syph.*
Dislocated, legs were—*Thuj.*
  –legs would be—*Raph.*
  –joints were—*Agn., Carb. s.*
  –right thigh bone were—*Aspar.*
  –hip joint were—*Agar., Ang., Caust., Kreos., Linar., Psor., Puls.*
  –in left hip joint—*Laur.*
  –on sitting down, femur were—*Ip.*
  –above the knee—*Arum t.*
  –patella would be—*Cahin.*
  –knee were—*Arn.*
  –in right knee—*Carb. s.*
  –in left foot—*Arum t., Hyper.*
  –metatarsal bones were—*Bell.*
  –ankles were—*Bry., Calc. p., Verat. v.*
  –especially when walking, ankles were—*Bry.*
  –right ankle were—*Dros.*
Dislocation in hip joint, when walking—*Bry.*
Distended, limbs were—*Chim. mac.*
Distorted, ankles were—*Verat. v.*
Double up on himself in tibia, he would—*Pin. s.*
Draft of air blowing on feet at night, must get up and tuck in bed-
    clothes—*Maland.*
Drag a heavy burden on stepping out, she had to—*Chel.*
Drawing in bones—*Aloe*
 ⋮ –from sole of foot through bones of leg, tendon were—*Crot. h.*
  –with needles in foot—*Nux v.*

Drawn together, hips were—*Polyg.*
–up on leg, flesh would be—*Crot. h.*
–down in left thigh on walking in open air, a string were—*Nux v.*
–up and would never be straightened again, left leg were—*Pyrus*
–downward, leg were too long and—*Aster.*
–up, thigh were—*Hep.*
–together, thigh were—*Cann. s.*
–out, tendons of patella were, and then let return—*Thuj.*
–cords of legs behind knee were—*Phys.*
–inward, toes were—*Sars.*
–down, toes had been—*Staph.*
–through bone of leg when walking in street, tendon were—*Crot. h.*
Dried up, veins of feet had—*Ham.*
Drop off, thighs would—*Am. c., Fago.*
–off limbs, flesh would—*Rhus t.*
–off, legs would, > motion—*Dios.*
Dropping off, legs were—*Tab.*
–through valve and bubbling in calf, blood were—*Spig.*
Drops of cold water trickling over anterior thigh—*Acon.*
Drunk in legs—*Hyper.*
Elastic stocking, legs were enclosed in—*Pic. ac.*
Electric current passed from head into limbs—*Ail.*
–shocks in legs—*Cic., Nux v.*
–shock from left hip to head—*Dios.*
Electricity in legs, followed by soreness of muscles—*Mag. p.*
Elongated, legs were—*Thuj.*
Elongation of right leg, at night on lying down—*Carb. an.*
Emptiness in great toes—*Daph. o.*
Enclosed in an elastic stocking, legs were—*Pic. ac.*
Enlarged, legs were—*Ced.*
Escape from patella, lower end of femur were about to—*Cahin.*
Exarticulated in hip joint—*Ang.*
Exhausted by fatigue, limbs were—*Verat. a.*
Expansion of legs—*Sep.*
Explode, femur would—*Lac. ac.*
Fall from bones of legs, flesh would—*Rumx.*
–from him, all limbs would—*Merc.*
–asunder, bones were broken and about to—*Ther.*

Falling off the bones, muscles were—*Eup. per.*
  –to pieces, hips and small of back were—*Tril.*
Fanned, legs were cold from being—*Agar.*
Fastened to os innominatum with iron claws, femur were—
    Coloc.
Fatigued, over, and could not keep them still, legs were—*Ferr.*
Feather, legs were as light as—*Nux m.*
Feathers, feet were made of—*Stict.*
Filled with lead, feet were—*Nat. m.*
  –with needles in the legs—*Conv.*
Fire were coursing through body from left foot to head—*Zinc.*
  –parts were on—*X-ray*
Fit, bones did not—*Wild.*
Flea bites on anterior thigh, at night—*Dulc.*
  –were biting above the knee—*Pall.*
  –bite on inner side of right knee—*Zinc.*
Floating in the air, legs were—*Stict., Verat. a.*
Flowing down legs, warm water were—*Bor.*
Fluid, a stream of warm, started at the feet and rushed to the
    head, followed by heaviness and dull pain in the head—
    Camph.
Foot on the leg, there were no—*Cot.*
Forced out of socket when walking, head of femur were—*Pall.*
  –apart, bones of legs would be—*Sep.*
  –asunder, left knee were being—*Calad.*
Fracture in legs—*Mag. p. Arct.*
Frostbite, feet were burning as if recovering from—*Helod.*
Frostbitten, feet were—*Pic. ac.*
  –toes were—*Carb. v.*
  –soles were—*Bor.*
Frosted in left great toe—*Cast.*
  –toes had been—*Staph., Zinc.*
Frozen, feet were—*Pic. ac., Puls.*
  –toes were—*Nux v.*
  –great toe had been—*Nit. ac., Zinc.*
  –in little toes—*Asar.*
Full and distended, limbs were—*Chin.*
  –limbs were—*Spire.*
  –legs and feet were too—*Osm.*
Fur, feet were—*Hyper.*

Furred, feet were—*Ars.*

Fuzzy in limbs—*Sec.*

Galvanic current passed through extremities—*Polyg.*

  –current passed through right leg—*Dor.*

  –current passed through feet while sitting—*Gels.*

Garters were too tight and legs would become stiff and go to sleep—*Chin.*

Gave way beneath feet, ground—*Tep.*

Give way, legs would—*Phos.*

  –way, knees would—*Ambr., Bell., Carb. v., Kreos., Laur.*

  –way after emission, knees would—*Nat. p.*

Given way, muscles and ligaments in hips had—*Arg. m.*

  –way in ankle—*Coca*

Giving way, thighs were—*Glon.*

  –way in knees and legs—*Ovi g. p.*

Gnawing flesh and bones of legs, deep in, dogs were—*Nit. ac.*

Gooseflesh covered right thigh—*Spig.*

Gout, rheumatic, would set in, in foot—*Merc. sul.*

Grasped, thigh were—*Ruta*

  –above the knee, left limb were severely—*Chim. umb.*

  –by someone in anterior part of right knee—*Nux m.*

  –by both hands in evening, knee were—*Sulph.*

Ground gave way beneath feet—*Atrop., Dign., Hyos., Tep.*

Growing into flesh, left great toe nail were—*Colch.*

Grown into flesh of right great toe, nail were—*Mar.*

  –to the flesh on side of great toe, nail had—*Mag. p. Aust.*

Gum, stocking feet were full of, with sweat—*Sanic.*

Gurgling from below upward, when sitting, in lower legs—*Arn.*

Hair were pulled on first phalanx of great toe—*Bapt.*

Hairs were being pulled out on inside of left knee—*X-ray*

Hand were lying about head of tibia and fibula, warm—*Agar.*

Hands slowly over thigh downward, someone were drawing icy—*X-ray*

Hanging on legs, lead were—*Agar.*

  –on the lower extremities, a weight were—*Chel., Verb.*

  –on end of tibia, a weight were—*Spong.*

  –from left leg when rested on right, weight were—*Stann.*

  –to feet, weight were—*Rhod.*

Heavy, thigh were too—*Lyss.*

  –calf of leg were too—*Lyss.*

  –weight on crest of ilium—*Kreos.*

Heavy—*Continued*
   —weight in each instep—*Arn.*
   —weight hanging to feet—*Rhod.*
Heels, he had jumped too hard on—*Samars.*
   —were crowding through the boots—*Eup. pur.*
Holding back sudden, when walking, stopping her; with electric
      shocks in the legs—*Nux v.*
Ice, bones were made of—*Aran.*
   —cold needles prickled all over legs—*Agar.*
   —feet had been in, with tingling—*Sanic.*
   —soles of feet were pressed upon—*Samars.*
Icy cold, legs were, as from a wintry wind—*Cinch. b.*
   —spots on thighs—*Berb.*
   —hands were drawn over thighs—*X-ray*
Impaired, mobility of limbs were—*Cyc.*
Impeded when walking, steps were—*Con.*
Independent, legs were—*Coniin.*
Inflamed, left great toe were—*Colch.*
Iron bar were pressing on hip joint—*Sol. t. æ.*
   —clamps, hip joint were fastened by—*Coloc.*
   —bars around foot—*Ferr.*
   —hot, went into ulcer on right little toe, on raising foot—*Cocc.*
Insects were creeping on legs—*Helod.*
   —were creeping on limbs, millions of—*Mez.*
Insensible, legs were—*Meph.*
Jammed, > hanging down, leg were—*Bell.*
   —in tendo Achillis, place were—*Mur. ac.*
Jerking and releasing, sciatic nerve were—*Tub.*
Journey, weariness from a long foot—*Kreos., Thuj.*
Jump, leg were going to—*Morph.*
Jumped too hard on heels, he had—*Samars.*
Jumping of a mouse in right border of left foot—*Sulph.*
Kneeling a long time, he had been, in right knee—*Bry.*
Knife were suddenly thrust into pudendum or from pudendum
      into right thigh—*Croc.*
   —bones of lower limbs scraped with a—*Phos. ac.*
   —stuck in left leg, a penknife were—*Elæis guin.*
   —right knee were ripped with—*Bar. c.*
   —pierced calf of leg and blood trickled down—*Nat. c.*
   —stepping on a sharp, left great toe were—*Am. c.*
   —penknife in soles of feet—*Caust.*

Knocked from under him, legs had been—*Agar.*
  –together, legs were—*Con.*
Lacerated by dull instrument, heel were—*Lat. k.*
Lame in walking, legs were—*Calc. p.*
  –foot were—*Thuj.*
Lameness in the muscles of the thigh—*Ang.*
  –in bones of limbs—*Cocc.*
Lance pierced through inside of left ankle joint—*Verb.*
Large and swollen in toes, too—*Apis*
  –as whole body, left foot were—*Daph. o.*
  –as whole body in great toes—*Daph. o.*
Larger, right thigh were growing—*Coll.*
  –knees were—*Merc.*
Lead, limbs were made of—*Bry.*
  –limbs were heavy as—*Nux v.*
  –were in limbs—*Op., Valer.*
  –were hanging on legs—*Agar.*
  –several pounds of, in each tibia—*Lyss.*
  –feet were filled with—*Nat. m.*
Ligature around ankles—*Acon., Bell.*
Light as a feather, legs were—*Nux m.*
  –limbs were—*Asar., Stict., Valer.*
  –legs and feet did not touch the ground, they were so—*Tep.*
Lightness in all the limbs—*Asar., Stict.*
Liquid moving in left thigh—*Op.*
Loaded, feet were—*Ind.*
Long, legs and arms feel about two miles, < eyes closed—
    Cann. s.
  –and drawn downward, legs were too—*Aster.*
  –if he stands on the other, left foot were too—*Kreos.*
  –on standing, left leg were too—*Kreos.*
  –and broken, toe nails were too—*Lyss.*
Longer than common, legs were—*Stram.*
  –than natural, at night on lying down, right leg were—*Carb. an.*
Loose on legs, flesh were—*Sulph.*
  –on thighs, flesh were—*Lyc.*
  –on thighs and arms, flesh were—*Nat. m.*
  –from tibia, flesh were—*Stann.*
  –ankles or knee joints were—*Wild.*
  –in joints, hands and feet were—*Stram.*
  –toe nails were—*Apis*

Looseness of joints—*Wild.*

Loosened from bones of hip joint, flesh were—*Zinc.*

–internal ligaments in right knee were—*Sumb.*

–in joints, hands and feet were—*Stram.*

Lose the use of her limbs, she would—*Lac c.*

Losing marrow of bones—*Carb. v.*

Luxated, left hip joint were—*Kreos.*

Marrow, pain were in—*Ruta*

Misstep in foot, taking a—*Hep.*

Molasses, feet had been in—*Sanic.*

Molten metal or boiling water under the skin in the hollow of knee and down back of leg—*Bar. c.*

Mouse were creeping in the limbs—*Arn., Aur., Bell., Calc. c., Nit. ac., Rhod., Sep., Sil., Sulph.*

–jumping in right border of left foot—*Sulph.*

–running through limbs or from solar plexus to stomach—*Sil.*

–running in lower limbs—*Sep.*

–running up and down limbs—*Sep.*

–running along legs—*Calc. c.*

Move limbs but he cannot, he must—*Valer.*

Moving, legs were, must look and see—*Kali br.*

–upward in thighs, something were—*Vip.*

–in left thigh, liquid were—*Op.*

Mummified, feet were—*Ars.*

Nail were driven into flesh of right great toe—*Mar.*

Nails, blunt, shooting in at root of great toe nail—*Sulph.*

–or tacks pricking in heels—*Puls.*

–would come off—*Nat. c.*

–running under skin of heels—*Rhus t.*

Needle sticking into left thigh and vulva—*Goss.*

–prick of, in fatty portion of great toe—*Tong.*

–thrust deep into forepart of right great toe—*Ran. s.*

Needles, sitting on, in nates—*Guaj.*

–pierced the thigh—*Plb.*

–pricking with, in right thigh—*Lob. c.*

–pricking in legs—*Lach., Pic. ac.*

–red hot, in limbs—*Lith.*

–prickled in legs from ice cold—*Agar.*

–drawing in feet—*Nux v.*

–pricking in feet with, seems pithy—*Hyper.*

Needles—*Continued*

—pricking in feet—*Cob.*

—were pricking in dorsum of feet—*Cupr. s.*

—were stitching in sole of right foot—*Nat. c.*

—when rising in morning, stepping on—*Berb.*

—walking upon—*Eupi., Rhus t.*

—soles of feet and palms of hands punctured with—*Syph.*

—in sole of right foot—*Nat. c.*

Nerves were pulled in sole of foot—*Arn.*

Nervous, feet were—*Puls. n.*

Net, right sole were stepping in a—*Tax.*

No limbs, he had—*Stram.*

—feet, she had—*Sec.*

Numb in feet—*Hyper.*

Nutshells, he were walking on—*Plb.*

Out of joint, knee were—*Arg. m., Arn.*

Overheated, limbs were—*Vacc., Vario.*

Overfatigued, he cannot keep them still, legs were—*Ferr.*

Own, legs were not her—*Sumb.*

Painful stripe inside of thigh—*Nux v.*

Paralysis extends from above knee down lower leg—*Kali n.*

—extends from above knee to foot—*Petr.*

—of right knee—*Chr. ac.*

—in left big toe—*Kali p.*

Paralyzed, thigh were—*Agar., Aur., Caust., Cocc., Crot. t., Verat. a.*

—extending to knees, thighs were—*Thuj.*

—extending to calves and knees, thighs were—*Ferr. i.*

—because wounded, thighs were—*Lyc.*

—legs were—*Acon., Amyg., Atrop., Azad., Bell., Both., Brom., Camph., Carb. ox., Carb. v., Card. b., Chel., Chin., Chlor., Chr. ac., Kali i., Kali t., Lath., Mag. c., Manc., Morph., Nat. p., Phos., Phos. ac., Rhus v., Sars., Sep., Sil., Stann., Stront., Tab., Tart. ac., Vip.*

—and heavy, legs were—*Kali c., Nat. p.*

—weakness of legs—*Sacc.*

—legs would be—*Raph.*

—right leg were—*Chel.*

—left leg were—*Amph.*

—left leg were from knee to hip—*Med.*

Paralyzed—*Continued*
  –arms and knees were—*Tab.*
  –limbs and feet were—*Sil.*
  –ankles were—*Nat. m.*
  –feet were—*Asar., Chel., Ip., Lipp.*
  –in extensors of toes—*Bad.*
Penetrated by spikes, soles were—*Cann. i.*
Pieces, hips and small of back were falling to—*Tril.*
Pierced through inside left ankle, lance—*Verb.*
  –by needles in thigh—*Plb.*
  –by a knife in calf of leg—*Nat. c.*
  –right sole, splinters—*Agar.*
Piercing all joints, a cutting instrument were—*Vesp.*
Pincers, flesh were torn away by hot—*Visc.*
Pinched by shoes though no shoes on—*Ran. b.*
  –by too narrow shoes, feet and heels had been—*Chel.*
  –off, big toe were being—*Meph.*
  –out little pieces of flesh all over body, especially the feet—
    Lac c.
Pin, right thigh were torn with a—*Merl.*
Pins in knees—*Tab.*
  –in both feet—*Eup. per.*
  –pricking in heels—*Spong.*
  –feet were full of—*Dor.*
  –sticking in feet, at beginning of chill—*Eup. per.*
  –in heels, stepping on—*Rhus t.*
  –walking on—*Nit. ac., Rhus t.*
Pithy in feet—*Hyper.*
  –extending from feet to knees—*Ang.*
  –sole were—*Cham.*
Plaster pulled off outer side of right sole, tingling—*Arn.*
Plug in left gluteal muscle—*Anac.*
  –on outer side of thigh—*Agar.*
  –pressed against inner side of calf—*Prun.*
  –dull, pushing in ankle joints—*Lac c.*
Plunged into boiling hot water, limbs were—*Culx.*
  –into boiling water, feet were—*Arund.*
Pointed body between thighs, stitches from—*Asaf.*
Position, muscle of thigh were not in the right—*Led.*
  –limbs were kept long in an unusual—*Staph.*
Pounds of lead in tibia—*Lyss.*

Pounded, feet were—*Lil. t., Polyp. p.*
  –hands and feet were—*Lil. t.*
  –heels were—*Polyp. p.*
Poured over side from shoulder to thigh, cold water were—*Verb.*
  –over legs, cold water were—*Lac c.*
  –on feet, cold water were—*Verat. a.*
Power in legs, loss of—*Form., Sil.*
  –in legs, sudden loss of—*Nux v.*
Perspire, foot wanted to—*Sal. ac.*
Pressed against inner side of calf, a plug were—*Prun.*
  –into lower part of left foot, blood were forcibly—*Ol. an.*
  –by shoe in great right toe—*Pæon.*
  –while walking, little toe were—*Ther.*
  –upon ice, soles of feet were—*Samars.*
Pressing on hip joint, an iron bar were—*Sol. t. æ.*
  –on thighs, a weight were—*Sep.*
  –in ankle joint, dull plug were—*Lac c.*
  –in ankle, a stone were—*Spig.*
  –foot to the ground, ankle were asleep when—*Gamb.*
Pressure in shoe when walking—*Sil.*
  –of a hand above left external malleolus—*Gamb.*
  –in left little toe—*Pæon.*
Prick of a needle in fatty portion of great toe—*Tong.*
Pricked in feet with needles, seems pithy—*Hyper.*
  –heels, tack—*Puls.*
Pricking with needles in right thigh—*Lob. c.*
  –as from needles in legs—*Pic. ac.*
  –of needles in all the limbs—*Lach.*
  –in feet, needles were—*Cob.*
  –with needles in feet and legs—*Cupr. s., Pic. ac.*
  –of needles in feet—*Cob.*
  –of needles in dorsum of feet—*Cupr. s.*
  –in heels from tacks or nails—*Puls.*
  –in heels from pins—*Spong.*
Prickled all over with ice cold needles in legs—*Agar.*
Prickles from needles in dorsum of feet—*Cupr. s.*
  –from needles in feet and legs—*Cupr. s., Pic. ac.*
Pulled from their sockets, head of hip bones were—*Agar.*
  –out of joint, shoulders and hips were—*Fl. ac.*
  –up in lower extremities, sinews were being—*Nit. ac.*
  –in legs, skin were—*Laur.*

30

Pulled—*Continued*

    —inside of left knee, hairs were being—*X-ray*

    —inward by little cords when walking, left big toe and adjoining parts were—*Psor.*

    —out, big toe were—*Prun.*

    —on first phalanx of right great toe, a hair were—*Bapt.*

    —in sole of foot, nerves were—*Arn.*

Pulling, muscles and tendons in thigh were too short and—*Merc.*

    —by a cord during pregnancy, foot were—*Plb.*

    —in right leg—*Agar., Mez.*

    —skin on left leg—*Laur.*

Punctured with needles in soles and palms—*Syph.*

Pushed something against ovary, legs—*Med.*

Pushing out on a spot large as the hand on inner side of right thigh—*Pulx.*

    —in ankle joints, dull plug were—*Lac c.*

Raise the limbs but he could, could not—*Sulph.*

Rat running up the legs—*Ail.*

Restrained in limbs, motor power were—*Tarax.*

Rheumatic in legs—*Ham., Kalm., Lith., Ostrya*

    —gout would set in, in foot—*Merc.*

Riding horseback, he had been—*Nux m.*

Ring or band encircled joints—*Lyc.*

Ripped with a knife, right knee were being—*Bar. c.*

Rising up while the head remained still, feet were—*Phos. ac.*

Running down leg when hanging down, hot water were—*Mag. p. Aust.*

    —up the leg, a rat were—*Ail.*

    —from clavicles to toes in a narrow line, cold water were—*Caust.*

    —away with him, feet were—*Pip. m.*

    —into feet, icy cold water were—*Verat. a.*

    —nails under the skin of heels—*Rhus t.*

Sand under the skin—*Coca*

Sausages, he were stepping on round—*Plb.*

Sawed bones with a dull saw, someone—*Syph.*

Scalded, toes were—*Nat. c.*

    —and itched, toes were—*Sanic.*

    —toes were, and itch terribly on under surface—*Maland.*

Scraped with a knife, bones were—*Phos. ac.*
  –bones near joints were—*Spig.*
Scraping over long bones, something were—*Ars.*
Scratched by a toothed instrument, soles of feet were—*Zinc.*
Screw were moving through right leg, on walking—*Ferr.*
Screwed in a vise, lower limbs were—*Coloc.*
Separated from the body, legs were—*Stram.*
  –from each other, all parts of limbs were—*Stram.*
  –joints were—*Stram.*
Set in, in foot, rheumatic gout would—*Merc.*
Severed from body and belonged to somebody else, lower limbs
    were—*Op.*
Shoes were too tight—*Chel., Merc., Nux v., Sep., Sulph.*
Shock, electric, in legs—*Cic., Nux v.*
  –electric, extending from thigh to top of head—*Dios.*
  –galvanic, in limbs—*Verat. v.*
  –galvanic, passing through extremities—*Polyg.*
Shooting under nail of right toe, blunt nails were—*Sulph.*
Short in right side of psoas magnus, lower extremities were too
    —*Coloc.*
  –legs were too—*Ambr., Anac.*
  –when rising, leg were too—*Caust.*
  –tendons in legs were too—*Cimx., Juncus, Lyc., Nux v., Puls.,*
    Rhus t., Sep., Spig., Syph.
  –muscles in legs were too—*Sabin., Spong.*
  –tendons in left hip were too—*Am. m.*
  –thighs were—*Ambr., Berb., Guaj., Nux v.*
  –muscles of thigh were too—*Guaj., Merc., Sulph., Til.*
  –tendon of thigh were too—*Euph., Merc.*
  –hamstring were too—*Am. m., Rhus t.*
  –knees were too—*Rhus t.*
  –muscles in bend of knees were too—*Zinc.*
  –cords of knee were too—*Nat. p.*
  –under the knees, tendons were too—*Calc. p.*
  –in popliteal space, were too—*Sulph.*
  –calves were too—*Arg. m., Sil.*
  –foot were—*Spig.*
  –muscles and tendons of foot were too—*Zinc.*
  –too, in tendo Achillis—*Gamb., Juncus*
  –heel were too—*Sulph.*
  –when sitting, tendon in sole were too—*Ind.*

Shortened, limbs were—*Mez.*
   –right leg from hip to heel were—*Crot. c.*
   –or drawn tight in right thigh, in neuralgia—*Bar. c.*
   –on ascending steps, thigh were—*Hyos.*
   –cords of knees were—*Nat. p.*
   –foot were—*Vip.*
Shortening of the right leg on rising—*Caust.*
   –of left leg when walking—*Cinnm.*
Shorter, right leg were—*Ambr.*
   –right leg were, during menses—*Tub.*
   –left leg were—*Caust., Cinnb., Cinnm., Lycps.*
   –left leg were, on walking—*Cinnm.*
Shrinking, legs were—*Trios.*
Sink under her, knees would—*Ferr.*
Sitting in ice water—*Tub.*
   –on needles in nates—*Guaj.*
Sleep in legs, gone to—*Ambr., Merc. c., Nat. m., Stram.*
   –limbs were going to—*Gels., Mill., Rheum*
   –feet had gone to—*Elect.*
   –foot had gone to—*Lac. ac.*
Slip out of their sockets, hip bones would—*Lyss.*
Small, leg were too—*Kali c.*
   –feet were—*Kali c., Raph.*
Smarting, a wound on right hip joint were—*Sabin.*
Smashed to pieces, pains in both legs as if they were—*Nux m.*
Snow-water, at night, legs were cold from—*Verat. a.*
Soaring during menses, feet were—*Eupi.*
Soft when walking, soles of feet were too—*Carb. v., Sulph.*
   –when stepping, soles were—*Alum.*
   –when touching ground, soles were—*Plb.*
   –in soles, walking on something—*Xanth.*
Sore and beaten, limbs were—*Dros.*
   –and beaten in knees—*Led.*
   –on inner surface of tibia—*Thuj.*
   –and stiff to move, patella would be—*Carb. ac.*
   –corns were—*Lac. ac.*
   –from walking, heel were—*Bor.*
Space, stepped on empty—*Dub.*
Sparks, electric, in limbs—*Phyt.*
Spasms in ankles—*Sil.*

Spikes, he trod on a number of, which penetrated soles and ran upward through limbs to hips—*Cann. i.*

Spilled over thigh, alcohol had been—*Lob. s.*

Splinter of bone sticking in right fibula just above outer malleolus—*Asaf.*

–under nail of left middle toe—*Ars. h.*

–stuck into toe—*Nit. ac.*

–in great toe—*Agar.*

–sticking in great toe when touched—*Pæon.*

–in heel—*Petr.*

Splinters in lower extremities—*Nit. ac.*

–pierced right sole—*Agar.*

Sponges, walking on—*Helod.*

Sprained, hip were—*Arg. m., Euph., Nat. m., Nit. ac., Pall.*

–thighs were—*Am. c.*

–right thigh were—*Caps.*

–left thigh were—*Euph.*

–legs were—*Agar., Euph., Rhus v.*

–when walking, legs were—*Am. c., Crot. t.*

–in joints of legs—*Rhus t.*

–above knee—*Ambr.*

–knees were—*Calc. p., Hipp., Lach., Nat. m., Spig.*

–when walking, tibial muscles were—*Calc. c.*

–feet were—*Bar. c., Bry., Chr. ox., Kalm., Rhus t., Sil., Zinc.*

–left foot were—*Calc. c., Crot. t., Cyc.*

–in joints of feet—*Camph.*

–in tarsal joints—*Merc.*

–ankle were—*Asc. t., Led., Nat. m., Phos., Prun., Zinc.*

–left ankle were—*Anac., Inul.*

–in toe joints—*All. s.*

–great toe were—*Aloe, Crot. t.*

–heel were—*Cyc.*

–in tendo Achillis—*Tetrad.*

–bottom of foot were—*Cham., Cyc., Mur. ac.*

Squeezed in a vise, legs were—*Alum.*

–together in bones of limbs—*Alum.*

–in marrow of bones—*Goss.*

–thigh were—*Kali i., Ruta*

Stabbed in the heel—*Eup. per.*

Stagnated in thigh after walking, blood—*Nit. ac.*

–in left leg, blood were—*Zinc.*

Stand for weakness of thighs, unable to—*Pip. m.*

Standing long or walking, aching in calves from—*Rumx.*

  –on oil cloth—*Morph.*

  –in cold water, right leg were—*Sabin.*

  –in cold water over the ankles—*Lyc.*

Step, he had taken a—*Thuj.*

  –out, she could not—*Chel.*

  –as long as the other, one leg will not take a—*Samars.*

Stepped on a hard body in ball of foot, one had—*Brom.*

  –on empty space—*Dub.*

Stepping on cushions, in soles and balls of toes—*Apis*

  –in a net, sole of right foot were—*Tax.*

  –on sharp knife, left great toe were—*Am. c.*

  –on nut-shell—*Plb.*

  –on needles when rising in the morning—*Berb.*

  –on pins in heels—*Rhus t.*

  –on round sausages—*Plb.*

  –soles were soft when—*Alum.*

Steps, she could take ten as easily as one, when walking—*Pulx.*

Sticking into left thigh and vulva, a needle were—*Goss.*

  –in right fibula just above outer malleolus—*Asaf.*

  –in feet at beginning of chill, pins were—*Eup. per.*

  –in great toe when touched, splinter were—*Pæon.*

Stiff, limbs were without joints and—*Petr.*

Stiffness in hollows of knees from a long walk, < morning on rising—*Lyc.*

Sting of a wasp at knee and elbow—*Arg. m.*

Stitches from a pointed body between thighs—*Asaf.*

Stitching of needles in sole of right foot—*Nat. c.*

Stockings, she had on damp—*Puls., Saponin.*

  –were cool and damp—*Calc. c., Ign., Sanic.*

  –legs were encircled in elastic—*Pic. ac.*

Stone, a heavy, were tied to feet and knees—*Verat. a.*

  –pressing in ankles—*Spig.*

  –or hard body with pain in middle of left foot, stepped on—*Brom.*

  –pressure from a stone on the hollow of soles—*Aur.*

  –pressure of hard, on bottom of right foot near toes—*Plat.*

  –or pebble lodged under heel when walking, pressure of—*Hep.*

  –little, under heel when treading on it—*Aur., Brom., Cann. i., Hep., Lyc., Rhus t.*

Stonebruise on ball of left foot—*Chin. s.*
  –in sole of left foot > stepping—*Lact.*
Stood for a long time, he had—*Cina*
  –in cold water up to ankles all day, he had—*Sep.*
Strained, limbs were—*Dub.*
  –muscles in limbs were—*Form.*
  –left foot were—*Hyper.*
  –in right ankle—*Valer.*
Strength, tendo Achillis had lost its—*Valer.*
  –in limbs, there were no—*Staph.*
Stretch limbs, wanted constantly to—*Rhus t.*
Stretched, muscles in left thigh were—*Nat. s.*
  –limbs were forcibly—*Rhus t.*
  –in muscles of calf—*Kali bi.*
  –along legs, threads were—*Lach.*
String were drawn down in thigh, on walking in open air—
    Nux v.
  –tied around thighs—*Am. br., Lyc., Manc.*
Struck by a blow on outer side of calf—*Euph.*
Strumming in legs—*Ambr.*
Stuck in left leg, penknife were—*Elæis guin.*
  –into toes, splinter were—*Nit. ac.*
Subluxation, partial, of patella—*Gels.*
Support the body, legs could not—*Euph., Thuj.*
  –the body, knees would not—*Thea*
Suppurate at roots of nails, about to—*Mag. p. Aust.*
Suppurating in nates—*Phos.*
  –in ankles—*Hep.*
  –left foot were—*Grat.*
  –in ball of right foot—*Lyc.*
  –in soles—*Calc. c., Kali n., Prun., Spig.*
  –in right heel—*Euph.*
Surging in legs while sitting—*Olnd.*
Sweat would break out on lower extremities in morning—*Lyc.*
  –on foot—*Lac. ac.*
Swelled, limbs were—*Guaj.*
  –arms and legs were suddenly—*Tanac.*
Swelling, thigh were—*Prun.*
  –soles were—*Coloc.*
  –on stepping, soles were—*Alum., Zinc.*

Swollen, limbs were—*Guaj., Kali br.*

–and heavy, legs were—*Lyc.*

–left leg were—*Prim.*

–knees were—*Carb. v., Pyrus*

–knees were, immensely—*Pyrus*

–in bends of knees—*Nit. ac.*

–and heavy, feet were—*Phos.*

–and too large in toes—*Apis*

–toes feel, immensely—*Pyrus*

–in tendo Achillis—*Juncus*

Tacks pricked heels—*Puls.*

Tendons were too short in hollow of knee—*Calc. p., Graph.*

–were too short in lower extremities—*Am. m., Cimx., Euph., Gamb., Graph., Juncus, Nat. p., Nux v., Puls., Sep., Syph., Zinc.*

–were drawing from sole to foot through bone of leg—*Crot. h.*

Tense as from cramps when walking, calves were—*Sil.*

–skin of ankles were—*Rhus t.*

Tension in thighs and legs—*Alum.*

Thick, bones of legs were too—*Sarr.*

–sole of shoe were too (below extremities of right metatarsus) —*Menth.*

Threads stretched along legs—*Lach.*

Thrilling in legs—*Phys., Stry.*

Thrust deep in great toe, needle were—*Ran. s.*

–suddenly into pudendum or right thigh, knife were—*Croc.*

Tickled arms and legs, someone suddenly—*Staph.*

Tied together, legs were—*Syph.*

–as with a ligature, ankles were—*Acon., Bell.*

–around leg under knee, cord were—*Alumn.*

–tightly below the knees—*Ant. c.*

Tight on limbs after walking, clothes were—*Chin.*

–about knee, something were—*Mag. c.*

–a few inches below the knee, pantaloons were too—*Card. m.*

–garters were too—*Chin., Raph.*

–shoe were too—*Chel., Merc., Nux v., Sep., Sulph.*

Tightness at bend of knee—*Anag.*

Tingling, limbs were—*Trios.*

–as if frozen in little toe—*Pyrog.*

–from plaster pulled off in outer side of sole—*Arn.*

Tired in legs—*Macrot.*

–legs and feet were—*Xanth.*

Tired—*Continued*
  –limbs were, when at repose—*Acon., Mag. c., Rhus t.*
  –from walking—*Rhod.*
Torn from her, hip would be—*Caust.*
  –with a pin, right thigh were—*Merl.*
  –from bones at back of thigh, muscles were—*Eupi.*
  –loose between thighs, flesh were—*Juncus, Led.*
  –out, limbs were—*Cham.*
  –off tibia, periosteum were—*Mez.*
  –apart when treading, metatarsal bones were—*Carb. v.*
  –out, great toe would be—*Lyc.*
  –from socket, left great toe were—*Pyrus*
  –off, tendo Achillis would be—*Prun.*
  –out, nails were being—*Phos.*
Touching ground, soles were soft when—*Plb.*
Treading on hard surface—*Nux m.*
Trembling in limbs—*Rhus t.*
Trickled down calf of leg, blood—*Nat. c.*
Trickling down front of thigh, drops of water were—*Acon.*
  –over joints, water were, in open air—*Nat. m.*
Trip, foot would—*Nux v.*
Tripped by a backward thrust in popliteal space—*Stram.*
Trod on a number of spikes—*Cann. i.*
Turned outward only during walking, right knee joint and leg
      below the knee were—*Lac c.*
  –outward, arms and feet were—*Graph.*
Tweezers were plunged into left thigh, turned and pulled out
      bringing up a nerve which let go before coming out—*Rhus t.*
Twisted around or off, legs and knees would be—*Zinc.*
  –off, three toes on left foot would be—*Trom.*
Twitching suddenly from worm crawling over thigh—*Nat. c.*
Ulcer, burning, were forming on leg—*Agar.*
  –on the ankle—*Ruta*
  –would form on foot—*Puls.*
  –would develop at margin of nails—*Tetrad.*
Ulcerate when walking, knee would—*Ruta*
  –in right great toe, it would—*Olnd.*
Ulcerated inside of thighs—*Arg. m.*
  –above knee while standing and walking—*Ruta*
  –muscle of left leg were—*Iodof.*

Ulcerated—*Continued*

   —knees were—*Am. c., Berb.*

   —extending from ball of left foot to ankle—*Til.*

   —in heel bone—*Am. c.*

   —heels and soles were—*Graph.*

Ulcerating in great toe—*Sil.*

Unjointed, left great toe and two adjoining toes were—*Am. c.*

Use of limbs on attempting to walk, he would lose—*Colch.*

   —of limbs would go—*Fil.*

Vise, legs were squeezed in—*Alum.*

   —parts about hips were screwed in a—*Coloc.*

Walk, stiffness in hollow of knees, from a long walk, < morning on rising—*Lyc.*

   —straight because of trembling of legs, one could not—*Phys.*

Walked too much, he had (in left thigh)—*Mez.*

   —a long journey, she had—*Eup. pur.*

   —too much, pain in soles of feet, he had—*Phos.*

   —too rapidly, weakness of legs, he had—*Rhus t.*

Walking or standing long, aching in calves from—*Rumx.*

   —on needles—*Rhus t.*

   —on nut-shells—*Plb.*

   —on pins—*Nit. ac.*

   —on sponges, and feet were swollen—*Helod.*

   —soles were soft when—*Sulph.*

Walks on knees—*Bar. c.*

Water trickling over joints, in open air—*Nat. m.*

   —limbs had been long time in hot—*Sec.*

   —boots were full of—*Ars.*

   —cold, were running from clavicles to toes in a narrow line—*Caust.*

   —cold, poured over one side from shoulder to thigh—*Verb.*

   —cold, were circulating in parts of lower extremities—*Verat. a.*

   —sitting in ice—*Tub.*

   —legs were cold from snow—*Verat. a.*

   —cold, poured over legs—*Lac c.*

   —cold, poured on feet—*Verat. a.*

   —drops of, were trickling down front of thighs—*Acon.*

   —right leg were standing in cold—*Sabin.*

   —feet were in cold—*Gels., Meny.*

   —feet were in cold, up to knees—*Meny.*

   —feet were dipped into cold—*Carb. v.*

   —standing in cold, over the ankles—*Lyc.*

Water—*Continued*
  –he stood in cold, up to the ankles all day—*Sep.*
  –icy cold, were running into feet—*Verat. a.*
  –she had put her cold feet into hot—*Raph.*
  –limbs were plunged into boiling—*Culx.*
  –foot were plunged into boiling—*Arund.*
  –boiling or molten metal under skin in hollow of **knee and**
     down back of leg—*Bar. c.*
  –hot, were running down leg when hanging down—*Mag. p.*
     Aust.
  –warm, were flowing down legs, leucorrhœa—*Bor.*
Waving, in right thigh—*Rat.*
Weak, capsules of hip joints were—*Thuj.*
  –thigh were—*Ruta*
Weakness of thighs, unable to stand because of—*Pip. m.*
  –of legs, he had walked too rapidly—*Rhus t.*
Weary and bruised in belly, loins and thighs—*Bov.*
Weight, heavy, on crest of ilium—*Kreos.*
  –in all limbs—*Hep.*
  –hanging on lower extremities—*Chel., Verb.*
  –pressing on thighs—*Sep.*
  –were hanging from left leg if rested on the other—*Stann.*
  –were hanging on lower end of tibia—*Spong.*
  –were attached to ankles—*Lyss.*
  –heavy, in each instep—*Arn.*
  –heavy, were hanging to feet—*Rhod.*
  –of sheet on feet would crush the toes—*Thea*
Wind, a cold, on legs—*Lil. t., Samb., Sulph.*
  –legs were blown upon by a wintry, icy cold—*Chin.*
  –cold, makes knees cold—*Cimx.*
  –were blowing on the knees—*Cimx.*
  –freezing cold, blowing on him from bend of the knees—*Helod.*
  –cold, were blowing up limbs from heel to popliteal space—
     Helod.
Wood, legs were made of—*Arg. n., Kali i., Kali n., Nux v., Phos.,*
     Rhus t., Thuj.
  –right leg were made of—*Kali i.*
  –bones were made of—*Crot. h.*
  –muscles of calves were made of—*Sulph.*
  –feet were made of—*Plb.*
  –soles were made of—*Ars.*
Working its way beneath the nail, something were—*Fl. ac.*

Worm were crawling over thigh, causing sudden twitching—*Nat. c.*

–moved about on external malleolus—*Laur.*

–were crawling in left heel—*Lach.*

Worms in legs, there were—*Morph.*

Worn out, feet were suddenly—*Cham.*

Wound in nail of great toe—*Mag. p. Aust.*

Wounded, thighs felt paralyzed—*Lyc.*

Wrapped too tightly, thighs were—*Plat.*

Wrenched, left hip joint were—*Iris*

–when going upstairs, right knee were—*Nux m.*

–her foot, she had—*Phos.*

–by misstep in left metatarsal bones—*Carb. s.*

SLEEP AND DREAMS

See also MIND AND SENSORIUM

Dazed on waking—*Plat.*

Dreamed of had really happened, things—*Anac.*

Fall asleep while walking in street, he would—*Ars. m.*

Falling a great distance in sleep—*Sol. n.*

Frightened, starting up from sleep—*Nit. ac., Psor.*

   –by a sound on waking—*Sars.*

   –in sleep—*Arum t.*

Hard, bed were—*Verat. a.*

Large in sleep, he had grown exceedingly—*Ferr. i.*

Lost several nights' sleep, he had—*Sol. n.*

Narcotized in sleep—*Cund.*

Position, she could get to sleep if she could find the right—*Form.*

Prolonged sleep, after—*Bapt.*

Short, sleep were—*Ars., Carb. an., Con., Dig., Dros., Euphr., Glon., Grat., Kali bi., Kali c., Mos., Myric., Ostrya, Phos., Til., Trif. p., Vio. t.*

Slept all night, he had—*Linar., Nux v.*

   –all night when he had not—*Fl. ac.*

   –enough, frequent waking—*Dros.*

   –enough, he had not—*Aur., Luna, Nit. ac., Phos., Stann., Sulph.*

   –long when waking at 3 a. m., he had not—*Form.*

   –at all in morning, he had not—*Eucal.*

Suffocating in dreams—*Agar.*

   –on falling asleep—*Valer.*

Tied up on falling asleep—*Tub.*

Wakened from sleep, one had just—*Cyc.*

   –from a dream, one had just—*Atro.*

Walking up and down room in dreams—*Agar.*

SKIN

For SKIN SYMPTOMS see also INDIVIDUAL PARTS

Acrid had been secreted under cuticle, something—*Cupr. ar.*

Adherent to bones, skin were—*Kali i., Phos.*

Alive in skin, insects or something were—*Brom.*

–were creeping under skin, something—*Sec.*

–beneath skin of abdomen, something were—*Spong.*

Ant, bitten by an—*Tarent.*

Ants were crawling around waist—*Tab.*

–were biting—*Gamb., Lach.*

–covered with—*Mag. p. Arct., Zinc.*

–were crawling over surface—*Anan., Phos. ac., Pic. ac.*

–were crawling in skin—*Saba.*

–were tingling and crawling—*Ign.*

–were creeping all over body—*Aran.*

Asleep in places when touched, skin were—*Nux v.*

Bath, he were in a vapor—*Acon.*

Bite of insect on spot touched—*Anthox.*

–of fleas—*Arg. m., Cact., Mar., Merc., Nux v., Pulx., Sil., Tell.*

Bites of flea on abdomen, arms and legs—*Thuj.*

Biting of ants—*Gamb., Lach.*

–her, fleas were—*Arg. m., Dulc., Mar., Nuph.*

–over whole body, flea were—*Nat. c.*

–above knee, a flea were—*Pall.*

–insects were—*Cop., Luna*

–leeches were—*Carb. s.*

–nettles were—*Pæon.*

–vermin were—*Atro.*

Bitten by an ant—*Tarent.*

–by bugs—*Syph.*

–by insects—*Cop., Lycps.*

–by something on abdomen—*Carb. ac.*

Bladder rose under skin and burst—*Sil.*

Blood would start through skin—*Aml. n.*

Blowing out from skin, cold wind were—*Cupr.*

Body, foreign, were under skin—*Bomb.*

Bodies, small foreign, were under skin—*Cocaine*

Boring and crawling on body, worms were—*Tarent.*

470

Bound, he were hide- —*Crot. t.*
Break out, old scar would—*Juncus*
Bruised, skin of head were—*Nux v.*
Bubbling of water were coming up through skin—*Berb.*
Bugs, he were bitten by—*Syph.*
Burned by heat of sun, he had been—*Lach.*
Burning of flea bites—*Merc.*
  –from contact with live coals—*Galvan.*
  –vapor were emitted from pores of body—*Fl. ac.*
Burst, skin would—*Tarent. c.*
Bursting on moving about, skin were—*Ars.*
Cap, skin of head were covered with—*Berb.*
Chill under skin—*Ip.*
Coal, bright, lay on rash—*Mez.*
Coals, skin were burning from contact with live—*Galvan.*
Coming out on body, pimples were—*Cinnb.*
Compressed between two fingers, skin of neck were—*Spong.*
Contracted, skin of head were—*Carb. v.*
  –skin on middle of forehead had—*Gels.*
Cord, thin, lay under skin—*Euph.*
  –were around skin of occiput—*Psor.*
Covered with a cap, skin of head were—*Berb.*
  –with ants—*Mag. p. Arct., Zinc.*
  –with gooseflesh in fever—*Crot. t.*
Crawling over surface, ants were—*Anan., Phos. ac., Pic. ac.*
  –of ants in skin—*Saba.*
  –and tingling, ants were—*Ign.*
  –around waist, ants were—*Tab.*
  –beneath skin on right knee and back—*Rat.*
  –of fleas on skin—*Pall.*
  –over skin, flies were—*Calad., Cench., Cod., Gymn., Laur.*
  –of insects on skin—*Arund., Dulc., Helod., Lac c., Nat. c.,
    Phos. ac., Sec., Tab.*
  –over skin, insects were rapidly—*Dulc.*
  –on shoulders, neck and hands, insect were—*Lac c.*
  –on him, millions of insects were—*Mez.*
  –and creeping on body, insects were—*Tarent.*
  –on skin, lice were—*Led.*
  –under skin, a mouse were—*Ign.*
  –up legs under skin from feet to uterus, something were—
    Tarent.

Crawling—*Continued*
　　—on body, spider were—*Dulc.*
　　—over back and scrotum, worms were—*Staph.*
　　—on body, worms were boring and—*Tarent.*
Creeping all over, evening—*Gent. c.*
　　—all over body, ants were—*Aran.*
　　—underneath skin, mice were—*Sec.*
　　—and crawling on body, insects were—*Tarent.*
　　—under skin, something alive were—*Sec.*
Crowded into a skin several times too small, he were—*Meny.*
Cut or sliced with a knife, skin were being—*Bell.*
Denuded, one were—*Sulph.*
Drawing in spots on skin, leeches were—*Coc. c.*
　　—downward under skin, weight were—*Spong.*
Drawn into wrinkles, skin were thick and could not be—*Par.*
　　—inward, skin were—*Rat.*
　　—tight and stiff, skin on bridge of nose were—*Petr.*
　　—over skin, woolen were—*Staph.*
　　—tight, skin of face were—*Cann. i.*
　　—tight on head, skin were—*Med.*
　　—together in center of forehead, skin were—*Rat.*
　　—up on face and nose, skin were—*Com.*
　　—upward, skin on temples were—*Sep.*
　　—up in center of chest, skin were—*Syph.*
Dried, skin had—*Tub.*
Eruption would appear—*Lachn.*
　　—would appear on chin—*Spong.*
　　—were appearing on right malar bone—*Coloc.*
　　—would make an appearance across abdomen—*Com.*
　　—would break out on skin—*Samb.*
　　—would come to surface—*Pop.*
Excoriated, skin were—*Canth.*
　　—when touched, skin were—*Ferr.*
Fast to skull, skin were—*Sabin.*
Fæcal matter passed through skin, itching—*Graph.*
Fingers, skin of neck were compressed between—*Spong.*
Fire falling on different parts of body, sparks of—*Sec.*
Flea on skin—*Spong.*
　　—were biting knee—*Pall.*
　　—were biting over whole body—*Nat. c.*

Flea—*Continued*
   –bites—*Arg. m., Cact., Mar., Merc., Nux v., Pulx., Sil., Tab., Tell.*
   –bites, itching were from—*Myric., Olnd.*
   –bites on abdomen, arms and legs—*Thuj.*
   –bites, burning—*Merc.*
Fleas were biting—*Arg. m., Dulc., Mar., Nuph.*
   –he were in a bag full of—*Ars.*
   –were crawling on skin—*Pall.*
   –on skin—*Gent. c., Nat. c., Nicc., Ptel., Pulx.*
   –itching were from—*Inul., Myric., Nicc., Puls.*
   –prickling were from—*Merc.*
Flies were crawling over skin—*Calad., Cench., Gymn., Laur.*
Fly were on chest, not > by scratching—*Cod.*
Foreign body under skin—*Bomb.*
   –bodies under skin—*Coca, Cocaine*
Frostbitten in many parts—*Colch.*
Furuncles would form here and there—*Kalm.*
Glass on skin, splinters of—*Calad.*
Gooseflesh in fever, one were covered with—*Crot. t.*
Grasped by hand, skin were—*Aconit., Ther.*
Hair were here and there on skin—*Laur.*
Hairs were prickling skin—*Merc.*
Heat of skin came from a stove—*Sel.*
   –in spots—*Tub.*
Hide-bound, he were—*Crot. t.*
Hot, skin were—*Calc. ar.*
Ice had touched skin, piece of—*Agar., Carb. ac.*
Icicle, skin were touched from time to time by an—*Caust.*
Immovable and tense, skin were—*Ars. m.*
Insect on spot touched, bite of—*Anthox.*
   –crawled over body—*Arund.*
   –were crawling on shoulders, neck and hands—*Lac c.*
Insects were here and there on skin—*Chlor.*
   –were biting parts—*Luna*
   –bitten by—*Cop., Lycps.*
   –were crawling on body—*Dulc., Lac c., Nat. c., Phos. ac., Sec., Tab.*
   –were crawling on skin—*Helod.*
   –were creeping and crawling on body—*Tarent.*

31

Insects—*Continued*
 —were rapidly crawling over skin—*Dulc.*
 —crawling on him, millions of—*Mez.*
 —or something alive were in skin—*Brom.*
Itching would return if he ceased rubbing—*Com.*
 —came from an eruption—*Olnd.*
Knots, skin were full of—*Hyper.*
Leeches were drawing in spots on skin—*Coc. c.*
 —were biting—*Carb. s.*
Lice were crawling on skin—*Led.*
Living were under skin of face, something—*Til.*
Loosened from flesh, skin would be—*Coc. c.*
Mice were creeping under skin—*Sec.*
Mold over whole body, sweat were forming—*Sil.*
Mouse were crawling under skin—*Ign.*
Mustard plaster were on various places—*Kali c.*
Needle were pricking in skin—*All. c., Apis*
 —on forearms, skin were raised by a—*Sulph.*
 —-like stitches in skin of throat—*Chin.*
Needles and pins in different parts, with eruption—*Bry.*
 —itching skin were pierced with hot—*Rhus t.*
 —skin were pierced with red-hot—*Vesp.*
 —all over, pricked by ice-cold—*Agar.*
 —skin were pricked with—*Celt., Thuj.*
 —in different places, pricked with—*Chel., Helod.*
 —a thousand, were pricking skin from within outward—*Lob.*
 —sticking all over body—*Culx., Dulc.*
 —skin were touched with—*Anthox.*
Nettles were biting—*Pæon.*
 —skin were pricked with—*Thuj.*
Parboiled, skin were—*Ars.*
Passed through skin, itching; fæcal matter—*Graph.*
Pasted on, skin were—*Agar.*
Pierced with hot needles, itching skin were—*Rhus t.*
 —with red-hot needles, skin were—*Vesp.*
Pimples would break out—*Cinnb., Gran.*
 —would form on skin—*Sel.*
Pin were pricking skin of abdomen—*Kali p.*
Pinched, skin were—*Bell., Caust., Gas.*
 —skin of cheek and chin were—*Sul. ac.*

Pins and needles in different parts with eruption—*Bry.*

    —extending downward from right side of chest to scrotum, pricking of—*Antip.*

Points were inserted into skin—*Æsc.*

Pressed on parts, sponge of cold water were (while other parts actually burning hot)—*Pim.*

Pricked with needles in different places—*Chel., Helod.*

    —with needles, skin were—*Celt., Thuj.*

    —by ice-cold needles all over—*Agar.*

    —with nettles, skin were—*Thuj.*

Pricking of needles in skin—*All. c., Apis*

    —skin from within outward, a thousand needles were—*Lob.*

    —skin of abdomen, pin were—*Kali p.*

    —of pins extending downward from right side of chest to scrotum—*Antip.*

Puffed all over—*Tarent.*

Raised by a needle on forearms, skin were—*Sulph.*

Ran through carbuncles, splinters—*Nit. ac.*

Rose under skin and burst, a bladder—*Sil.*

Rough, skin were—*Ars.*

Rubbed sore, skin were—*Lyc.*

    —with a woolen cloth, skin were—*Rhus t.*

    —off at anus, skin were—*Carb. ac.*

Rubbing, the itching would return if he ceased—*Com.*

Running between skin and muscle, something were—*Am. m.*

    —over body, vermin were—*Aloe, Mez.*

Sand under skin, grain of—*Coca, Cocaine*

Scratched off arms, skin were all—*All. c.*

Scorched, skin were—*Urt. u.*

Secreted under cuticle, something acrid had been—*Cupr. ar.*

Separated from cutis by an intervening layer, epidermis were—*Acon.*

Short, skin were too—*Eupi.*

Sliced with a knife, skin were being cut or—*Bell.*

Sodden, skin were—*Muscn.*

Sparks of fire falling on different parts of body—*Sec.*

Spider were crawling on body—*Dulc.*

Spiders were crawling over skin—*Laur.*

Splinters of glass on skin—*Calad.*

    —ran through carbuncles—*Nit. ac.*

Sponge of cold water were pressed on parts (while other parts
    actually burning hot)—*Pim.*

Start through skin, blood would—*Aml. n.*

Sticking all over body, needles were—*Culx., Dulc.*

Stiff, skin were swollen and—*Apis*
    –skin on bridge of nose were drawn tight and—*Petr.*
    –skin on upper lips were—*Sin.*

Stitches of needle in skin of throat—*Chin.*

Streaming through skin, warmth were—*Coc. c.*

Stroked across skin with something cold—*Sulph.*
    –with delicate fingers, skin were—*Med., Thuj.*

Stung it, an insect flitted over skin and—*Chlor.*

Sun, skin had been burned by—*Lach.*

Suppurate on skin of face, something would—*Rhus t.*

Sweat were forming mold over whole body—*Sil.*

Swell, skin of face were beginning to—*Sulph.*

Swelling, skin were—*Atro.*

Tear skin with her nails, she would—*Graph.*

Tense, skin were immovable and—*Ars. m.*
    –skin of ankles were—*Phos.*

Thick and could not be drawn into wrinkles, skin were—*Par.*

Tight on body, skin were too—*Graph.*
    –on parts, skin were too—*Rhus t.*
    –skin on face were too—*Phos., Sumb.*
    –on abdomen, skin were too—*Calc. s., Rhus t.*
    –skin of hands were—*Gins.*
    –skin in groins were too—*Rhus t.*

Tightened over whole body, skin were—*Graph.*

Torn, skin were being—*Tab.*

Touched with a piece of ice, skin were—*Agar., Carb. ac.*
    –by an icicle, skin were—*Caust.*
    –with needles, skin were—*Anthox.*

Ulcerated, skin were—*Kreos.*
    –on leg, skin were—*Thuj.*

Vapor bath, he were in a—*Acon.*
    –a burning, emanated from all pores—*Fl. ac.*

Vermin were biting—*Atro.*
    –were running over body—*Aloe, Mez.*

Warmth were streaming through skin—*Coc. c.*

Washed in acrid water, skin were—*Sumb.*

Water were bubbling up through skin—*Berb.*

Weight were drawing downward under skin—*Spong.*
Wind, cold, blowing out of skin—*Cupr.*
Woolen cloth, skin were rubbed with a—*Rhus t.*
  –were against skin—*Sul. ac.*
  –were drawn over skin—*Staph.*
Worm under skin which ran away when touched—*Coca*
Worms were crawling and boring on body—*Tarent.*
  –were crawling over back and scrotum—*Staph.*

GENERALS

Absent, parts of body were—*Cocaine, Cot.*

Ached with a constant desire to sit, bones—*Rhus t.*

Adherent to a woolen sack, body were—*Coc. c.*

Agitated by unpleasantness—*Alumn.*

Air, cold, were blowing on one—*Canth., Chel., Graph., Lac d., Mag. p. Aust., Mosch., Nux v., Olnd., Puls., Rhus t., Sabin., Spig., Squill., Stram., Tub.*

–cold, blowing on covered parts—*Camph.*

–cold, blowing on her even though covered warmly—*Lac d.*

–she must be in open—*Puls.*

–cold, penetrated the system—*Cimic.*

–cool, blowing on uncovered parts—*Mosch.*

–too great heat in the—*Verat. a.*

–just in front of her were hot—*Sulph.*

–were piercing marrow of bone—*Pip. n.*

Alive in muscles, something were—*Berb.*

Anguish were in the blood—*Sep.*

Animal, large, were running over body—*Cyc.*

Animals, creeping as of little—*Agn., Alum., Arg. m., Bar. c., Bor., Cann. s., Caust., Chin., Dulc., Kali c., Lach., Laur., Nux v., Plb., Ran. b., Ran. s., Rhod., Rhus t., Saba., Sec., Staph., Sulph., Tarax., Thuj.*

Ants were running through whole body—*Cist.*

Asleep all over—*Dub.*

Ball internally—*Acon., Asaf., Calc. c., Cann. i., Caust., Coloc., Con., Crot. t., Graph., Ign., Kali c., Lach., Mag. m., Nat. m., Par., Phyt., Plat., Plb., Ruta, Sep., Sil., Staph., Stram., Sulph., Valer.*

Band—*Acon., Alum., Alumn., Ambr., Am. br., Am. m., Anac., Ant. c., Ant. t., Arg. n., Arn., Ars., Asaf., Asar., Aur., Bell., Benz. ac., Bism., Brom., Bry., Cact., Calc. c., Cann. i., Carb. ac., Carb. s., Carb. v., Caust., Chel., Chin., Cinch., Cocc., Coc. c., Colch., Coloc., Con., Croc., Dig., Dros., Ferr., Gels., Graph., Hell., Hyos., Ign., Iod., Kali c., Kreos., Laur., Lyc., Mag. m., Mag. p., Manc., Merc., Merc. i. r., Mosch., Nat. c., Nat. m., Nit. ac., Nux m., Nux v., Olnd., Op., Petr., Phos., Phos. ac., Plat., Plb., Puls., Rhod., Rhus t., Ruta, Saba., Sabin., Sars., Sil., Spig., Stann., Sulph., Sul. ac., Tarent., Til., Thuj., Zinc.*

Band—*Continued*

-tight, around different parts—*Saba., Sulph.*

-iron, prevented normal motion—*Cact.*

-about body—*Phos.*

-parts were bound with a tight—*Alumn.*

-drawn tight about body—*Mag. p.*

-or hoop about part—*Anac.*

Bathed in sweat which it was not, body were—*Podo.*

-in cold water, shuddering as if—*Verb.*

Beaten—*Ars. h., Ars. m., Lith., Merc. i. f., Sil.*

-joints were—*Puls.*

-from bone, flesh were—*Thuj., Zinc.*

-in parts—*Calend.*

-in muscles—*Agar., Arg. m.*

-or bruised, parts were—*Acon.*

-with menses—*Goss.*

-wounds were—*Calend.*

-tired as if—*Arn.*

Beating, paralyzed with—*Am. m.*

Bed-clothes were about to crush one—*Pic. ac.*

-were too hard—*Arn., Bapt., Bry., Lac c., Laur., Merc., Pyrog., Rhus t., Til.*

-were not large enough to hold him—*Sulph.*

-would break down unless supported, too heavy and—*Ovi g. p.*

Bee had stung her in various parts of body—*Gels.*

-had stung her—*Apis*

Belong to her, divided into halves and left half did not—*Sil.*

Bend double, he must—*Lil. t.*

Bent yet < doing so, he must sit—*Kalm.*

-forward when walking, he were—*Asc. t.*

-outward, cartilages were—*Sabin.*

Blew clear through marrow, wind—*Tub.*

Blighted with old age, suddenly—*Arn.*

Blowing on body, cold wind were—*Mag. p. Aust.*

-on covered parts, cold air were—*Camph.*

-on her, cold air were—*Canth., Chel., Cor. r., Graph., Lac d., Mag. p. Aust., Mosch., Nux v., Olnd., Puls., Rhus t., Sabin., Spig., Squill., Stram., Tub.*

-on her even though covered up warm, cold air were—*Lac d.*

-on parts, cold wind were—*Camph., Croc., Hep., Laur., Lil. t., Mosch., Rhus t., Samb., Sep.*

Blowing—*Continued*

–through holes in garments and freezing him, a frosty wind were—*Helod*.

–on uncovered parts, cool air were—*Mosch*.

Board, lying on a—*Bapt., Sanic*.

–had been lying on a—*Ars. m.*

Body were elastic and stretched itself out—*Xanth*.

–were scattered about in bed—*Bapt*.

Bound, numbness as if—*Plat*.

–with a tight band or cord, parts were—*Alumn*.

–tightly—*Asaf*.

Bones would break—*Cupr., Rhus v.*

Break down unless supported, too heavy and bed would—*Ovi g. p.*

–if she lay too long in one position, she would—*Pyrog*.

–down with sudden weakness, she would—*Arg. m.*

–out but does not, sweat would—*Ign*.

–out, perspiration would—*Ferr., X-ray*

Breaking, all bones were—*Sars*.

Broken, bones were—*Aur., Bry., Cupr., Eup. pur., Hep., Merc., Nat. m., Puls., Ruta, Sep., Ther., Vario., Verat., Vip.*

–parts were—*Ang., Cham., Chel., Cocc., Dros., Ign., Phos., Pyrog., Ruta, Verat. a.*

–every bone had been—*Eup. per., Lyss., Tub.*

–from head to foot, bones were—*Ther*.

–body were frail and easily—*Thuj*.

–with hæmorrhage, bones were—*Tril*.

–joints were—*Par*.

–whole body had been—*Sil*.

Bruised—see the GENERAL REPERTORIES

Bruised all over—*Lyc., Nux v., Uva*

–or beaten—*Acon., Æsc., Arn.*

–aponeuroses of muscles were—*Pæon*.

–muscles were—*Macrot*.

–at night, all parts of body were—*Ruta*

–in bed, whole body were—*Sol. t. æ.*

–in outer parts—*Nux v.*

–in all bones—*Ip*.

–in joints—*Mur. ac.*

–on waking—*Lepi*.

Burning—see the GENERAL REPERTORIES

Burning hot, sponge full of cold water were pressed over cold spots on body, other places were—*Pim.*

–like small transient flames in spots here and there—*Viol. o.*

–like sparks of fire over parts of body—*Sec.*

–up with heat—*Syph., Tub.*

–vapor emitted from all parts of body—*Fl. ac.*

–whole body were—*Rhus t.*

Burst, body would—*Coff.*

–parts of body would—*Ran. b.*

–he were bound up and would—*Lyc.*

–enlarged and puffed all over as if skin would—*Tarent. c.*

Bursting, whole body were enlarged to—*Cench.*

Buzzing—*Caust., Kreos., Nux m., Nux v., Olnd., Op., Puls., Rhus t., Sep., Spig., Sulph.*

Caged, each wire being twisted tighter and tighter, whole body were—*Cact.*

Capable of carrying body, one were not—*Arn.*

Car moving and jarring her, she were in a railroad—*Sang.*

Carried a great load, he had—*Euph.*

–a weight, he had—*Xanth.*

Carrying a weight, he were—*Raph.*

Cavity or emptiness of whole inner body (with weakness)—*Aur.*

Chill would come on—*Onos., Sac. lac.*

–he would have a—*Malar., Onos.*

–ice-cold wet handkerchief caused—*Berb.*

Chilly, parts of body touched were—*Spig.*

Chopped in half at waist—*Stry.*

–all over with an ax, joints were being—*Phyt.*

Clothes were too heavy—*Euph.*

Clothing were too tight—*Arg. m.*

–whole body were enveloped in cold damp—*Verat. v.*

Coat of skin were drawn over inner parts—*Caust., Cocc., Dros., Merc., Nux m., Phos., Puls.*

Cold, he had taken—*Ars. i., Bapt., Carb. ac., Conv., Eucal., Myric., Nux v., Plan., Phys., Sabin., Sin. n., Sulph., Uran.*

–he had taken a severe—*Ars., Dios., Malar., Meli., Sep., Still.*

–she were continually taking—*Ol. j.*

–beginning of a—*Raph.*

–in affected parts—*Merc.*

Cold—*Continued*
   –after exertion, he had taken—*Tell.*
   –in various spots of body—*Helod.*
   –would come on—*Phyt.*
   –damp clothing, whole body were enveloped in—*Verat. v.*
   –thin body, touched here and there with a—*Ran. b.*
   –when approaching warm stove—*Laur.*
   –wounds were—*Led.*
   –yet it is not, weather were—*Lob. c., Syph.*
   –whole alimentary tract were—*Mit.*
Collapsed—*Sul. ac.*
Comminution, bones were undergoing process of—*Vacc., Vario.*
Compressed, nerves were—*Phys.*
Contracted, muscles were firmly but not spasmodically—*Acon.*
   –internal parts were—*Par.*
Constriction—see the GENERAL REPERTORIES
Control all parts of body at same time, could not—*Dub.*
Cord or ligature about body—*Ail., Alum., Sil.*
   –parts were bound with a tight—*Alumn.*
Cords in any part of body during pregnancy, pulling down of—
      Plb.
Cramped position, lying in a—*Nat. s.*
Cramps, he must hop about with—*Sec.*
Crawling through whole body when knocking against anything—
      Spig.
   –in all parts—*Ign.*
Creeping as of little animals—*Agn., Alum., Arg. m., Bar. c.,*
      Bor., Cann. s., Caust., Chin., Dulc., Kali c., Lach., Laur.,
      Nux v., Plb., Ran. b., Ran. s., Rhod., Rhus t., Saba., Sec.,
      Staph., Sulph., Tarax., Thuj.
   –about in muscles, mouse were—*Bell.*
   –of internal heat over body—*Saba.*
   –things throughout body—*Med.*
   –through parts, worm were—*Rhod.*
Crush through flesh, bones would—*Ind.*
Crushed, joints were—*Dig.*
   –marrow of bones were being—*Coloc.*
   –with bed-clothes, about to be—*Pic. ac.*
Current, electric, tingling as of an—*X-ray*
Cut in all bones—*Saba.*
   –in two—*Plat.*

Damp clothing, whole body were enveloped in cold—*Verat. v.*
 –sheets were—*Lac d.*
Darting through muscles, fire were—*Mez.*
Dashed to pieces, body were—*Calc. c.*
 –with cold water—*Chin., Croc., Mag. c., Rhus t., Saba., Tub., Verat. a.*
 –with cold water, single parts were—*Mez.*
 –with warm water, he were—*Rhus t.*
 –with hot water, he were—*Puls.*
Debauch, after a night's—*Gran.*
Decline, she were going into a—*Sil.*
Desire to sit, bones ached with a constant—*Rhus t.*
Difficult to locate, symptoms are like phantoms—*Stront.*
Dislocated, joints would be easily—*Puls.*
 –joints were—*Agn.*
 –parts lain upon were—*Mosch.*
Dissolution, whole system were in a state of—*Crot. h.*
Distended, inner parts were—*Olnd.*
 –without being, everything were—*Coch.*
Distending within him, something were suddenly—*Coc. c.*
Done up after hard work—*Staph.*
Drawing in marrow of bones—*Rhod.*
 –in bones—*Aloe*
 –in muscles (shifting) < night with warmth—*Puls.*
 –through marrow of bone—*Crot. h.*
Drawn tight about body, a band—*Mag. p.*
 –back and forth, something in muscles were—*Nux v.*
 –through body, threads had been—*Meph.*
 –out, harpoon sticking deep in and being—*Vesp.*
 –together, organs were—*Naja*
 –through shafts of bones, thread were—*Bry.*
Drenched with hot water, she had been—*Calc. c., Puls.*
 –with water—*Mez., Puls.*
Driven into side, stone were—*Paull.*
Drop asunder, she would—*Lil. t.*
Dropping within, water were—*Chin. s.*
Dwindled to nothing, whole body—*Agar.*
Elastic, parts were not sufficiently—*Sul. ac.*
Electric current, tingling as of an—*X-ray*
 –shock in whole body on dozing off to sleep—*Arg. m.*

Electric—*Continued*

  —shock, cutting instrument were piercing all joints like an— *Vesp.*

  —shock passed through her—*Euph., Stram.*

  —shock passed from head through whole body—*Mag. p.*

  —shocks in different spots—*Cimic., Thea*

  —shocks, he fell suddenly from—*Clem.*

  —shocks over body—*Vip.*

  —shocks in many parts—*Cic.*

  —shocks in all joints—*Paraf.*

  —shocks over body, from pricking of—*Xanth.*

  —shocks, twitching as from—*Ter.*

Electricity had been applied to limbs going up **back giving a** shock—*Saponin.*

Electrified when touching anything—*Alum.*

  —he had been—*Nux m.*

Emitted from all parts of body, burning vapor were—*Fl. ac.*

Emptiness—*Acon., Agar., Alum., Am. c., Am. m., Ant. c., Ant. t., Apoc., Arg., Arn., Aur., Bar. c., Bry., Calad., Calc. c., Calc. p., Caps., Carb. v., Caust., Cham., Chin., Cina, Coca, Cocc., Coff., Colch., Coloc., Croc., Crot. t., Cupr., Dig., Dulc., Euph., Ferr., Gamb., Gels., Glon., Graph., Guai., Hep., Hydrs., Ign., Iod., Ip., Kali c., Kali n., Lach., Laur., Lyc., Mag. c., Mang., Mar., Meny., Merc., Mez., Mur. ac., Nat. c., Nat. m., Nux v., Olnd., Op., Par., Petr., Phos., Plat., Plb., Podo., Puls., Rhus t., Ruta, Saba., Sang., Sars., Seneg., Sep., Spig., Squill., Stann., Stram., Sulph., Sul. ac., Tab., Verat. a., Verb., Vib., Zinc.*

  —and hollowness in various cavities of body, especially chest— *Cocc.*

  —or cavity of whole inner body with weakness—*Aur.*

Empty or hollow, whole body were—*Kali c.*

Enlarged all over—*Caj.*

  —joints were—*Caj.*

  —and puffed all over as if skin would burst—*Tarent. c.*

  —body, or part of it, were greatly—*Bell.*

  —to bursting, whole body were—*Cench.*

Enveloped in cold damp clothing, whole body were—*Verat. v.*

Everything about body were too tight—*Puls.*

Exhalation, vaporous, from body were constant—*Grat.*

Expanding, some part of body were—*Arg. n.*
Failing, all strength were—*Coloc.*
Fall out of bed, one would—*Arg. n., Ars.*
–from him, all limbs would—*Merc.*
–asunder, pain in all bones as if they would—*Ther.*
Falling to pieces, whole body were—*Xanth.*
–on different parts, sparks of fire were—*Sec.*
–inner parts were—*Bell.*
Fanned—*Camph., Canth., Chel., Cor. r., Croc., Fl. ac., Graph., Lac d., Laur., Mosch., Nux v., Olnd., Puls., Rhus t., Sabin., Samb., Spig., Squill., Stram., Zinc.*
Fatigue in going upstairs—*Lyss.*
–from a long journey—*Nux m.*
Fat internally, she were getting—*Conv.*
Fatigued, system were over—*Lycps.*
Feel every muscle and fiber from right shoulder to feet, she could —*Sep.*
Fell on different parts, sparks—*Sec.*
Felt, objects touched were covered with fine—*Ign.*
Fever though normal temperature, he had a—*Pyrog.*
Feverish, he would become—*Malar., Vichy*
Filled with cold water passed here and there over surface, a sponge—*Pim.*
Fire were darting through muscles—*Mez.*
–were falling on different parts, sparks of—*Sec.*
–were coming through body—*Zinc.*
–he were on—*Visc.*
Flabby—*Acon., Agar., Ambr., Am. m., Ant. t., Arg., Arn., Ars., Asar., Bar. c., Bell., Bov., Bry., Calc. c., Canth., Caps., Carb. an., Carb. v., Caust., Cham., Chel., Chin., Cic., Cina, Coff., Croc., Cyc., Dig., Euph., Euphr., Graph., Hep., Ign., Iod., Ip., Kali c., Kali n., Laur., Lyc., Mag. c., Mag. m., Mar., Meny., Merc., Mosch., Mur. ac., Nat. c., Nit. ac., Nux m., Nux v., Olnd., Par., Petr., Phos., Plat., Puls., Rhod., Rhus t., Saba., Sabin., Seneg., Sil., Spong., Staph., Stront., Sulph., Tar., Thuj., Verat. a., Zinc.*
–internally—*Calc. c., Kreos., Sep.*
Flame, small transient, burning here and there—*Viol. o.*
Flesh were falling from bones—*Eup. per.*
–were torn by rough ends of bones—*Symph.*

Flesh—*Continued*

 −on bones were loose—*Ign., Lyc.*

 −over body, < feet, pinched out little pieces of—*Sac. lac.*

 −were torn from bones—*Nit. ac.*

Flint, had been lying on—*Mag. p. Aust.*

Flowed through different parts, hot water—*Sumb.*

Flowing through body, warmth were—*Chlf.*

Fluid, hot, were running along over affected part—*Arg. n.*

Flying round and round, tendons were—*Eup. pur.*

Food contained neither juice nor strength—*Ferr.*

Forming from sweat, mold were—*Sil.*

Fracture in joints—*Mag. p. Ambo*

Freezing him, a frosty wind were blowing through holes in garments and—*Helod.*

Frozen to death, from within outward, he were being—*Helod.*

Full of cold water—*Pyrus*

Fullness in external parts—*Cyc.*

 −in inner parts—*Rhus t.*

Gather all her strength, she had to—*Nux m.*

Give way, joints would—*Mez.*

Gnawing in marrow of bones—*Mang., Stront.*

 −her, two dogs with sharp teeth were—*Lyc.*

Gnawed, bones were—*Plb., Rhod.*

Grating in bones, sudden sharp painful—*Cinnb.*

Growing larger or swollen, parts were—*Kali br.*

 −longer and longer, body were—*Plat., Stram.*

Grown taller, he had—*Pall.*

 −together, inner parts were—*Rhus t.*

Gushing forward when stooping, water were—*Ars. m.*

Hand all over body, being stroked with—*Carb. v.*

Handkerchief caused chill, ice-cold wet—*Berb.*

Hard, bed were too—*Acon., Arn., Bapt., Bry., Caust., Con., Dros., Graph., Kali c., Lac c., Laur., Mag. c., Mag. m., Nux m., Nux v., Phos., Plat., Pyrog., Rhus t., Saba., Sil., Stann., Sulph., Tarax., Thuj., Til., Verat. a.*

Harpoon were sticking deep in and being drawn out—*Vesp.*

Heat in air were too great—*Verat. a.*

 −over body, creeping of internal—*Saba.*

 −radiating from eyes, ears, vertex, palms and **soles**—*Blatta*

 −as in reaction after a bath—*Pim.*

Heavy, were too—*Caj.*
  –as a ton—*Elect.*
  –limbs could not carry, body so—*Euphr.*
  –for bed and it would break down unless supported, one were too—*Ovi g. p.*
Holding a heavy weight, weakness from—*Plat.*
Hollow or empty, whole body were—*Kali c.*
Hollowness or emptiness in various cavities of body, especially chest—*Cocc.*
Hook were pulled out—*Vesp.*
Hoop or band around part—*Anac.*
Hop about with cramps, he must—*Sec.*
Hot air just in front of her—*Sulph.*
  –pains were lightning—*Æsc.*
  –parts were internally—*Staph.*
Hovering or sinking down—*Bry., Lach.*
Ice, pointed, touched or pierced body—*Agar.*
  – -cold wet handkerchief caused chill—*Berb.*
  –bones were made of—*Aran.*
  –lying on—*Lyc.*
Ill a long time, he had been—*Echi.*
Immersed in hot water—*Phos.*
Instrument, cutting, were piercing all joints like an electric shock—*Vesp.*
Itching in bones—*Kali c.*
Jarring and moving her, she were in a railroad car—*Sang.*
Jelly, whole body were made of—*Eupi.*
Jerked about, some part of body were—*Cot.*
Joint, all bones were out of—*Med.*
Joints were loose, all—*Wild.*
Jumped under skin like a mouse under a cloth, muscles—*Merc. n.*
Knife, interior of bones were scraped with a—*Saba.*
  –bones were scraped with a—*Chin., Phos. ac.*
Knives, stabbed with—*Thuj.*
  –were running through her—*Sil.*
Knocking against anything, crawling through whole body when —*Spig.*
Laced tightly together, parts were (but changing place often)— *Mag. p.*

Lain in an uncomfortable position, he had—*Psor., Puls., Rhus t., Sil., Sulph.*

　–in a wrong position, he had—*Ran. b.*

　–in a wrong position and parts had gone to sleep—*Sep.*

　–on blocks of wood, whole body feels as if he had—*Saba.*

Lame, joints were—*Seneg.*

Large, internal organs, especially of left side, were too—*Jug. c.*

　–parts of body had become—*Alum.*

　–parts were becoming—*Coll.*

Larger and larger, body were growing—*Aur., Plat., Stram.*

　–single parts became thicker and—*Cann. i.*

　–or swollen, parts were growing—*Kali br.*

　–and longer, body grew—*Plat.*

Lay too long in one position, she would break if she—*Pyrog.*

　–in a bad position—*Nat. s.*

Lightning, hot—*Æsc.*

Load, he had carried a great—*Euph.*

Longer and larger, body grew—*Plat.*

Loose, flesh on bones were—*Ign., Lyc.*

　–bones were—*Arg. n.*

Looseness of joints—*Stram.*

Lying on a hard bed, one had been—*Acon., Arn., Bapt., Bry., Caust., Con., Dros., Graph., Kali c., Lac c., Laur., Mag. c., Mag. m., Nux m., Nux v., Phos., Plat., Pyrog., Rhus t., Saba., Sil., Stann., Sulph., Tarax., Thuj., Til., Verat. a.*

　–in a cramped position—*Nat. s.*

　–on a board—*Bapt., Sanic.*

　–on a board, she had been—*Ars. m.*

　–on flint, he had been—*Mag. p. Aust.*

　–on her, weight were—*Pyrog.*

　–on ice—*Lyc.*

　–on a stone—*Plat.*

Marrow of bones, drawing through—*Crot. h.*

　–of bone, drawing in—*Rhod.*

　–of bone, air were piercing—*Pip. n.*

　–of bones, hot water ran through—*Hydrc.*

　–of bones were stiff—*Ang.*

　–in bones, there were no—*Lyc., Sulph.*

　–of bones, gnawing in—*Mang., Stront.*

　–of bones were being crushed—*Coloc.*

　–of bones, symptoms were in—*Stront.*

Motion, iron band prevented normal—*Cact.*

   –was no relief, he must move yet—*Puls.*

Mouse creeping about in muscles—*Bell.*

   –under cloth, muscles jumped under skin like a—*Merc. n.*

Move, too lazy to—*Eucal.*

   –yet motion was no relief, he must—*Puls.*

   –about, he had to—*Ars. h., Mosch.*

   –about, weak and unable to—*Podo.*

   –yet > by moving, she could not—*Homar.*

   –even a finger, unable to—*Iber.*

Moving, he had more power when—*Arg. m.*

   –and jarring her, she were in a railroad car—*Sang.*

Needle pricked here and there, a very fine—*Spong.*

   –points on body, a thousand—*Cann. s.*

Needles, pain from—*Eup. per.*

   –pain as from red-hot—*Ars., Ol. an.*

   –pain as from cold—*Agar.*

   –pricking as from—*Arg. n., Hep., Nit. ac.*

   –pricking in right side of body with headache—*Lach.*

   –pricking of red-hot—*Lith., Ol. an., Vesp.*

   –thousand, sticking all over body—*Cann. s.*

   –stick all over body, large sharp—*Thlaspi*

   –parts were punctured by a great number of—*Syph.*

   –pricking in bones—*Kali bi.*

   –sticking with—*Dulc., Kali br., Mez.*

Nerve, every, were unstrung—*Phys.*

Nerves were violently torn—*Zinc.*

   –were tense—*Gent. c.*

Noise, every, penetrated whole body—*Ther.*

Nothing, good for—*Arn.*

Numb—see the GENERAL REPERTORIES

Numbness as if bound—*Plat.*

Oiling, all joints wanted—*Sabal*

Oppression with swelling of whole body—*Bufo*

Overexertion, as from—*Meph.*

Overstrained—*Tell.*

Pain from a blow—*Phos.*

   –would give a twist while running up body—*Corn.*

   –in all bones as if they would fall asunder—*Ther.*

   –from needles—*Eup. per.*

   –as from red-hot needles—*Ars., Ol. an.*

Painful, sudden sharp grating in bones—*Cinnb.*

Pains occupy small spots as if hard pressure with ends of fingers —*Lil. t.*

Paralyzed—*Cist., Phys., Saba., Sang.*

–about to be—*Syph.*

–in inner parts—*Olnd.*

–joints were—*Plb.*

–muscles were—*Colch.*

–right side were—*Arn., Ars., Bell., Colch., Elaps, Phos.*

–with beating—*Am. m.*

Penetrated parts, warmth—*Euphr.*

–system, cold air—*Cimic.*

–whole body, every noise—*Ther.*

Pepper, cayenne, sprinkled on parts—*Caps.*

Perspiration would break out—*Ferr., X-ray*

Phantoms and difficult to locate, symptoms are like—*Stront.*

Pieces, all bones of body were being torn to—*Ip.*

–and it were only by a great effort that she kept herself together, it would be a relief to fall to—*Sac. lac.*

–body had been dashed to—*Calc. c.*

Pierced body, pointed ice touched or—*Agar.*

–by hot iron—*Alum., Cann. i.*

Piercing all joints like an electric shock, a cutting instrument were—*Vesp.*

–marrow of bone, air were—*Pip. n.*

Pinched out little pieces of flesh over body, < feet—*Sac. lac.*

Pins or needles on right side of body with headache, pricking of —*Lach.*

–pricking in different places—*Sil.*

–pricking in whole body, thousands of—*Vip.*

Plug internally—*Acon., Agar., Aloe, Ambr., Am. br., Am. c., Anac., Ant. c., Arg. m., Arn., Asaf., Aur., Bar. c., Bell., Bov., Calc. c., Caust., Cham., Chel., Cocc., Coc. c., Coff., Con., Croc., Crot. t., Dros., Ferr., Graph., Hell., Hep., Ign., Iod., Kali bi., Kali c., Kreos., Lach., Led., Lyc., Merc., Mez., Mur. ac., Nat. m., Nux v., Olnd., Par., Plat., Plb., Ran. s., Rhod., Ruta, Saba., Sabin., Sang., Sep., Spig., Spong., Staph., Sulph., Thuj.*

–in various parts—*Anac.*

Plunged into cold water, she had just—*Lyss.*

Poison, she had taken—*Caj., Euph.*

Position, he had lain in an uncomfortable—*Psor., Puls., Rhus t., Sil., Sulph.*

–he had lain in a wrong—*Ran. b.*

–she had lain in a wrong, and parts had gone to sleep—*Sep.*

–she would break if she lay too long in one—*Pyrog.*

–lying in a cramped—*Nat. s.*

Pounded all over—*Phyt.*

Poured over body from shoulder to thigh, water were—*Verb.*

–water over him—*Ant. t.*

–over her, ice-water were being—*Lyss.*

–over parts, boiling water were—*Verat. v.*

–over one, hot water were—*Ars., Bar. c., Cann. s., Cimx., Led., Merc., Sep.*

Pouring over parts, cold water were—*Led.*

Power when moving, he had more—*Arg. m.*

–were going, all—*Colch., Phys.*

Pressed asunder, body would be—*Zinc.*

–full, whole body were—*Ruta*

–over cold spots on body, other places burning hot; sponge full of cold water were—*Pim.*

–down by weight—*Eup. per., Merl.*

–downward on right side of body and came up on left side of body, something—*Chim. mac.*

–on parts, dull stick—*Merc. sul.*

Pressing in spots, a hard blunt tool were—*Valer.*

Pressure with ends of fingers, pains occupy small spots as if by hard—*Lil. t.*

–with a dull point especially near a bone—*Lith.*

–lame, in periosteum—*Cyc.*

Prevented normal motion, an iron band—*Cact.*

Pricked here and there, a very fine needle—*Spong.*

–by little sticks or splinters in folds of mucous membranes—*Æsc.*

Pricking, needles were—*Hep., Nit. ac.*

–red-hot needles—*Lith., Ol. an., Vesp.*

–electric shocks over body—*Xanth.*

–needles, in bones—*Kali bi.*

–of needles or pins on right side of body with headache—*Lach.*

–in whole body, thousands of pins—*Vip.*

–in different places, pins were—*Sil.*

Process of comminution, bones were undergoing—*Vacc., Vario.*

Prostrated, not real, extremely—*Eup. per.*

Puffed and enlarged all over as if skin would burst—*Tarent. c.*

Pulled and torn into threads—*Plat.*

Pulling on motion, very fine wire were—*Cocc.*

  –down of cords of any part during pregnancy—*Plb.*

Punctured by a great number of needles, parts were—*Syph.*

Quick-silver, living, were in different parts of body—*Agar.*

Quivering with tingling—*Med.*

Radiating from ears, eyes, vertex, palms, and soles, heat were—
    Blatta

Raised, cartilages and muscles were being—*Sabin.*

Ran through marrow of bones, hot water—*Hydrc.*

Recovering from a long illness—*Ars. h., Asc. t., Bapt., Conv.*

Removed from one position to another, anatomical structures
    were being—*X-ray*

Rested upon him, the world—*Tab.*

Rise again after stooping, she could not—*Rhus t.*

Round and round, tendons were flying—*Eup. pur.*

Running through her, knives were—*Sil.*

  –over body, large animal were—*Cyc.*

  –down part, hot water were—*Mag. p. Aust.*

  –through tube in nerve, hot water were—*Ter.*

  –from clavicle down to toes in narrow line, cold water were—
    Caust.

  –from vulva up to mouth, boiling water were—*Sec.*

  –up body, pain would give a twist while—*Corn.*

  –down body, hot sweat were—*Stann.*

  –along over affected part, hot fluid were—*Arg. n.*

  –through whole body, ants were—*Cist.*

Sack, woolen, body were adherent to—*Coc. c.*

Salt were put on a wound—*Sars.*

Sawed through, bones were—*Stram.*

  –in bones—*Syph.*

Scorched by sun, he had been—*Pop.*

Scraped, bones were being—*Berb., Phos. ac., Rhus t.*

  –with a dull knife, periosteum were—*Chin., Phos. ac.*

  –with a knife, interior of bones were—*Saba.*

Scratched him, clothes did not fit and—*Verat. v.*

Scream, had not sufficient strength to—*Calad.*

Separated from one another, parts of body were—*Daph. o.*

Severed, connection of different parts were in danger of being—
Thuj.

Shaken inwardly, whole body were—*Agar.*

  —nerves were—*Cean.*

Sharp sudden painful grating in bones—*Cinnb.*

Shock, electric—*Acon., Agar., Ail., Alum., Ambr., Anac., Ang., Apis, Arg. m., Arg. n., Arn., Ars., Art. v., Bar. c., Bar. m., Bell., Bufo, Calad., Calc. c., Calc. p., Camph., Cann. s., Carb. ac., Carb. v., Caust., Cic., Cimic., Cina, Clem., Cocc., Colch., Con., Croc., Cupr., Dig., Dulc., Fl. ac., Graph., Hell., Hep., Kali c., Kreos., Laur., Lyc., Mag. m., Manc., Mang., Mez., Mur. ac., Nat. a., Nat. c., Nat. m., Nat. p., Nit. ac., Nux v., Olnd., Ol. an., Phos., Plat., Puls., Ran. b., Ruta, Sep., Spig., Squill., Stram., Stry., Sulph., Sul. ac., Sumb., Tab., Thal., Verat. a., Xanth., Zinc.*

  —electricity had been applied to limbs going up to back giving a
—*Saponin.*

  —electric, passed through her—*Euph., Stram.*

  —electric, in all joints—*Paraf.*

  —electric, a cutting instrument were piercing all joints like a—
Vesp.

  —under influence of a galvanic—*Cahin.*

Shocks, he fell suddenly from electric—*Clem.*

  —electric, over body—*Vip.*

  —electric, of whole body on dozing off to sleep—*Arg. m.*

  —over body, pricking of electric—*Xanth.*

  —electric, in different spots—*Cimic., Thea*

Short, muscles were too—*Bov., Eupi., Macrot.*

  —tendons were too—*Bar. c., Cimx., Mang., Ran. b.*

Shudder through whole frame, touch of body sent—*Spig.*

Sick, about to be—*Vichy*

Sitting on something hard, or wrinkles in clothes—*Arn.*

  —in ice-water—*Tub.*

Sleep, parts had gone to—*Caps., Ign.*

  —parts of body were going to—*Acon.*

  —she had lain in wrong position and parts had gone to—*Sep.*

  —joints had all gone to—*Ip.*

  —anywhere, he could not—*Samars.*

Small, body were too—*Tarent.*

Smaller, body were—*Acon., Agar., Calc. c., Carb. v., Croc., Euphr., Glon., Kreos., Saba., Tarent.*

Snow, parts were in—*Sec.*

Someone were poking him with fingers in various parts of body —*Inul.*

Something pressed downward on right side of body and came up on left side of body—*Chim. mac.*

    –were distending within him, suddenly—*Coc. c.*

    –in muscles were drawn back and forth—*Nux v.*

Soreness of parts lain upon—*Ruta*

Sparks fell on different parts of body—*Sec.*

Splinter sticking in parts—*Arg. n., Hep., Nit. ac.*

Splinters—*Æsc., Agar., Alum., Arg. n., Bar. c., Carb. v., Cic., Colch., Coll., Dol., Fl. ac., Hep., Nit. ac., Petr., Plat., Ran. b., Sil., Sulph.*

    –or sticks were pricking in folds of mucous membranes—*Æsc.*

Sponge full of cold water were pressed over cold spots on body; other places burning hot—*Pim.*

Sprinkled on parts, cayenne pepper were—*Caps.*

Squeezed narrower, bones were—*Alum.*

Stabbed with knives—*Thuj.*

Stick, dull, pressed on parts—*Merc. sul.*

    –flesh were struck with a—*Lyc.*

    –all over body, large sharp needles—*Thlaspi*

Sticking in parts, splinters—*Arg. n., Hep., Nit. ac.*

    –from all sides at once—*Eug.*

    –with needles—*Dulc., Kali br., Mez.*

    –all over body, thousand needles were—*Cann. s.*

    –in bones—*Con.*

    –deep in and were being drawn out, a harpoon were—*Vesp.*

Sticks or splinters were pricking in folds of mucous membranes —*Æsc.*

Stiff, marrow of bones were—*Ang.*

    –all over in going upstairs—*Calc. p.*

Stiffened with cramp-like pains, she would be—*Stry.*

Stiffness, internal, from head to abdomen—*Caust.*

Stone, lying on a—*Plat.*

    –were driven into side—*Paull.*

Straighten up, he could not—*Cob.*

Strain herself easily, she could—*Sep.*

Strained in left side—*Vib.*

Stream, sweat so profuse he were in a warm—*Fl. ac.*

Streaming through skin, warmth were—*Coc. c.*
  –through bones, icy-cold water were—*Verat. a.*
Strength—*Agar., Bufo, Coff., Fl. ac., Op., Stram.*
  –she had to gather all her—*Nux m.*
  –to breathe, there were not—*Cyc.*
Stretched, all tendons were—*Ang.*
Stroked with a hand all over body, one were being—*Carb. v.*
Struck with a stick, flesh were—*Lyc.*
Strumming through body—*Meph.*
Stuffed, body were—*Anac., Coc. c.*
Stung her in various parts of body, bee had—*Apis, Gels.*
Sudden sharp painful grating in bones—*Cinnb.*
Sun, he had been out in hot—*Glon.*
Surged through body like a vapor, hot wave—*Lyss.*
Sweat would break out—*Bapt., Cimx., Cop., Croc., Gels., Glon.,*
    Nicc., Pop., Raph., Spong., Stann., Sulph., Thuj., Zinc.
  –hot, were running down body—*Stann.*
  –would break out but does not—*Ign.*
  –anxious, would break out—*Plat.*
  –general, would break out—*Croc.*
  –which it were not, body were bathed in—*Podo.*
  –cold, trickled down to foot—*Croc.*
Sweaty parts, cold wind on—*Croc.*
Sweets, body were made of—*Merc.*
Swell, parts would—*Puls.*
Swollen, body were—*Pop., Prim.*
  –or larger, parts were growing—*Kali br.*
  –almost anywhere or all over—*Aml. n.*
  –after washing—*Æth.*
Symptoms were in marrow of bones—*Stront.*
Tearing in bones—*Ang.*
Tense, nerves were—*Gent. c.*
Thicker, parts became larger and—*Cann. i.*
Thread drawn through shaft of bones—*Bry.*
Threads, pulled and torn into—*Plat.*
  –had been drawn through body—*Meph.*
Thrill all through body—*Tanac.*
Thrust in spots—*Thuj.*
Tickled, one were being—*Merc. i. f.*
Tight cord, parts were bound with a—*Alumn.*
  –clothing were too—*Arg. m., Nux v.*

Tight—*Continued*

  –band around different parts—*Saba., Sulph.*

  –whole body were—*Arn., Bar. c., Graph., Sulph.*

  –around body, band were drawn—*Mag. p.*

Tightly together, parts were laced—*Mag. p.*

Tingling as of an electric current—*X-ray*

  –with quivering—*Med.*

Tired—*Calend.*

  –as after hard work or as if beaten—*Arn.*

  –and weak—*Chr. ac.*

Together, joints would not hold—*Psor.*

  –he could not get himself—*Caj.*

  –and it would be a relief to fall to pieces, only by a great effort she kept herself—*Sac. lac.*

  –inner parts had grown—*Rhus t.*

Ton, she weighed a—*Elect.*

Tool pressing in spots, a hard blunt—*Valer.*

Torn to pieces, all bones of body were being—*Ip.*

  –from their attachments, muscles were—*Ip.*

  –from bones, muscles were—*Eupi., Nat. m.*

  –and pulled into threads—*Plat.*

  –by rough ends of bones, flesh were—*Symph.*

  –nerves were violently—*Zinc.*

  –from bones, flesh were—*Nit. ac.*

  –out, everything were—*Phos.*

Touch of body sent shudder through whole frame—*Spig.*

Touched or pierced body, pointed ice—*Agar.*

  –here and there with a cold thin body—*Ran. b.*

  –seemed thicker than natural, everything—*Coc. c.*

  –were chilly, part of body—*Spig.*

Touching anything, electrified when—*Alum.*

Trembling like jelly all over—*Eupi.*

  –inside, all nerves were—*Sol*

  –without trembling, she were—*Carb. s., Homar., Med., Sul. ac., Zinc.*

Tremor all over body—*Sul. ac.*

Trickling over joints in open air, water were—*Nat. m.*

Tumult in whole body, there were—*Coc. c.*

Turned about, everything in body were—*Op.*

Twist while running up body, pain would give a—*Corn.*

Twisted tighter and tighter, whole body were caged, each wire being—*Cact.*

Ulcerating on whole side lain upon—*Sil.*

Undulating all over body—*Trios.*

Unstrung, every nerve were—*Phys.*

Vacuity of whole body—*Aur.*

Vapor, hot wave surged through body like—*Lyss.*

  –burning, emitted from all parts of body—*Fl. ac.*

Vaporous, exhalation from body were constantly—*Grat.*

Vibrating through whole body—*Carb. s., Clem.*

Vise, one were in a—*Æth., Quer.*

Wabbled in upper part of body—*Eupi.*

Walked a great distance, he had—*Lac. ac., Merc. i. f., Sal. ac., Stann.*

Walking, body were light when—*Thuj.*

  –he were bent forward when—*Asc. t.*

Warm, room were too—*Still.*

Warmth penetrated parts—*Euphr.*

  –were streaming through skin—*Coc. c.*

  –were flowing through body—*Chlf.*

Washed out, all—*Pic. ac.*

Water, cold, were pressed over cold spots on body, other spots burning hot; sponge full of—*Pim.*

  –full of cold—*Pyrus*

  –cold, running down from clavicle to toes in a narrow line—*Caust.*

  –parts in cold—*Sec.*

  –dashed with cold—*Chin., Croc., Mag. c., Mez., Rhus t., Saba., Verat. a.*

  –drenched with—*Mez., Puls.*

  –were dropping within—*Chin. s.*

  –were gushing forward when stooping—*Ars. m.*

  –she had just plunged into cold—*Lyss.*

  –ice-, were being poured over her—*Lyss.*

  –poured over him—*Ant. t.*

  –were poured over body from shoulder to thigh—*Verb.*

  –cold, pouring over parts—*Led.*

  –passed here and there over surface, a sponge filled with cold—*Pim.*

  –sitting in—*Morph.*

Water—*Continued*

   —sitting in ice- —*Tub.*

   —icy-cold, were streaming through bones—*Verat. a.*

   —were trickling over joints in open air—*Nat. m.*

   —warm, between flesh and bones—*Ox. ac.*

   —hot, ran through marrow of bones—*Hydrc.*

   —immersed in hot—*Phos.*

   —hot, were running down parts—*Mag. p. Aust.*

   —hot, she had been drenched with—*Calc. c., Puls.*

   —hot, were running through tube in nerves—*Ter.*

   —warm, he were dashed with—*Rhus t.*

   —hot, flowed through different parts—*Sumb.*

   —boiling, were poured over parts—*Verat. v.*

   —hot, were poured over one—*Ars., Bar. c., Cann. i., Cann. s., Cimx., Led., Merc., Sep.*

   —hot, he were dashed with—*Puls.*

   —boiling, running from vulva up to mouth—*Sec.*

Wave-like sensation as if he would break out in perspiration—*X-ray*

Weak and tired—*Chr. ac.*

   —and unable to move about—*Podo.*

Weakness, great—*Viol. t.*

   —he would die from—*Vinc.*

   —from holding a heavy weight—*Plat.*

Wearied by too great an effort—*Zinc.*

Weighed a ton—*Elect.*

Weight in sides—*Sep.*

   —he had carried a—*Xanth.*

   —carrying a—*Raph.*

   —were lying on her—*Pyrog.*

   —pressed down by a—*Eup. per., Merl.*

   —incapable of raising slightest—*Gnaph.*

   —weakness from holding a heavy—*Plat.*

Weighted down with general indisposition, everything were—*Plb.*

Wet ice-cold handkerchief caused chill—*Berb.*

Wind—*Canth., Chel., Cor. r., Graph., Lyss., Mosch., Nux v., Olnd., Puls., Rhus t., Sabin., Spig., Squill., Stram.*

   —blew clear through marrow—*Tub.*

   —cold—*Camph., Croc., Lac d., Laur., Lyss., Mosch., Rhus t., Samb.*

Wind—*Continued*
    –cold, blowing on parts—*Hep., Lil. t., Sep.*
    –cold, blowing on entire body—*Mag. p. Aust.*
    –frosty, blowing through holes in garments and freezing him
        —*Helod.*
    –cold, on sweaty parts—*Croc.*
Wires, whole body were caged in—*Cact.*
Worm were creeping through parts—*Rhod.*
Wood, parts were made of—*Kali n., Petr., Thuj.*
    –whole body feels as if he had lain on blocks of—*Saba.*
Woolen sack, body were adherent to—*Coc. c.*
Worked hard, he had—*Apis*
Wound, salt were put on—*Sars.*
Wounds were beaten—*Calend.*
    –were cold—*Led.*
Wrinkled, sitting on something hard or—*Arn.*

LIST OF REMEDIES AND ABBREVIATIONS

Abies c.—Abies Canadensis
Abies n.—Abies nigra
Abrot.—Abrotanum artemisia
Absin.—Absinthium
Acal.—Acalypha Indica
Acet. ac.—Acetic acid
Acon. a.—Aconitum anthora
Acon. c.—Aconitum cammarum
Acon. f.—Aconitum ferox
Acon. l.—Aconitum lycoctonum
Acon.—Aconitum napellus
Aconit.—Aconitinum
Cimic.—Actæa racemosa (Cimicifuga)
Act. sp.—Actæa spicata
Adren.—Adrenalin
Æsc. g.—Æsculus glabra
Æsc.—Æsculus hippocastanum
Æth.—Æthusa
Agar. em.—Agaricus emeticus
Agar.—Agaricus muscarius
Agar. p.—Agaricus phalloides
Agn.—Agnus castus (Vitex)
Ail.—Ailanthus glandulosa
Alco.—Alcohol
Alet.—Aletris farinosa
All. c.—Allium cepa (Cepa)
All. s.—Allium sativum
Aloe—Aloe socrotina
Alst.—Alstonia constricta
Alumn.—Alumen
Alum.—Alumina
Alum. sil.—Alumina silicata
Ambr.—Ambra grisea
Ambro.—Ambrosia artemisæfolia
Ammc.—Ammoniacum
Am. ac.—Ammonium aceticum
Am. be.—Ammonium benzoicum

Am. br.—Ammonium bromatum
Am.c.—Ammonium carbonicum
Am. caust.—Ammonium causticum
Am. m.—Ammonium muriaticum
Am. n.—Ammonium nitricum
Am. phos.—Ammonium phosphoricum
Amph.—Amphisbæna
Amyg.—Amygdalæ amaræ aqua
Aml. n.—Amylenum nitrosum
Anac.—Anacardium orientale
Anag.—Anagallis arvensis
Anan.—Anantherum muricatum
Ang.—Angustura vera
Angel.—Angelica atropurpurea
Anil.—Anilinum
Ill.—Anisum stellatum (Illicum)
Anth.—Anthemis nobilis
Anthr.—Anthracinum
Anthox.—Anthoxanthum
Anthro.—Anthrokokali
Antif.—Antifebrinum
Ant. a.—Antimonium arsenicosum
Ant. c.—Antimonium crudum
Ant. ox.—Antimonium oxydatum
Ant. s.—Antimonium sulphuratum aureum
Ant. t.—Antimonium et potass. tartaricum
Antip.—Antipyrinum
Aphis—Aphis chenopodii glauci
Apis—Apis mellifica
Ap. g.—Apium graveolens
Apoc.—Apocynum cannabinum
Apom.—Apomorphinum
Aqua m.—Aqua marina
Aqua pet.—Aqua petra
Aral.—Aralia racemosa
Aran.—Aranea diadema (Diadema)
Aran. s.—Aranea scinencia
Aran. t.—Aranearum tela
Arg. c.—Argentum cyanatum
Arg. m.—Argentum metallicum
Arg. mur.—Argentum muriaticum

Arg. n.—Argentum nitricum
Coch.—Armoracea sativa (Cochlearia)
Arn.—Arnica montana
Ars.—Arsenicum album
Ars. h.—Arsenicum hydrogenisatum
Ars. i.—Arsenicum iodatum
Ars. m.—Arsenicum metallicum
Ars. s. f.—Arsenicum sulphuratum flavum
Ars. s. r.—Arsenicum sulphuratum rubrum
Arist. m.—Aristolochia milhomens
Art. v.—Artemisia vulgaris
Arum d.—Arum dracontium
Arum m.—Arum maculatum
Arum t.—Arum triphyllum
Arund.—Arundo mauritanica
Asaf.—Asafœtida
Asar.—Asarum europœum
Asc. c.—Asclepias cornuti (Syriaca)
Asc. t.—Asclepias tuberosa
Asim.—Asimina triloba
Aspar.—Asparagus
Astac.—Astacus fluviatilis (Cancer fluviatilis)
Aster.—Asterias rubens
Atham.—Athamantha
Atro.—Atropinum
Aur. a.—Aurum arsenicicum
Aur. i.—Aurum iodatum
Aur.—Aurum metallicum
Aur. m.—Aurum muriaticum
Aur. m. n.—Aurum muriaticum natronatum
Aur. s.—Aurum sulphuratum
Azad.—Azadirachta Indica

Bad.—Badiaga
Bapt.—Baptisia tinctoria
Bart.—Bartfelder
Bar. ac.—Baryta acetica
Bar. c.—Baryta carbonica
Bar. i.—Baryta iodata
Bar. m.—Baryta muriatica
Bell.—Belladonna

Bell. p.—Bellis perennis
Benz.—Benzinum
Benz. n.—Benzinum nitricum
Benz. ac.—Benzoicum acidum
Berb. a.—Berberis aqui
Berb.—Berberis vulgaris
Bism.—Bismuthum
Bol.—Boletus laricis (Polyporus officinalis)
Bomb.—Bombyx processionea
Bon.—Bondonneau
Bor. ac.—Boracicum acidum
Bor.—Borax
Both. a.—Bothrops atrox
Both.—Bothrops lanceolatus
Bov.—Bovista
Brach.—Brachyglottis repens
Brom.—Bromium
Bruc.—Brucea antidysenterica
Bry.—Bryonia alba
Bufo—Bufo rana and sahytiensis
Thlaspi—Thlaspi bursa pastoris

Cact.—Cactus grandiflorus
Cadm. br.—Cadmium bromatum
Cadm. s.—Cadmium sulphuratum
Cahin.—Cahinca (or Cainca)
Caj.—Cajuputum
Calad.—Caladium
Calc. ac.—Calcarea acetica
Calc. ar.—Calcarea arsenicosa
Calc. br.—Calcarea bromata
Calc. c.—Calcarea carbonica
Calc. caust.—Calcarea caustica
Calc. f.—Calcarea fluorata
Calc. i.—Calcarea iodata
Calc. ox.—Calcarea oxalica
Calc. p.—Calcarea phosphorica
Calc. sil.—Calcarea silicata
Calc. s.—Calcarea sulphurica
Calend.—Calendula officinalis
Camph.—Camphora

Camph. br.—Camphora bromata
Cann. i.—Cannabis Indica
Cann. s.—Cannabis sativa
Canth.—Cantharis
Caps.—Capsicum
Carb. an.—Carbo animalis
Carb. v.—Carbo vegetabilis
Carb. ac.—Carbolicum acidum
Carb. h.—Carboneum hydrogenisatum
Carb. o.—Carboneum oxygenisatum
Carb. s.—Carboneum sulphuratum
Card. b.—Carduus benedictus
Card. m.—Carduus marianus
Carl.—Carlsbad
Casc.—Cascarilla
Cast. eq.—Castor equi
Cast.—Castoreum
Caul.—Caulophyllum thalictroides
Caust.—Causticum
Cean.—Ceanothus Americanus
Cedr.—Cedron
Celt.—Celtis
Cench.—Cenchris contortrix
Cent.—Centaurea tagana
Cere. b.—Cereus bonplandii
Cere. s.—Cereus serpentinus
Cham.—Chamomilla
Chel.—Chelidonium majus
Chen. a.—Chenopodium anthelminticum
Chen. v.—Chenopodium vulvaria
Chim. mac.—Chimaphila maculata
Chim. rotund.—Chimaphila rotundifolia
Chim. umb.—Chimaphila umbellata
Chin. b.—China Boliviana
Chin.—China officinalis
Chin. a.—Chininum arsenicosum
Chin. m.—Chininum muriaticum
Chin. s.—Chininum sulphuricum
Chion.—Chionanthus Virginica
Chlol.—Chloralum
Chlf.—Chloroformum

Chlor.—Chlorum
Chol.—Cholesterinum
Chr. ac.—Chromicum acidum
Chr. ox.—Chromicum oxidatum
Cic.—Cicuta virosa
Cich.—Cichorium
Cimx.—Cimex
Cimic.—Cimicifuga actæa racemosa
Cina—Cina
Cinch. b.—Cinchona Boliviana
Cinch. s.—Cinchoninum sulphuricum
Cinnb.—Cinnabaris
Cinnm.—Cinnamomum
Cist.—Cistus canadensis
Cit. ac.—Citric acid
Cit. l.—Citrus limonum
Cit. v.—Citrus vulgaris (Aurantium)
Clem.—Clematis erecta
Cob.—Cobaltum
Coca—Coca
Cocaine—Cocaine
Cocc.—Cocculus indicus
Coc. c.—Coccus cacti
Cocc. s.—Coccinella septempunctata
Coch.—Cochlearia armoracea (Armoracea sativa)
Cod.—Codeinum
Coff.—Coffea cruda
Coff. t.—Coffea tosta
Colch.—Colchicum autumnale
Coll.—Collinsonia canadensis
Coloc.—Colocynthis
Colocn.—Colocynthinum
Colos.—Colostrum
Com.—Comocladia
Coniin.—Coniinum
Con.—Conium maculatum
Conv.—Convallaria majalis
Cop.—Copaiva
Cor. r.—Corallium rubrum
Cori. r.—Coriaria ruscifolia
Corn. a.—Cornus alternifolia

Corn.—Cornus circinata
Corn. f.—Cornus Florida
Corn. s.—Cornus serica
Cot.—Cotyledon umbilicus
Crat. ox.—Cratægus oxycantha
Croc.—Crocus
Crot. c.—Crotalus cascavella
Crot. h.—Crotalus horridus
Crot. t.—Croton tiglium
Cub.—Cubeba
Culx.—Culex musca
Cund.—Cundurango
Cupr. ac.—Cuprum aceticum
Cupr. ar.—Cuprum arsenicosum
Cupr.—Cuprum metallicum
Cupr. s.—Cuprum sulphuricum
Cur.—Curare
Cyc.—Cyclamen europæum

Daph.—Daphne Indica
Daph. o.—Daphne odorata
Datura a.—Datura arborea
Datura f.—Datura ferox
Delph.—Delphininum
Der.—Derris pinnata
Dict.—Dictamnus
Dig.—Digitalis
Dign.—Digitalinum
Digit.—Digitoxinum
Dios.—Dioscorea villosa
Diph.—Diphtherinum
Dirc.—Dirca palustris
Dol.—Dolichos pruriens
Dor.—Doryphora
Dros.—Drosera
Dub.—Duboisinum
Dulc.—Dulcamara solanum

Echi.—Echinacea angustifolia
Elæis guin.—Elæis guineensis
Elaps—Elaps corallinus

Elat.—Elaterium
Elect.—Electricity
Ephed.—Ephedra vulgaris
Epig.—Epigea repens
Epiph.—Epiphegus
Equis.—Equisetum
Erech.—Erechthites
Erig.—Erigeron canadense
Eriod.—Eriodictyon glutinosum
Ery. a.—Eryngium aquaticum
Ery. m.—Eryngium maritimum
Ether.—Etherum
Eth. n.—Ethyl nitrate
Eucal.—Eucalyptus
Eug.—Eugenia jambos (Jambos eugenia)
Euon. atrop.—Euonymus atropurpurea
Euon.—Euonymus Europæus
Eup. per.—Eupatorium perfoliatum
Eup. pur.—Eupatorium purpureum
Euph. amyg.—Euphorbium amygdaloides
Euph.—Euphorbium officinarum
Euphr.—Euphrasia
Eupi.—Eupion
Exal.—Exalgin

Fago.—Fagopyrum
Fel t.—Fel tauri
Ferr. ac.—Ferrum aceticum
Ferr. ar.—Ferrum arsenicosum
Ferr. i.—Ferrum iodatum
Ferr. ma.—Ferrum magneticum
Ferr.—Ferrum metallicum
Ferr. p.—Ferrum phosphoricum
Ferr. pic.—Ferrum picricum
Ferr. s.—Ferrum sulphuricum
Ferr. t.—Ferrum tartaricum
Fer. g.—Ferula glauca
Fil.—Filix mas
Fl. ac.—Fluoricum acidum
Form.—Formica
Franc.—Franciscea uniflora

Franz.—Franzenbad
Frax.—Fraxinus Americana
Fuc. ves.—Fucus vesiculosus

Gad.—Gadus morrhua
Gal. ac.—Gallicum acidum
Galvan.—Galvanismus
Gamb.—Gambogia
Gels.—Gelsemium
Gent. c.—Gentiana cruciata
Gent. l.—Gentiana lutea
Genist.—Genista
Ger.—Geranium maculatum
Get.—Gettysburg water
Gins.—Ginseng
Gland.—Glanderine
Glon.—Glonoinum
Gnaph.—Gnaphalium
Goss.—Gossypium herbaceum
Gran.—Granatum
Graph.—Graphites
Grat.—Gratiola
Grin.—Grindelia robusta
Gua.—Guaco
Guai. or Guaj.—Guaiacum
Guan.—Guano
Guar.—Guarana
Guare.—Guarea
Gymn.—Gymnocladus canadensis

Hæm.—Hæmatoxylon
Ham.—Hamamelis
Hecla—Hecla lava
Hedo.—Hedeoma
Helia.—Helianthus
Helio.—Heliotropium
Hell. f.—Helleborus fœtidus
Hell.—Helleborus niger
Helod.—Heloderma
Helon.—Helonias
Hep.—Hepar sulphuris calcareum

Hepat.—Hepatica
Herac.—Heracleum
Hipp.—Hippomanes
Homar.—Homarus
Hura—Hura Brasiliensis
Hydrang.—Hydrangea arborescens
Hydrs.—Hydrastis
Hydrc.—Hydrocotyle Asiatica
Hydr. ac.—Hydrocyanicum acidum
Hyos.—Hyoscyamus niger
Hyper.—Hypericum

Iber.—Iberis
Ictod.—Ictodes fœtida (Pothos fœtidus)
Ign.—Ignatia
Ill.—Illicum anisatum (Anisatum stellatum)
Indg.—Indigo
Ind.—Indium metallicum
Inul.—Inula
Iodof.—Iodoformum
Iod.—Iodium
Ip.—Ipecacuanha
Irid.—Iridium
Iris fl.—Iris florentina
Iris fœ.—Iris fœtidissima
Iris t.—Iris tenax
Iris—Iris versicolor
Itu—Itu

Jab.—Jaborandi
Jac.—Jacaranda
Jalap.—Jalapa
Jatr.—Jatropha
Jug. c.—Juglans cinerea
Jug. r.—Jugland regia
Juncus—Juncus effusus
Juni.—Juniperus Virginianus

Kali a.—Kali aceticum
Kali ar.—Kali arsenicosum
Kali bi.—Kali bichromicum

Kali br.—Kali bromatum
Kali c.—Kali carbonicum
Kali chl.—Kali chloricum
Kali chlo.—Kali chlorosum
Kali cy.—Kali cyanatum
Kali fer.—Kali ferrocyanatum
Kali i.—Kali iodatum
Kali ma.—Kali manganicum
Kali m.—Kali muriaticum
Kali n.—Kali nitricum
Kali ox.—Kali oxalicum
Kali per.—Kali permanganicum
Kali p.—Kali phosphoricum
Kali pic.—Kali picricum
Kali s.—Kali sulphuricum
Kali t.—Kali tartaricum
Kalm.—Kalmia latifolia
Kaol.—Kaolin
Kiss.—Kissengen
Kreos.—Kreosotum

Lac c.—Lac caninum
Lac f.—Lac felinum
Lac v.—Lac vaccinum
Lac d.—Lac vaccinum defloratum
Lach.—Lachesis
Lachn.—Lachnanthes
Lac. ac.—Lacticum acidum
Lact.—Lactuca virosa
Lappa a.—Lappa arctium (Arctium lappa—Lappa officinalis)
Laps. c.—Lapsana communis
Lath.—Lathyrus
Lat. k.—Latrodectus katipo
Lat. m.—Latrodectus mactans
Laur.—Laurocerasus
Led.—Ledum palustre
Leon.—Leonurus cardiaca
Lepi.—Lepidium bonariense
Lept.—Leptandra Virginica
Lil. sup.—Lilium superbum
Lil. t.—Lilium tigrinum

Linar.—Linaria
Linum—Linum
Lipp.—Lippspringe
Lith.—Lithium carbonicum
Lith. m.—Lithium muriaticum
Lob. c.—Lobelia cardinalis
Lob. d.—Lobelia dortmanna
Lob. e.—Lobelia erinus
Lob.—Lobelia inflata
Lob. s.—Lobelia syphilitica (cœrulia)
Lol. tem.—Lolium temulentum
Lonic.—Lonicera xylosteum
Luna—Luna
Lycpr.—Lycopersicum
Lyc.—Lycopodium clavatum
Lycps.—Lycopus Virginicus
Lyss.—Lyssin (Hydrophobinum)

Macrot.—Macrotinum
Mag. c.—Magnesia carbonica
Mag. m.—Magnesia muriatica
Mag. p.—Magnesia phosphorica
Mag. s.—Magnesia sulphurica
Mag. p. Ambo—Magnetis poli Ambo
Mag. p. Arct.—Magnetis polus Arcticus
Mag. p. Aust.—Magnetis polus Australis
Magnol. gl.—Magnolia glauca
Magnol.—Magnolia grandiflora
Maland.—Malandrinum
Malar.—Malaria officinalis
Manc.—Mancinella
Mand.—Mandragora
Mang.—Manganum
Mang. m.—Manganum muriaticum
Mar.—Marum verum (Teucrium marum verum)
Med.—Medorrhinum
Meli.—Melilotus
Menis.—Menispermum
Ment.—Mentha piperita
Ment. pu.—Mentha pulegium
Meny.—Menyanthes

Meph.—Mephitis
Merl.—Mercurialis perennis
Merc.—Mercurius (sol et vivus)
Merc. b.—Mercurius biniodatus
Merc. c.—Mercurius corrosivus
Merc. cy.—Mercurius cyanatus
Merc. d.—Mercurius dulcis
Merc. i. f.—Mercurius iodatus flavus
Merc. i. r.—Mercurius iodatus ruber
Merc. m.—Mercurius methylenus
Merc. n.—Mercurius nitricus
Merc. p.—Mercurius protoiodatus
Merc. sul.—Mercurius sulphuricus
Mez.—Mezereum
Mill.—Millefolium
Mim.—Mimosa
Mit.—Mitchella repens
Momor.—Momordica
Morph.—Morphinum
Mosch.—Moschus
Murx.—Murex
Mur. ac.—Muriaticum acidum
Musa—Musa
Muscn.—Muscarin
Mygal.—Mygale lasiodora
Myric.—Myrica cerifera
Myris.—Myristica sebifera
Myrt. c.—Myrtus communis

Nabalus—Nabalus
Naja—Naja
Naph.—Naphthalinum
Narcot.—Narcotinum
Narz.—Narzan
Nat. ac.—Natrum aceticum
Nat. a.—Natrum arsenicatum
Nat. c.—Natrum carbonicum
Nat. h.—Natrum hypochlorosum
Nat. m.—Natrum muriaticum
Nat. n.—Natrum nitricum
Nat. ntrs.—Natrum nitrosum

Nat. p.—Natrum phosphoricum
Nat. sal.—Natrum salicylicum
Nat. s.—Natrum sulphuricum
Nicc.—Niccolum
Nicot.—Nicotinum
Nit. s. d.—Nitri spiritus dulcis
Nit. ac.—Nitricum acidum
Nitro. o.—Nitrogenium oxygenatum
Nit. m. ac.—Nitroso-muriaticum acidum
Nuph.—Nuphar luteum
Nux m.—Nux moschata
Nux v.—Nux vomica
Nym.—Nymphæa odorata

Œna.—Œnanthe crocata
Olnd.—Oleander
Ol. an.—Oleum animale
Ol. j.—Oleum jecoris aselli
Onos.—Onosmodium
Op.—Opium
Opun.—Opuntia
Ornith.—Ornithogalum
Osm.—Osmium
Ostrya—Ostrya
Ovi g. p.—Ovi gallinæ pellicula
Ox. ac.—Oxalic acidum
Oxygen.—Oxygenium
Oxyt.—Oxytropis lamberti

Pæon.—Pæonia
Pall.—Palladium
Pana.—Panacea
Par.—Paris quadrifolia
Paraf.—Paraffinum
Pareir.—Pareira brava
Passi.—Passiflora
Paull.—Paullinia pinnata
Pedi.—Pediculus
Pen.—Penthorum sedoides
Peti.—Petiveria
Petr.—Petroleum

Petros.—Petroselinum
Phal.—Phallus impudicus
Phaseo.—Phaseolus
Phel.—Phellandrium
Phos. ac.—Phosphoricum acidum
Phos.—Phosphorus
Phys.—Physostigma
Phyt.—Phytolacca
Pic. ac.—Picricum acidum
Picrot.—Picrotoxinum
Pim.—Pimenta
Pimp.—Pimpinella
Pin. s.—Pinus sylvestris
Pip. m.—Piper methysticum
Pip. n.—Piper nigrum
Plan.—Plantago
Plat.—Platinum
Plect.—Plectranthus
Plumb.—Plumbago littoralis
Plb.—Plumbum
Podo.—Podophyllum
Polyg.—Polygonum hydropiperoides
Polyp. o.—Polyporus officinalis (Boletus laricis)
Polyp. p.—Polyporus pinicola
Pop.—Populus
Ictod.—Pothos fœtidus (Ictodes fœtida)
Prim.—Primula veris
Prun. p.—Prunus padus
Prun.—Prunus spinosa
Psor.—Psorinum
Ptel.—Ptelea trifoliata
Pulx.—Pulex irritans
Puls.—Pulsatilla
Puls. n.—Pulsatilla nuttaliana
Pyrog.—Pyrogenium
Pyrus—Pyrus Americana

Quass.—Quassia
Quer.—Quercus

Rad.—Radium
Ran. b.—Ranunculus bulbosus

Ran. g.—Ranunculus glacialis
Ran. r.—Ranunculus repens
Ran. s.—Ranunculus sceleratus
Raph.—Raphanus
Rat.—Ratanhia
Rheum—Rheum
Rhod.—Rhododendron
Rhus a.—Rhus aromatica
Rhus g.—Rhus glabra
Rhus r.—Rhus radicans
Rhus t.—Rhus toxicodendron
Rhus v.—Rhus venenata
Ricin.—Ricinus
Rob.—Robinia
Rumx.—Rumex crispus
Ruta—Ruta graveolens

Saba.—Sabadilla
Sabal—Sabal serrulata
Sabin.—Sabina
Sacc.—Saccharum album
Sac. lac.—Saccharum lactis
Sal. ac.—Salicylicum acidum
Salam.—Salamandra
Salic.—Salicinum
Salix p.—Salix purpurea
Samb. c.—Sambucus canadensis
Samb.—Sambucus nigra
Sang.—Sanguinaria canadensis
Sang. n.—Sanguinarinum nitricum
Sanic.—Sanicula aqua
Sant.—Santoninum
Saponin.—Saponinum
Sarr.—Sarracenia
Sars.—Sarsaparilla
Schinus—Schinus
Scroph.—Scrophularia
Scut.—Scutellaria
Sec.—Secale cornutum
Sel.—Selenium
Semp.—Sempervivum tectorum

Senec.—Senecio aureus
Senec. j.—Senecio Jacobœa
Seneg.—Senega
Senn.—Senna
Sep.—Sepia
Serp.—Serpentaria
Sil.—Silica
Sin.—Sinapis (not defined; see below)
Sin. a.—Sinapis alba
Sin. n.—Sinapis nigra
Slag—Slag
Sol—Sol (Helios)
Sol. m.—Solanum mammosum
Sol. n.—Solanum nigrum
Sol. o.—Solanum oleraceum
Sol. t. æ.—Solanum tuberosum ægrotans
Solid. or Sol. v.—Solidago virgaurea
Sphin.—Sphingurus (Spiggurus Martini)
Spig.—Spigelia
Spira.—Spiranthes
Spire.—Spiræa ulmaria
Spong.—Spongia tosta
Squill.—Squilla
Stach.—Stachys betonica
Stann.—Stannum
Staph.—Staphisagria
Stel.—Stellaria media
Stict.—Sticta pulmonaria
Still.—Stillingia sylvatica
Stram.—Stramonium
Stront.—Strontium carbonicum
Stroph.—Strophanthus
Stry.—Strychninum
Sulph.—Sulphur
Sul. i.—Sulphur iodatum
Sul. ac.—Sulphuricum acidum
Suls. ac.—Sulphurosum acidum
Sumb.—Sumbul
Syph.—Syphilinum
Symph.—Symphytum officinale

Tab.—Tabacum
Tanac.—Tanacetum
Tan.—Tanninum
Tarax.—Taraxacum
Tarent.—Tarentula Hispanica
Tarent. c.—Tarentula Cubensis
Tax.—Taxus baccata
Tell.—Tellurium
Tep.—Teplitz
Ter.—Terebinthina
Tetrad.—Tetradymite
Mar.—Teucrium marum verum
Thal.—Thallium
Thea—Thea
Ther.—Theridion
Thlaspi—Thlaspi bursa pastoris
Thuj.—Thuja
Thyroid.—Thyroidinum
Til.—Tilia
Tong.—Tongo
Trades.—Tradescantia
Trif. p.—Trifolium pratense
Trif.—Trifolium repens
Tril.—Trillium pendulum (erectum or cernuum)
Trios.—Triosteum
Trom.—Trombidium muscæ domesticæ
Tub.—Tuberculinum
Tub. lar.—Tuberculin laryngis
Tus. f.—Tussilago fragrans
Tus. p.—Tussilago petasites

Upas—Upas
Uran.—Uranium nitricum
Urea—Urea
Urt. u.—Urtica urens
Usn. bar.—Usnea barbata
Ust.—Ustilago
Uva—Uva-ursi

Vacc.—Vaccininum
Valer.—Valeriana

Vario.—Variolinum
Verat. a.—Veratrum album
Verat. v.—Veratrum viride
Veratn.—Veratrinum
Verb.—Verbascum
Vesp.—Vespa
Vib.—Viburnum opulus
Vichy—Vichy
Vinc.—Vinca minor
Viol. o.—Viola odorata
Viol. t.—Viola tricolor (Jacea)
Vip.—Vipera
Vip. l. f.—Vipera lachesis fel
Visc.—Viscum album

Wies.—Wiesbaden
Wild.—Wildbad
Wye.—Wyethia

Xanth.—Xanthoxylum

Yuc.—Yucca

Zinc. ac.—Zincum aceticum
Zinc. cy.—Zincum cyanatum
Zinc.—Zincum metallicum
Zinc. m.—Zincum muriaticum
Zinc. s.—Zincum sulphuricum
Zinc. val.—Zincum valerianicum
Zing.—Zingiber
Ziz.—Zizia